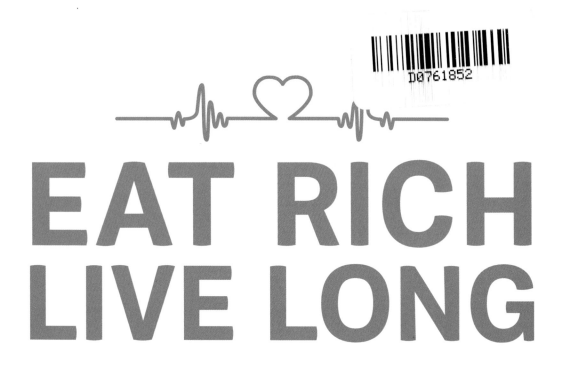

EAT RICH LIVE LONG

USE THE POWER OF LOW-CARB AND KETO FOR WEIGHT LOSS AND GREAT HEALTH

IVOR CUMMINS & JEFFRY GERBER, MD

RECIPES BY RYAN TURNER

VICTORY BELT PUBLISHING

LAS VEGAS

D0761852

First Published in 2018 by Victory Belt Publishing Inc.

ISBN-13: 978-1-628602-73-9

The information included in this book is for educational purposes only. It is not intended or implied to be a substitute for professional medical advice. The reader should always consult his or her health-care provider to determine the appropriateness of the information for his or her own situation or if he or she has any questions regarding a medical condition or treatment plan. Reading the information in this book does not constitute a physician-patient relationship.

Recipes created by Ryan Turner and edited by Jordan von Trapp

Recipe photos by Ryan Turner

Author photos by Leonard Photography and Truth Photography, LLC

Interior design by Justin-Aaron Velasco

Printed in Canada

TC 0218

CONTENTS

In memory of my father, Nicholas J. Cummins, one of the countless secret diabetics who were never diagnosed. He passed away at seventy-two following many years of poor health—long before the knowledge in this book could have saved him. Also in memory of Dr. Joseph R. Kraft, who half a century ago could have told my father all that he needed to know.

—IVOR CUMMINS

In memory of Dr. Alexander C. Szabo Jr., a family physician and dear friend who devoted his life to helping others. Like so many, he thought he was healthy, yet he was suddenly lost to us at the age of sixty-two due to a massive heart attack.

—JEFF GERBER

FOREWORD

You may wonder how it came about that a third of us are outright obese, half of us are overweight, diabetes is at epidemic proportions, and many of us are taking statins. Strangely enough, this sorry state we find ourselves in came about as a consequence of intense focus on a single molecule: cholesterol.

Everyone has heard of cholesterol, but what really is it? Cholesterol is a waxy molecule essential for life. So important, in fact, that virtually every cell can make it. It is the main structural component for all the cells and tissues in the human body. Without it, the body would, in the words of Shakespeare, "melt, thaw and resolve itself into a dew." It plays a major role in bone building, is the main building block for adrenal and reproductive hormones, and is needed to synthesize the bile salts required for proper digestion, and the brain and nervous system are both highly dependent upon it for optimal function. The list of cholesterol's virtues goes on and on. Because it is necessary for life, the body itself manufactures around 80–85 percent of the cholesterol it requires, with the other 15–20 percent coming from the diet.

Given the enormous importance of this single molecule, it beggars belief that it is also the most maligned molecule in the body, accused of causing heart disease, stroke, and a host of other problems. How did an indispensable molecule, made by the body itself, get such an horrific reputation? More importantly, how did fear of cholesterol lead to the epidemics of obesity and diabetes we're in the midst of today?

Largely thanks to the efforts of just one man.

More than a half century ago a research scientist named Ancel Keys concluded that heart disease was caused by elevated cholesterol in the blood. It wasn't such a far-fetched notion, because the plaque in diseased coronary arteries contains a fair amount of cholesterol, so it was a reasonable hypothesis that cholesterol in the diet would end up in the blood and could then find its way into the lining of arteries. But after careful study, Keys concluded the fat in the diet, not cholesterol, was the real culprit. Keys dominated the field of nutritional research, especially where dietary fat, cholesterol, and heart disease were concerned. It is impossible to overestimate the influence his theories exert on us still today. His influence was such that Keys appeared on the cover of *Time* magazine in 1961. By this time, the battle against saturated fat was fully engaged, and "heart-healthy" polyunsaturated fats were the new darlings of the nutritional world. Fifteen years later, the McGovern Committee formulated the first Dietary Goals of the United States, which hewed closely to the ideas put forth by Ancel Keys: keep the fat low and keep it polyunsaturated. "Saturated fat" became a dirty word. In fact, it became not just a dirty word but a dirty word grouping. It was almost never written as "saturated fat" but instead as "artery-clogging saturated fat."

So how did all this create the obesity and diabetes epidemics now flourishing?

It did so by completely changing the dietary patterns people had followed for generations. At the time the first nutritional guidelines came out, people in the United States had been following the same diet for decades with fairly stable levels of obesity and diabetes. The new standards exhorted people to reduce fat intake to 30 percent of calories and bump carbohydrates to between 50 and 60 percent. The assumption was that reducing fat, especially saturated fat, would reduce the incidence of heart disease.

But heart disease didn't really go down. What happened instead is that body weight went up and people started developing obesity and diabetes at epidemic rates.

Despite the epidemic burgeoning before their eyes, most physicians and dietitians still focus on cholesterol levels. And in their misguided way—thanks to the legacy of Ancel Keys—they encourage their patients to cut the fat, especially saturated fat, and increase the carbohydrates to try to drive their cholesterol levels ever lower. The sad, but predictable, result is an inexorable increase in weight and perhaps the onset of diabetes.

But though most medical and nutritional practitioners continue these ineffectual and counterproductive practices, there are a growing number who have veered from the crowd-think majority and are actually turning their patients' lives around.

The two authors of this book, both amateur athletes, initially fell victim to the antifat fervor but were ultimately able to break through the bias, see through the fallacies, and regain their health. Dr. Jeffry Gerber, a practicing physician in Denver, Colorado, who struggled with his weight, finally immersed himself in the science of weight gain and loss, and now he has a practice devoted to helping others achieve the success he himself found. Ivor Cummins, an engineer from Dublin, Ireland, decided to take a systems-based approach to figuring out his own cholesterol issues after his doctor couldn't explain them.

Jeff now shares his experience treating thousands of patients with other physicians, spreading the knowledge he's gained in treating lipids and other metabolic illnesses with a low-carb diet, and Ivor's in-depth analysis of every aspect of the lipid hypothesis has become an online legend in his Fat Emperor series of YouTube lectures. Both of them now lecture internationally on low-carb nutrition and its impact on lipids and the constellation of disorders related to insulin resistance and inflammation.

The book you hold is the outgrowth of their diverse experience. It contains an enormous amount of priceless information that is truly life changing. You will learn everything from a simple test for diabetes to an inexpensive procedure that actually visualizes the degree of any plaque you might have in your coronary arteries. And with the nutritional advice provided, you will be given a road map to ditch your excess weight, reverse your diabetes, and clean your coronary arteries—all while following a diet rich in all the foods you probably thought you could never eat again. You'll end up smarter, thinner, and with vastly improved health to carry you through a long and productive life.

Michael R. Eades, M.D.
Incline Village, Nevada

INTRODUCTION

No one wants to be fat—everyone wants to be slim. The vast majority of us are not lazy, nor are we mindless gluttons. People are overweight, despite their best efforts, because what they've been taught about the causes of obesity is simply wrong. In this book, we'll identify the real causes of obesity and ways to overcome it.

Both of us, Ivor and Jeff, struggled with weight control for decades. I, Ivor, should have known better. I have a degree in biochemical engineering and have specialized in leading complex problem-solving teams for more than twenty-five years, which led to my achieving the rare role of "technical master" in a huge corporation—so figuring out the ins and outs of complex systems (such as those involved in body weight) and how to optimize them is second nature to me. Jeff should also have worked it out sooner, with his enormous experience as an MD running a family-medicine practice for more than twenty years. He worked hard trying to manage the obesity explosion among his patients and identify addressable root causes. But in spite of our technical and medical experience, even we fell for the fake solutions: We exercised and systematically starved ourselves on many, many occasions. We dutifully lowered our dietary fat intake. We consumed complex carbohydrates like good boys. We ate more fruits and vegetables. We tried it all, and we failed, just like most of the population.

I competed in many Olympic-distance triathlons. These required a grueling regimen of intense training, which helped me to lose weight. But the weight always came back a few months later. The same thing happened for most of my friends. When I eventually researched the biochemistry of human metabolism and weight control, the situation at last became clear, and the fatal flaws in the official advice were unmasked. Fortunately, the actual fix was reasonably straightforward, and since then, I have been able to easily control my weight with minimal exercise, for the first time in my adult life.

Jeff had the exact same weight-off-weight-on experience with his chosen sport of competitive tennis. When he did his own research into the biochemistry of weight control, it changed the way he ate and the way he treated his patients. You'll find stories of patients who've had immense success under Jeff's guidance throughout this book.

For fifty years, we've all been taught that eating a low-fat diet and burning more calories are the keys to losing weight and getting healthy. This dogma has failed. The data indicating why has been misinterpreted or ignored for decades, protecting the low-fat emperor from embarrassment. One reason for this speaks directly to human nature itself. Health authorities and researchers simply couldn't accept that they had made an enormous error—especially when the error had negative implications for millions of people. As a result, most people are still not clear on the best science-based strategy for health and weight loss.

In this book, we will lay out the reality of what science really says. We are all machines—complex biochemical machines. Engineers know that all complex machines rely on many feedback loops, some of which are critical for proper functioning. Appetite and weight control have several of these crucial loops, and you must identify and understand these feedback loops in order to fix your body. We will explain all of them in this book.

We will guide you to lower your intake of inflammatory carbohydrates and enable you to target the least-inflammatory fuels for the human machine. You will learn how to safely increase your intake of healthy fats from natural sources. All this is not just helpful but *necessary* for healthy weight loss. But even if you're not looking to lose weight, the steps we recommend will improve your health and productivity and help you achieve a longer life in which to enjoy your new vitality.

As we shall see in Chapter 1, our opportunity to embrace healthy fats was stolen from us by human folly. This book reverses many decades of bad nutritional science and sets the record straight on what science tells us will deliver optimum nutrition for weight loss and longevity.

HOW TO USE THIS BOOK

We've organized this book with the aim of building from an overview of health and nutrition to specific steps you can take to improve your health and finally to a more detailed explanation of the scientific truth about insulin and mortality, cholesterol and heart disease, important vitamins and minerals, and much more.

In Part 1, we focus on a clear-sighted explanation of where the world went wrong in understanding what dietary strategies prevent disease. We cover the main errors of the past so that you can understand where the mistaken low-fat (and hence high-carb) dogma came from. We then move on to identifying the real dietary culprits—what foods really promote disease and cause obesity (not to mention problems losing weight). We also summarize the dietary approach that will enable you to use food as medicine in order to lose weight, avoid or resolve chronic diseases such as heart disease and diabetes, and improve longevity.

With a firm grasp of how nutrition really works, you will be ready to implement the ten action steps laid out in Part 2. We have broken this part into chapters on the overall plan, the first week on the plan, and the second and third weeks on the plan. Focusing specifically on the first week helps you create a great foundation, and we've tried to ensure that this first week has a straightforward focus on the most important change—diet—without worrying too much about other factors, such as meal spacing and exercise (although these are also important, of course). After the first week, we'll focus more closely on these further measures in weeks two and three to complement the core dietary changes and propel your success.

Part 3 is a more detailed narrative of the science supporting all of the strategies outlined in Part 2. It is possible to use just Parts 1 and 2 to transform your health and weight. However, your success over the long term will be greatly enhanced by understanding *why* these strategies are so important. Part 3 tells the fascinating scientific story around dietary carbohydrate, fat, and protein. We will demystify all of the confusion of the past fifty years and give you the real scoop on why combining these dietary components in a certain way will increase your longevity. There is also crucially important information in Part 3 explaining how you can verify that your plan is working properly. For example, we explain what various cholesterol metrics mean and the power of the CAC scan to verify that you have successfully tackled the risk of heart disease. Part 3 continues with a comprehensive summary of important vitamins and supplements, and it closes with an overview of your long-term health strategy, with tips for success and troubleshooting advice for some pitfalls that you may encounter.

We also put particular care into the appendixes. There's a great section on books, websites, and other resources that talk about health and nutrition, and another on navigating sweeteners on a healthy diet. And if you're as fascinated by the science behind nutrition as we are, you'll want to make sure to take a look at appendixes C, D, and E. These include some fascinating science on cholesterol and lipoproteins, glucose, and polyunsaturated fats—it's not necessary to know all this in order to have great success with the Eat Rich, Live Long plan, but it will be of great interest to many of you who want to dig even deeper.

1

SICK AND TIRED OF BEING UNHEALTHY

"**Let me ask you something. If the rule you followed brought you to this—of what use was the rule?**"

—Cormac McCarthy,
No Country for Old Men

CHAPTER 1

WE'RE GETTING HEAVIER AND HEAVIER

For two hundred thousand years, our body's appetite and weight-control systems functioned well. They even worked during the US boom years from the 1940s through the 1970s, when food was just as abundant as it is today. And just like today, almost everyone had an automobile—we weren't walking everywhere—and jogging and gym-going were relatively rare. Our systems still worked. Then, for some reason, they failed: we started getting heavier and heavier.

Most people are now overweight. Only a third of American adults have escaped the obesity epidemic.[1] Shockingly, children have succumbed to the epidemic in huge numbers as well. But the obesity is only part of what has befallen us. We also have an epidemic of chronic disease to tackle. Diabetes, heart disease, cancer, and Alzheimer's are ramping up in spite of enormous advances in medical technology that tackle them. So, after twenty millennia, how was our species transformed in two short generations? After two decades of investigation, what answers has modern science given us? We have all heard the "experts" wrangling over the "key drivers of obesity": Animal fat. Sugar. Processed food. Television. Whatever.

Eventually, most of the so-called experts found a happy consensus. Conveniently, they blame the victims. It has been all about "calories in versus calories out." People simply need to "move more and eat less." It has centered for decades on "reducing your dietary fat." As we shall see, this was actually the worst advice that we could have been given. All through the years, the media faithfully repeated this message until we became numb. The bloated bodies all around us are testament to its failure.

Finally, today the failed dogma of the past is being subjected to rigorous scientific research. In this book, we will share the truth with you.

FITTING THE EMPEROR'S SUIT

Let's be honest with ourselves. In spite of massive improvements in medical technology, the health of our population is declining.[2] Millions of non-overweight people are now harboring hidden fat in their organs, which leads directly to countless surprise heart attacks every day and contributes to Alzheimer's disease, diabetes, many cancers, and most of the diseases of modernity. Today's generation of young people is the first in human history that may live shorter lives than their parents.[3] This is in spite of continued advances in medical technology. Heart disease rates are spiraling out of control.[4] Diabetic dysfunction is everywhere.[5] What's more, the vast majority of diabetic people go undiagnosed—whether they are slim or fat. And it can all be traced directly to the advice to consume a low-fat diet.

We'll look at the faulty research involved in the recommendations for a low-fat diet, going all the way back to the 1960s, in the next chapter. Here, let's take an overview of the role the government and other health authorities played in promoting a low-fat diet.

In the 1960s, during the era of heart disease investigation, it was theorized that fatty foods were to blame for heart disease because of fat's putative ability to raise cholesterol, which was associated with a higher risk of heart disease. No one really had a clue about how humans metabolized healthy natural fats back then, but they barged ahead as if they did. While researchers wrestled with the question, the low-fat diet gained some powerful proponents in the 1970s.

In 1977, a Senate committee led by George McGovern issued *Dietary Goals for the United States*, which would become the *Dietary Guidelines for Americans* that we know today. The report was driven and supported by the American Heart Association and many other respected parties. It promulgated low-fat guidelines primarily, despite questioning by some notable experts. For instance, Philip Handler, the president of the National Academy of Science, asked a pivotal question: "What right has the federal government to propose that the American people conduct a vast nutritional experiment, with themselves as subjects, on the face of so little evidence?" No answer came forth. The politicians and publicists of the day decided that there was no time to gather proof of the low-fat theory's correctness. So Handler was ignored by the Senate committee he addressed, and its report officially promoted a low-fat diet for all Americans. And then we embarked on a long, slow car crash. The whole world went down, since most other countries also adopted the American nutritional guidelines—even France, where *cuisine minceur* became popular, if only briefly.

In the early 1980s, hundreds of millions of dollars was spent on trials to prove the theory that fat is bad because it raises cholesterol. These trials failed spectacularly—dietary fat does not meaningfully raise cholesterol in the majority of humans.[6] The authorities, however, chose to ignore these results.[7] Low-fat had already been sold to the world, and the authorities were not inclined to admit that they were wrong. The emperor could not be exposed as naked.

Since the low-fat mistake was forged into policy, obesity rates have mushroomed, and type 2 diabetes is the signature disease resulting from the fatally flawed fat theory. The number of people with type 2 diabetes has gone from less than 1 percent of the US population in the 1960s to approximately 12 percent today. And for every person diagnosed with diabetes, there are several more people who are undiagnosed. The explosive growth of type 2 diabetes will collapse our health systems in the coming decades. Bad scientific methods, groupthink, and hubris have created a modern monster.

The researchers in the 1980s convinced themselves that something was wrong with these experiments showing that dietary fat doesn't meaningfully impact disease rates. This was not true, however—if dietary fat were related to chronic disease, these experiments would have shown it. But the misguided low-fat message had been parroted by every me-too nutrition "expert" for more than a decade, and it had been enthusiastically adopted by the heads of the processed food industry. The profit potential coming from low-fat fare was enormous, so our hormonal weight-control systems were about to take a serious beating. Unsurprisingly, the obesity and diabetes epidemics really began soon after the low-fat guidance was foisted on the population.

For decades, the American Heart Association (AHA) pushed the low-fat message. But today, the AHA is saying something quite different. In their massive 2015 report *Heart Disease and Stroke Statistics*, they buried a bombshell in the text.[8] It says that five huge randomized controlled trials have demonstrated that *total fat consumption does not affect rates of coronary heart disease or stroke.* Wow. The AHA is now acknowledging that there is no evidence to support the low-fat advice. They are finally coming clean.

But there is another bombshell in their report. They state that each 5 percent of saturated fat in your diet that you replace with carbohydrate is associated with a 7 percent higher risk of coronary heart disease.

So you don't even need us to convince you. The AHA itself has switched sides! And it is not just the AHA who are putting their gears into reverse. Other primary authorities are also quietly acknowledging their big mistake. In May 2015, the new *Dietary Guidelines for Americans* was revealed—and dietary cholesterol and natural fats had been dropped from the no-no lists. The Academy of Nutrition and Dietetics also pushed the low-fat fad with gusto for many decades, but now they too are waking up to the truth: "Saturated fat is to be *de-emphasized* from nutrients of concern, given the lack of evidence connecting it with cardiovascular disease." Cholesterol was also dropped from their list of "nutrients of concern."

After fifty years of delusional diet dogma, we are finally seeing the return of scientific sanity. It's about time—and it's not too late for us to improve our health.

DIANA'S STORY

Diana is a patient of Jeff's who suffered badly from all the low-fat advice. She had a long history of being overweight and had attempted countless diets to improve her situation. Many of these were fads that would create a small temporary loss. All of them included some element of reducing fat intake. Of course, Diana, like most people, gained the weight back in no time. On one occasion she drove herself to successfully lose a lot of weight with a low-fat, reduced-calorie regimen. She realized she would have to eat low-fat and starve herself for the rest of her life. Deep down, she knew that was never going to happen. She lost her will to stick with the diet, regaining all of the weight she'd lost and then some.

At 210 pounds and suffering from back and joint pain, she was too tired to enjoy any healthy exercise. So she went to Jeff for advice. Jeff quickly diagnosed her with prediabetes—her blood sugar was significantly elevated. Diana had a family history of diabetes and knew something had to be done. Then and there she resolved to try something completely new—to follow Jeff's advice and consume a high-fat diet. Jeff explained that this would address her prediabetes problem—and it would be highly appetizing and sustainable in the long term.

The results were dramatic and highly motivating. Diana lost more than 50 pounds in the following twelve months, with her appetite remaining under easy control. She is no longer driven by constant hunger, and she is no longer prediabetic. The joint pain that had plagued her has faded away. She was able to drop the melatonin she previously required for sleep, and she now gets eight hours of refreshing sleep nightly. Her constipation disappeared. Her periods became regular and her painful cramps went away. Other benefits she felt include mental acuity, improved energy levels, a settled stomach, and lack of breathlessness when exercising.

Jeff has countless patients who have transformed their health, weight, and productivity by dumping the low-fat obsession. Diana's experience is typical of the benefits that accrue. Jeff's primary health-care intervention is to switch people away from the official nutritional advice. He is having enormous success with this science-based strategy, saving hundreds of people from chronic health problems and early mortality.

CHAPTER 2

SEVEN WAYS TO TWIST THE TRUTH

The low-fat dietary confusion highlighted in the last chapter did not come about by chance. It was driven remorselessly by that most dangerous of things: an idea. The idea became a theory and then, over time, dogma. It is important to know how this occurred because we are being misled by this same theory to this very day. The theory was "proven" using some deceptive and unsound scientific methods. Truth became mangled as groupthink took over the world of nutrition. And it was all based on simplistic interpretations of how the food groups interacted with our bodies. So that's where we'll start, with some basic definitions of the elements in food and their characteristics.

All food is composed of three macronutrients: fat, carbohydrate, and protein. These are what provide us with energy, in the form of calories, and nutrients.

FATS

▶ Fats are energy-dense at 9 calories per gram.

▶ They are concentrated in many highly nutritious foods, including fatty meats, eggs, cheeses, nuts, avocado, olives, and coconut.

▶ Fats are also found in ingredients created through high-volume, industrial chemical processes; these are not at all good for you:

Vegetable oils, low-cost, supposedly healthy polyunsaturated fats that are extracted from seeds in a multistep industrial refining process

Hydrogenated fats, vegetable oils chemically altered to make them more solid at room temperature; often used in baked goods

▶ There are many essential fats that our body needs but cannot make—we have to consume them to be healthy. There are also many fat-soluble vitamins that our body requires fats to absorb. Fat is crucial for health!

▶ According to the Institute of Medicine, the minimum amount of dietary fat humans require is around 20 percent of dietary intake. That means that at least 20 percent of your calories each day *must* come from fat. If you approach zero, you will soon become ill.

PROTEIN

▶ Protein is low in energy density at 4 calories per gram.

▶ It is concentrated in many healthy whole foods, including meat and fish, eggs, cheese, nuts, and some vegetables and plant foods.

▶ Protein supplies the molecular building blocks our bodies use to make muscle and other tissues.

▶ The minimum human requirement for protein is around 15 percent of dietary intake, or 0.4 gram per pound of body weight. This equates to around 55 grams (2 ounces) per day for an adult weighing 150 pounds. If you approach zero protein intake, you will soon become very ill. Protein also affects our appetite: if we don't get enough, we tend to keep eating until we do.

CARBOHYDRATES

▶ Like protein, carbs are low in energy density at 4 calories per gram.

▶ All carbs are broken down into glucose, which the body either uses for fuel or stores—mostly as body fat.

▶ Carbs are abundant in many healthy whole foods, including vegetables, some nuts, fruits, and roots and tubers such as potatoes.

▶ Carbs are also abundant in wheat, which humans began using on a large scale approximately eight thousand years ago, making it a more recent addition to our diet than the foods listed above.

▶ More modern still are highly processed carbohydrates: refined sugar and refined wheat flour and all the foods they're found in—soft drinks, candy, chips, bread, pasta, baked goods of all types, breakfast cereal, and more.

▶ The three bullet points above on foods that contain carbs start with the more slowly digested carbs, which can have beneficial nutritional effects—they can assist the function of your gut. At the bottom of the list are sugary foods that can destroy the function of your gut. In terms of your health, this distinction matters a lot.

▶ The minimum human requirement for carbohydrate is effectively 0 percent of dietary intake. *That's right—zero—you don't have to eat any carbs at all.* Your body can easily synthesize all the glucose it requires. So—unlike with fats and protein—as your carbohydrate intake approaches zero, there is no known scientific reason for you to become ill. The exception is if the foods you're eating are all missing a key nutrient— vitamin C, for example, is classically associated with fruit. But you can get vitamin C from organ meats and low-carb vegetables, too. In short, unlike fat and protein, carbohydrate is not a necessary part of the human diet.

All that may be surprising. It certainly doesn't match what we've been told for decades about health and nutrition. So given that dietary fat is a key essential nutrient and carbohydrate is not, why did authorities decide that dietary natural fats could be the primary source of risk for heart disease and other diet-related health problems?

Unfortunately, they all fell for the low-fat theory that had been knocking around in the 1950s, although it was highly contested in the scientific community at the time. But what really planted the seeds for the low-fat era was a crucial event: the theory attracted a true champion, an extraordinarily influential champion, who was set to change the course of history. He took a complex issue and simplified it to the point that he created a lie.

THE ELEPHANT IN THE ROOM

There's an old parable about four blind men and an elephant. None of the men has encountered an elephant before, so each feels a different part of the elephant to try to determine what it is. One feels the trunk and thinks the elephant is like a snake; another feels its side and thinks it's a kind of wall; the third feels a leg and thinks it's a pillar; and the last feels the tail and thinks it's like a rope. Each man has a piece of information that's pretty convincing, and each feels that he has enough data to make a judgment. *But each blind man doesn't know what he doesn't know*. None of them have enough information to see the big picture, so each one gets what an elephant is like totally wrong.

In the 1960s, an influential blind man grasped onto a trunk and would not let go. He was absolutely, positively sure that he held a snake in his hands. He believed with fervor that his nutritional villain was causing the world's heart disease problems, and over time he convinced many people that his villain was the primary driver of heart disease.

This blind man's name was Ancel Keys. The villain he held onto was dietary fat, particularly saturated fat. He convinced the world that this dietary fat from natural sources was the thing we should all fear, thereby setting in motion the biggest mistake in the history of nutritional science. The world is only now beginning to recover from his mistake, and very slowly at that.

ANCEL KEYS AND HIS LOUSY RESEARCH

To verify that something actually causes a specified result and isn't just associated with it, there are three primary pillars of proof that must be demonstrated.

The first pillar is *associational evidence*. This is essentially some kind of indication that two things have an association. It is hardly even a pillar because it is so weak—it only suggests that there might be a relationship between two things; it doesn't prove that one thing causes the other. You've probably heard it said that "correlation does not imply causation," meaning that just because two things are linked doesn't mean one causes the other—for instance, the divorce rate in Maine correlates with the per capita consumption of margarine, but it would be absurd to suggest that one causes the other.[1] One should *never* say that X causes Y using associational evidence alone, and yet the vast majority of nutritional studies you see in the media are teetering on this one weak pillar of evidence.

The second pillar is *mechanism evidence.* Here you have to demonstrate that your cause makes *technical sense*—that it is physically probable that one thing should cause the other. But that alone doesn't prove it is significant, especially if there is bias to defend a prevailing theory. Mechanism evidence is regularly exaggerated to defend dogmas.

The third pillar is *experimental evidence*. When it comes to medicine, this refers to evidence obtained through a randomized controlled trial, the gold standard for determining cause and effect without bias. A randomized controlled trial changes a single factor and demonstrates a clear change in outcome, showing that that factor is a causal one. It is the only pillar that might

Figure 2.1. While the change in margarine consumption correlates with the divorce rate in Maine, obviously a change in one doesn't cause a change in the other. Source: Tyler Vigen, *Spurious Correlations*, www.tylervigen. com/spurious-correlations.

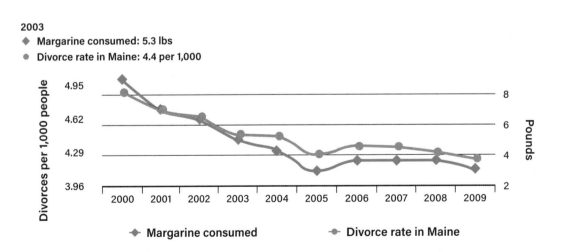

Divorce Rate in Maine Correlates with Per Capita Consumption of Margarine

2003
◆ **Margarine consumed: 5.3 lbs**
● **Divorce rate in Maine: 4.4 per 1,000**

◆ **Margarine consumed**   ●— **Divorce rate in Maine**

technically stand on its own, but the danger with using the third pillar alone is that the experiment might be poorly designed, some interactional factors may be missed and therefore not controlled for, or the experimenter may inappropriately change several things at once.

The strongest case for a cause-and-effect relationship is made when you have all three pillars of evidence solidly in agreement.

Of the three pillars required, the associational pillar is the most dangerous to lean on—it is the very lowest quality of evidence possible. And now we get to the problem with Ancel Keys: the evidence he used to blame dietary fat for cardiovascular disease was made up almost exclusively of associational data.

PILLAR ONE: AN ASSOCIATIONAL DISASTER

Ancel believed in his heart that dietary fat (particularly saturated fat) was a key cause of coronary heart disease (CHD). He bolstered this belief by highlighting *associations* between dietary fat and CHD. (Even though at the time, in the 1950s, CHD was associated as or more closely with many other things, like sugar and latitude/sun exposure.[2]) No scientist should ever come to a conclusion based primarily on associational evidence, but Ancel Keys did—and the whole world followed him into the void.

Ancel's offending theory is known as the diet-heart hypothesis, and it basically states that dietary saturated fat increases levels of cholesterol in the blood, and high blood cholesterol in turn increases the risk of coronary heart disease.

We will deal with the cholesterol part of this theory in Part 3. But what about the claim about saturated fat, which fooled the world for fifty years?

Embarking on his association fest, Ancel put together his Six Countries Study. In this statistical confection he observed a relationship between the percentages of dietary fat in the diets of six handpicked countries (the United States, Japan, Italy, England/Wales, Canada, and Australia) and their death rates from CHD.

This of course is merely a correlation, showing that fat content in the diet appears to associate or correlate with deaths from CHD. It is a near-meaningless pillar of nothing. Also, he had selected which countries to use in the study—the exact opposite of what happens in a randomized study, in which the participants are chosen at random to prevent researcher bias from affecting the outcome.

And what if we stood back and looked at all of the data available at the time of the study? Figure 2.2 on the following page shows the complete data available when Ancel began to mislead the world.

The Selected Six Countries

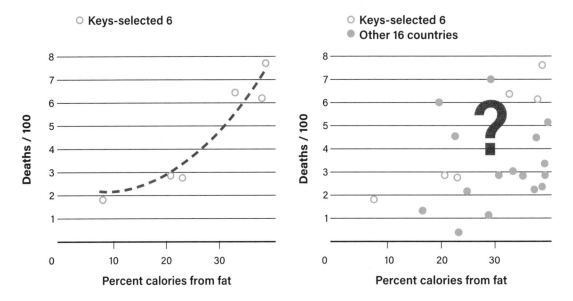

Figure 2.2. Source: J. Yerushalmy and H. E. Hilleboe, "Fat in the Diet and Mortality from Heart Disease: A Methodologic Note," *New York State Journal of Medicine* 57, no. 14 (1957): 2343–54.

Though an association between dietary fat and CHD in these particular countries would mean little, there wasn't a consistent association in the first place. But Ancel appeared to have bewitched himself with this contrived pillar of association. Justly, in spite of his personal passion, Ancel did not get very far in the scientific community with his Six Countries analysis—in fact, he was humiliated at a World Health Organization gathering of scientists, and an excellent paper was published in the *New York State Journal of Medicine* that eviscerated his correlational capers.[3]

Ancel was furious. So how did he proceed? He designed and executed the Seven Countries Study, which looked at the diets and disease rates of United States, Japan, Italy, Finland, Netherlands, Yugoslavia, and Greece. This study would artfully place dietary fat at the scene of the crime and seal its fate for decades.

Scientific studies and experiments can be constructed to tell whatever story you want to be told. If the initial results don't support your desired outcome, the data can always be statistically tortured to say what you want.

Ancel designed his experiment in such a way that he didn't need to torture things too much afterward, but he did strap the data into a chair and slap it around a bit. By personally choosing the regions for the Seven Countries Study, Ancel could largely predict the outcome of the study. It therefore *appeared* to deliver a real answer the way a proper experiment might. But nothing could be further from the truth.

We won't summarize the Seven Countries Study here. The bottom line is that it was simply another associational study, propped up with cherry-picked countries. It included only 12,700 men—no women—and it sampled only a percentage of the dietary information for these men.[4] So do we have a similar modern study that analyzes much larger numbers of both men *and* women? One that covers a much larger range of countries, to avoid the cherry-picking that creates misleading results? One that, although associational, is at least capable of *properly* analyzing the associations for our review? Luckily, we do.

In August 2017, the results of the Prospective Urban Rural Epidemiology (PURE) study were published.[5] This seven-year study used modern methods and technology to examine the very same questions around dietary fat and disease that Keys looked at. But in marked contrast to the Seven Countries Study, the PURE study tracked 135,335 men and women across eighteen countries. So it was essentially a massively more dependable test of the fat theories. You might say it was a huge modern upgrade of a sloppy old study. So what did this PURE analysis conclude?

It came to the opposite conclusion of Ancel Keys's Seven Countries Study.

PURE found that neither coronary heart disease nor mortality in general were associated with intake of overall fat or saturated fat. In fact, higher saturated fat intake was associated with benefits such as lower stroke rates. However, carbohydrate did not fare so well: higher carbohydrate intake tracked with increasing mortality. Which was exactly what the American Heart Association quietly acknowledged in their 2015 report *Heart Disease and Stroke Statistics*, based on statistics relating to 344,696 men and women.

But sadly, fifty years of fat phobia have done untold damage to our perceptions of diet and disease. The Seven Countries Study has a lot to answer for.

For anyone who wishes to enjoy a detailed account of the shenanigans in Ancel's Seven Countries Study, we highly recommend *The Big Fat Surprise* by investigative journalist Nina Teicholz. Deservedly a *New York Times* bestseller, it is a gripping historical account of how the world was cleverly duped into fearing fat, and it was one of the first mainstream publications to make a comprehensive argument that saturated fats have been unfairly maligned.

As we will discuss later, many recent studies have revealed that higher saturated fat in the diet is associated with lower heart disease rates. Does this mean that saturated fat could actually reduce heart disease? Maybe, maybe not. We cannot tell from associational data. Associational data is best used to disprove a theory or correct another, weaker associational study. Just as the PURE study has nicely demonstrated.

PILLAR THREE: IGNORING THE EXPERIMENT REALITIES

We'll be addressing elements of the second pillar in Part 3 of the book. For now, suffice to say that the mechanism evidence for the low-fat theory was based on mistaken beliefs around the importance of cholesterol and the idea that dietary fat had an important influence on it. So let's go straight to the third pillar here: the experimental evidence. Remember that this is the most powerful evidence. It can provide proof on its own, without associational or mechanism evidence. Experimental evidence supporting the low-fat diet would have been crucial to have before directing the world's population to jack up their carbohydrate intake.

There actually were good experiments—proper randomized controlled trials—on dietary fat and heart disease in the 1960s and 1970s. These trials were all carried out on human subjects, so their results are particularly important. Sadly, they were ignored.

The problem was that these experiments showed that dietary fat was not significantly linked to heart disease. These gold-standard experiments *disproved* the diet-heart hypothesis! The leaders who were pushing the low-fat theory did not like these results, so the experiments were ignored. (British researcher Zoe Harcombe published a paper in the esteemed *British Medical Journal* whose title says it all: "Evidence from Randomized Controlled Trials Did Not Support the Introduction of Dietary Fat Guidelines in 1977 and 1983.")

One notable trial in 1973 even had its results withheld from publication.[6] Eventually, the study was quietly published in a modest journal in 1989, a full sixteen years after its analysis was completed. The results were not published for so long because, as recounted by the principal investigator of the experiment, Ivan D. Frantz Jr., "We were just so disappointed in the way they turned out."[7]

More randomized controlled trials on the diet-heart hypothesis were run in the 1980s and 1990s. They had the desperate goal of showing even a tiny problem with dietary fat. Hundreds of millions of dollars were invested to get the required results. The trials all failed to change mortality outcomes, even though some were biased to "help" the hypothesis.

The most notable trial was carried out at enormous cost—several hundred million dollars—and ran for nearly ten years.[8] It reduced total fat intake significantly, to approximately 20 percent, and saturated fat down to a paltry 7 percent. This was a major achievement, as lower-fat diets like these are unpalatable for most people. So what resulted from this huge intervention? There was no improvement in heart disease rates, or any health outcome for that matter—it was a total failure. (It did manage to significantly reduce LDL cholesterol levels, but as we'll discuss in Chapter 11, LDL levels are a poor predictor of heart disease.)

There was also an interesting fact in the final report that speaks to the lack of any benefits seen from this reduction of fat: "Levels of high-density lipoprotein cholesterol, triglycerides, glucose, and insulin did not significantly differ in the intervention vs comparison groups." These are very important biometrics that should have been the focus all along. Instead, total cholesterol and LDL were the focus, even though they are weak and often misleading, as we'll see in Chapter 11. In focusing on improving these metrics over the important ones, the researchers made a serious error. This scientific error was one big reason why their experiments were doomed to fail.

Many other large trials had similarly useless results. Eventually researchers simply gave up trying to prove that a low-fat diet had any value—but they certainly did not give up *saying* it had value.

Dietary fat was never within a mile of being convicted as a cause of heart disease. None of this was acknowledged, and nothing was learned. Authorities went on promoting the low-fat lunacy in spite of having no worthy evidence. But let's now meet the substance that was used to replace natural dietary fat. A substance that is only now being fully banned as toxic for human consumption.[9]

FRANKENFATS: A TOXIC SOLUTION TO A NONEXISTENT PROBLEM

Natural saturated fat—the kind found in animal foods, nuts, olives, and other healthy whole foods—has been consumed by humans for millennia. It's an excellent ingredient in a huge range of tasty foodstuffs. But once natural fats started to be vilified by low-fat proponents, what substance was chosen by the industrial food complex to replace them?

In the face of fat phobia and with the ancestral saturated fats out of favor, industry had to find a solution they could sell. They would gladly have used cheap refined polyunsaturated oils—soybean and corn oils, among others—but polyunsaturated oils are unstable, which means they don't have a long shelf life, and they don't give foods the firm texture that their saturated cousins do. Luckily for industry, there was an available solution that perfectly fit the bill.

In the early 1900s, the food industry figured out how to convert cottonseed oil into a stable semisolid product through a process known as hydrogenation. This was achieved in huge industrial chemical plants. The high temperatures, pressures, and solvents used made this "vegetable shortening" rather toxic for humans, but nobody realized this at the time. The tortured molecules delivered the required properties of solidity and shelf life. And it was filthy cheap to produce. That was all that mattered.

And so, since 1911, we have been eating these industrially synthesized saturated fats known as partially hydrogenated oils. It turns out that hydrogenation creates molecules called trans fats that we now know are directly linked to coronary heart disease. So, ironically, these products contributed to the explosion of heart disease for which Ancel Keys and his acolytes blamed natural saturated fats. And yet, in the 1980s, their production was ramped up to replace natural saturated fats. Our food supply became flooded with these "frankenfats."

Attempting to beat evolution at its own game has had consequences. The effects of these mass-produced substances on heart disease and overall health is hard to quantify. Before they were largely banned, however, we all ate plenty of them for decades in "heart-healthy" margarines and spreads, low-fat foods, and all the copious sugar-laden junk foods of the era.

Trans fats have finally been deemed unfit for human consumption. The restrictions took place in a series of actions from the early 2000s on around the world, starting with Denmark.[10] As trans fats were removed from the food supply, however, natural fats were not given a pardon to replace them. So now industry is attempting to replace partially hydrogenated oils with some mixture of the following:

► modified hydrogenated seed oils

► genetically modified seed oils

► interesterified seed oils

The new frankenfats, in other words. All of the above are made through new industrial chemical processes. We'll see how harmful these are to humans, but we must be patient. Going from past experience, it may take decades before we discover exactly how much harm they cause us.

But even without the hydrogenation that makes them solid and shelf-stable, there are huge questions remaining around the health of vegetable oils. Should we be consuming them in any form, rather than simply eating real food? No, as we will see in Chapter 4 (and in even more disturbing detail in Appendix E).

THE FINAL INSULT: SWEET POISON DESCENDS

The other main replacement for natural fats truly planted the seeds for disaster.

In 1977, *Dietary Goals for the United States* officially told us to jack up the percentage of carbohydrate in our diet to 55–60 percent of our caloric intake. This gave the food industry the opportunity to provide a major new source of processed carbohydrate. What form did this mass of new carbohydrate take?

The food industry released an enormous mushroom cloud of refined wheat flour and sugar, including the especially odious high-fructose corn syrup. It entered most processed food products with frightening speed. With the delicious flavor and mouthfeel of natural fat banished, pretty much everything got a shot of refined grains or sugar to sweeten it or improve the texture. And without fat's natural satiating effects, refined carbohydrates created a new era of hunger—and a major business benefit to the food corporations. It wasn't just waistlines that started growing. The hunger that these products created drove food revenues also.

Another industry was also set for enormous revenue growth. The pharmaceutical industry massively exploited an explosion of chronic disease driven by the new food supply. Two of the biggest industries in the world made out like bandits from the low-fat diet fad. For we had unwittingly replaced an imaginary poison—natural fats—with very real ones—trans fats, refined grains, and sugar. However lacking in any robust science, the low-fat age began in earnest. Nothing would ever be the same again.

THE WILD-GOOSE CHASE

And that's how we embarked on a fifty-year wild-goose chase, before finally realizing that it was never really natural fats that caused our problems in the first place. Now we can start addressing the real issues. But our task ahead has been made extremely difficult because we are now burdened by the host of fake foods and carby trash littering the landscape.

Between food-industry marketing and the steady drumbeat of media messages explaining that red meat and eggs are deadly, Americans have gotten the message, all right. Apparently around 36 percent of Americans believe that UFOs are real, but only 25 percent believe that there's no link between natural fats and heart disease. We are more willing to believe that we've been visited by creatures from outer space than we are to believe that these foods full of natural, healthy fats are not harmful. These are foods that humans have been eating ever since we became human—foods that arguably are responsible for our *becoming* human.

DENNIS'S STORY

Jeff's patient Dennis has always struggled with being overweight. When he was a kid, his aunt would bring a grocery bag full of Entenmann's pastries to the house every Wednesday afternoon. They would never last until the following Wednesday whenever Dennis was around.

Although he was an active and athletic kid, Dennis was always borderline obese. He joined the Marine Corps when he was eighteen years old, 5'8" and 185 pounds. Boot camp quickly took 50 pounds off his frame, and after thirteen weeks of running, hiking, and other "fun" activities, he graduated at a trim 135 pounds. The problem really came when diet and exercise became his responsibility.

After his four-year tour ended, he went right back to nearly 200 pounds. He managed to control his weight at around 200 pounds until he married and had a son. With the stress of running his own business and taking care of his new family, combined with typical lunches of pizza or subs and potato chips, he ballooned. Within a couple of years he was weighing in at 260 pounds, and his blood pressure, triglycerides, and cholesterol numbers were astronomical. He was only thirty years old, but he looked and felt much older. He became depressed and desperate. A friend's wife was a nurse and recommended an experimental drug known as fen-phen. The drug enabled him to get back to 200 pounds, but its side effects and risks were starting to become known, and soon it was banned. Without the drug, the hunger crept back. Dennis gained back 40 pounds within a year. Although he now followed a "food pyramid" diet, he remained fat and hungry. He resigned himself to his fate, thinking that this was just how he was made.

Then he heard about Jeff and decided to give it one more go. He was taken aback by Jeff's unorthodox approach to weight loss. Jeff told him that breads, cereals, pasta, and sugar had to go. To Dennis, it sounded bizarre and hard to imagine. But then Jeff also told him to start eating bacon, real butter, eggs, and many other "forbidden" foods. As soon as he committed to this change, he started dropping weight without any effort. Within six months he was down to 173 pounds—67 pounds gone. What's more, he was now off blood pressure meds for the first time in twenty years.

Dennis still struggles with his old desires for New York–style pizza and Krispy Kreme—and pies, cakes, and candy during the holidays. He has even gone through some cheat periods when he gained back around 10 pounds. But the crucial thing is that he now knows how to get back on track with high-fat real food. He also finds that the low-carb books and websites that have become popular over the last few years make the low-carb lifestyle much easier and more enjoyable. Having dumped the high-carb food pyramid, he can ski all day with his boys—and they wear out before he does. He is also grateful to his wife for creating new and wonderful low-carb recipes that keep him from drifting. He keeps safely away from the high-carb fare that was ruining both his health and his enjoyment of life.

CHAPTER 3

RESPECT YOUR INSULIN:
WHY MOST WEIGHT-LOSS PLANS FAIL

> " Those with cardiovascular disease not
> identified with diabetes are simply undiagnosed. "
>
> —Dr. Joseph R. Kraft

Let's look at why most weight-loss plans fail. Importantly, we will also keep an eye on their long-term health implications. A diet for longevity and vitality is not all about weight loss. There are countless "normal weight" individuals who desperately need a corrected diet to avoid premature death. Perhaps not surprisingly, the ideal dietary regime for weight loss is the same one that will optimize health and longevity.

Any weight-loss diet must have two crucial elements. First, it must improve your body's existing appetite and weight control system. That is essentially why most orthodox dietary regimens fail: they ask you to restrict calories by eating less, tell you to burn away the calories you do eat by moving more, and often deprive you of fatty, protein-rich, and nutrient-dense foods—which would help return your appetite to a healthy level.

The other fundamental key to a successful diet is the ability to use fat as your body's preferred fuel. If a dietary regimen does not improve your ability to burn body fat efficiently, it will fail. The key is to switch from being a carbohydrate-burner to being a fat-burner. You will not achieve this transformation with a high-carbohydrate, low-fat diet—not even if the carbohydrates are so-called complex ones. As we'll explain later in this chapter, it simply doesn't work that way.

Let's start by looking at the two most common ways people are told to lose weight—follow a low-fat diet and "eat less, move more"—and why they don't work.

FOOL ME ONCE, SHAME ON YOU

Let's start with the first nutritional myth that's caused so many problems: that a low-fat diet is healthy and good for weight loss. When a low-fat diet was first proposed in the 1950s, it was under the misguided belief that it would reduce heart attacks. Since the 1970s, following a low-fat diet has also been the primary advice for weight loss and good health. Yet, as we talked about in the previous chapter, this advice is not based on sound evidence, and it's had very serious consequences. Low-fat ideology has contributed significantly to our current epidemics of obesity, diabetes, heart disease, and more. In a twist of irony, the low-fat diet was proposed as a solution to the obesity epidemic it helped create in the first place.

Here's how the story that a low-fat diet would help us lose weight was sold:

► Fat has 9 calories per gram, whereas carbohydrate has 4 calories per gram. Therefore, eating less fat and more carbohydrate will lower your caloric intake.

► Fat causes heart disease, and heart disease is linked to obesity, so fat probably causes obesity, too.

► Also, it's *called* "fat"—get it? So it stands to reason that it probably makes you fat.

We could go on, but the logic wouldn't get any better. So what was ignored in this overly simplistic thinking? The science of human metabolism, for starters. Body weight is controlled by an exquisite hormonal signaling system that includes everything from the food sensors in your gut to signals in your brain and other organs. The number of calories in fat is not relevant unless you are eating too much carbohydrate with it (for reasons we'll cover later)—a healthy human body will smoothly compensate for an increase in the number of calories consumed by increasing satiety signals. In other words, because fat has more calories per gram than carbohydrate, it also makes you feel full faster, so you end up eating less of it. The fact that it has more calories is the least relevant point.

There are many benefits to eating a higher-fat, lower-carbohydrate diet. It has overwhelmingly been shown to be better for weight loss than a lower-fat diet. This is not based on theory; it is based on direct experimental evidence from over fifty trials.[1] The reasons are many, but one important reason involves the master signaling hormone, insulin: unlike carbohydrate, dietary fat does not trigger a significant release of insulin, and controlling your insulin is the single best way to control your body weight—as we'll discuss later in this chapter. It is also the best way to achieve great health and longevity.

Even a slender person carries the vast majority of his or her energy stores in the form of body fat. It can keep you alive for many weeks or even months with no food. It is the master fuel our species evolved on. In contrast, our body's carbohydrate stores run out after a day or so.

We evolved to burn fat as a favored fuel. Carbohydrate is a flash fuel that must be constantly topped up. When almost no carbohydrate is available, however, we can get along just fine—we can smoothly burn dietary or body fat. For most of human existence, this was the evolutionary norm. The idea that natural fat sources could be toxic to humans was a false and contrived notion with no basis in evolutionary or physiological science. Avoiding fat in favor of carbohydrate will undermine your weight-loss efforts.

Fat is nutrient-dense in natural food sources. *But man-made fats and vegetable oils are not nutrient-dense.* Fat promotes satiety and minimizes inflammatory factors—if eaten in natural, whole foods that humans evolved eating.

FOOL ME TWICE, SHAME ON ME

The second primary concept for weight loss in the past couple of decades has been the "move more and eat less" dogma. It sounds plausible and feels sensible, just like the "lower your fat intake" paradigm. And yet it also ignores the realities of human metabolism.

Let's examine the proposition piece by piece.

Move more. Exercise has many health benefits, but weight control is not one of them.[2] Yes, if you move more you will burn more calories—great. But you will also increase your appetite. There is no escaping this fact. Even after long months of painfully rigorous training, many people who take up running to lose weight are still fat—because they are now ravenous. Back in the sixties, runners were not fat. Even most of the paper-pushers who spent their time behind a desk were not fat. The "move more" mantra only helps reduce weight in the long term *if you also chronically starve yourself.* Which, of course, is unsustainable.

Eat less. Mild starvation and self-denial has its benefits, but *sustainable* slimness is not one of them. Yes, if you eat little enough, you will lose weight—try eating nothing for a week to prove this obvious fact. But you will also unleash hunger, which in itself is a core driver of our obesity epidemic. Back in the sixties, hunger was not such a terrible threat. The kinds of foods we were eating did not drive hunger to problematic levels— they did not cut the wires on our hunger control system. The kinds of foods we're eating now do.

The "eat less, move more" theory assumes that humans are like simple steam engines rather than complex, hormone-controlled machines. In simple steam engines, the "energy in" matches the "work out"—it is a relatively straightforward calculation. In contrast, human machines are vastly more complicated, with myriad control-feedback loops that change everything. "Eat less, move more" ignores these most important body mechanisms—the crucial feedback loops of hormones that control appetite and weight loss and gain—and the pivotal effects of the *type* of food we eat. That is why the vast majority of calorie-counting diets fail over the long term.[3] They implement the unsustainable and entirely bypass the most important factors in the problem.

The same type of flawed and simplistic thinking led to the recommendations that placed "complex carbohydrates" like breads and pasta at the base of the food pyramid. Ignoring the hormonal systems has led to serious unintended consequences, from obesity to diabetes and more.

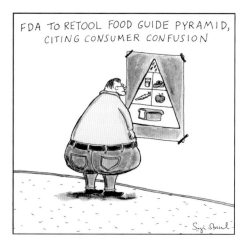

By Sage Stossel for TheAtlantic.com.

BEATING THE SPRING

So what is it about the body's feedback loops that's so important to weight loss and good health? It all comes down to hormones. Hormones are powerful signaling molecules that control many functions in the body. Many, many hormonal control loops govern appetite and body weight. Over the long run, the powerful effects of these hormones will beat willpower every time.

Imagine that you are stretching out a strong spring that's attached to a wall. You can hold it for quite a while, perhaps, but eventually your arm grows tired and the spring wins. Understanding this fact, you lock the spring with a hook or fastener, so it will stay put without your constant focus and effort.

In this analogy, the spring is your hormonal weight-control apparatus, which is ancient and remorseless. Your arm is your willpower. It may be robust when you start, but eventually it weakens. Maybe a difficult time in your life will undermine your willpower. Maybe time alone will weaken it. Regardless, slippage is almost inevitable. Willpower eventually fails. We will teach you how to beat the spring by restraining it with clever "hooks" that you can create in your body.

First, it is crucial to understand that *food is information*. What you put in your mouth sets off an explosive cascade of hormonal signaling throughout your body. The most trivial aspect of food is its calories. It is the *type* of food that is crucial to long-term weight-management success—as is the mixture of foods that make up your meals. What you eat determines how your body produces hormones that affect weight and health.

Many hormones work together and respond dramatically to the types of food you eat. Here's a short list of some major ones:

▶ Insulin (master regulator of glucose and fat-burning)

▶ Glucagon (controller of glucose release into your system, the yin to insulin's yang)

▶ Leptin (released by your fat cells to regulate appetite and more)

▶ Ghrelin (the hunger hormone, released by your empty stomach)

▶ GIP (stimulated by carbohydrate, released by your gut to trigger insulin and prime fat cells for energy take-up)

▶ GLP-1 (released in your gut to enhance the function of the pancreas, which makes insulin)

▶ PYY (released in your gut to control appetite and enhance pancreatic function)

AN INTRODUCTION TO INSULIN

Of all the hormones involved in weight control, insulin is the one to watch the most closely. Engineers live by the Pareto Principle, which says that 80 percent of a given problem is generally caused by 20 percent of the factors driving it. We need to focus on the *big* factors to be successful. Insulin signaling is one of those factors that can cause 80 percent of weight-control problems.

Insulin:

▶ rises rapidly based largely on signals emitted from your gut when you eat

▶ runs high in most people who are obese or have type 2 diabetes

▶ runs low in slim and healthy people (it may be high in slim people who are unhealthy)

▶ can be manipulated masterfully by the food choices you make

▶ is provoked most strongly by high carbohydrate intake—particularly refined carbohydrates

▶ is provoked to a lesser extent by protein intake

▶ is minimally provoked by fat intake

▶ can be badly disrupted by many nondietary factors, including poor sleep, stress, gut microbiome issues, smoking, and limited exposure to sunlight

Insulin is the master manager of glucose in the body: it moves glucose from the bloodstream into cells, which use glucose for energy. It also directly controls glucagon, which has an enormous effect on glucose production and release. Carbohydrate is essentially just glucose—a sugar molecule, or a bunch of them joined together. When you eat carbohydrate, your blood glucose levels rise, and insulin levels rise correspondingly. Insulin also tells the body not to burn fat—since more insulin means more glucose is available to use immediately as fuel. Insulin therefore dictates your ability to use fat as a fuel.

The most important goal you can have for weight loss or longevity is to *keep your insulin levels low.* This can be easy to do—when you eat the correct type of low-carb diet. Keeping insulin at low levels will enable this crucial hormone to perform its signaling functions optimally. Any dietary advice that doesn't account for insulin's effects will be deeply flawed.

Insulin in various molecular forms has existed for nearly a billion years. It has been doing its pivotal job in our bodies since the dawn of humanity. It manages the body's response to food, promotes fat storage, and prevents fat from being burned for energy when carbohydrate has been consumed. It is the last thing you want to provoke inappropriately.

For weight loss and longevity, you must respect your insulin!

WHAT YOU EAT MATTERS

All proper biochemistry textbooks acknowledge these fundamental properties of insulin. In spite of this fact, many of these textbooks still recommend a high-carbohydrate, low-fat diet for health and weight loss. This absurd contradiction is made possible by the fat-phobic lunacy that took over in the late 1970s and 1980s, as discussed in Chapter 1.

The supreme irony is that excessive glucose and excessive insulin can actually cause problems with the dietary fat you ingest. Many of the associations between fat and disease were created through this mechanism.

Remember that insulin prevents fat-burning. When insulin is driven higher by ingested carbohydrate, you cannot optimally burn any fat that you eat along with it. Insulin shuts down your fat-burning machinery. And with that machinery shut down, your body can't easily turn to stored fat for fuel when it's used up available glucose, resulting in more feelings of hunger. The spring will continue to exert its tireless pull.

What is the *worst* thing you can eat to provoke problematic amounts of insulin? A mixture of refined carbohydrate—for example, bread—and fatty foods: for example, a grass-fed meaty hamburger. Actually, it's never okay to eat bread. The hamburger could be okay if eaten on its own. In fact, bread can *cause* the hamburger to become problematic. There is a synergy between macronutrients. The mixture matters.

The higher-carb, lower-fat regimen has another major problem. Carbohydrate-rich foods raise blood sugar levels. Insulin must be promptly raised to manage this blood sugar. Particularly in people who need to lose weight, the insulin response can overshoot the mark. This will drive blood sugar levels down in the hour or two following a meal. The natural response to this blood sugar drop is the triggering of hunger signals. Carbohydrate-rich foods are also poorly satiating to begin with—they don't fill you up and keep you feeling full. The overall effect is that you feel hungry again soon after a meal. The spring is difficult to ignore—it will whisper in your ear, "You really need and deserve a snack."

RESISTANCE IS FUTILE

It is tragic that the people who really need to lose weight are generally the very people who have the greatest insulin-related problems, making it harder for them to lose weight. Overweight and unhealthy people normally have higher insulin levels, a condition known as hyperinsulinemia. Unfortunately, they also respond less well to insulin's orders, even though they have higher insulin levels—just as with any powerful drug, you can become resistant to the effects of insulin over time. This phenomenon is called insulin resistance. In fact, the majority of adult Americans now have an insulin resistance problem.[4] And a shocking proportion of our children have it, too.[5] A high level of insulin in the bloodstream with associated insulin resistance is the signature dysfunction of our modern age.

Anyone who needs to lose weight is highly likely to have some degree of insulin resistance. In contrast, slim, healthy people normally have low levels of insulin—they are insulin sensitive.

Most weight problems are underpinned by excessive insulin secretion. Moreover, type 2 diabetes is a manifestation of long-term insulin resistance. In type 2 diabetes, insulin resistance has progressed to the point that the body has lost control of blood glucose levels. Most heart disease is driven by diabetic vascular inflammation: high insulin and glucose levels damage the walls of your arteries, which leads to the buildup of materials in the artery walls. This process is called atherosclerosis, and it is the primary driver of heart attacks. Therefore, most heart disease is the result of being in a state of hyperinsulinemia and insulin resistance. Interestingly, even recent mathematical models based on very large data sets illustrate this point.[6] Many cancers are also tightly linked to hyperinsulinemia and its linked effects.[7] Shockingly, most primary care doctors don't measure insulin levels during a regular checkup.

Many population studies clearly show that insulin levels have been rising for decades, as of course you would expect given the diabetes epidemic.[8] In line with this rise, the decline in atherosclerosis rates since 1977, which was driven mainly by a reduction in smoking habits, stalled in 1994. Atherosclerosis rates then began to tilt upward again, in spite of continued smoking reduction.[9] One recent report predicts that the menace of diabetes-induced heart disease will sink our collective health.[10]

The first step in any health and weight-loss strategy should be to lower insulin levels. Whatever achieves this goal will tend to resolve insulin resistance and improve weight loss. This may not be a magic fix for everybody with weight issues, but it is the clear first step. Ignoring this step is one of the primary reasons why most diets fail.

BECOMING SENSITIVE

There will be more on the science of insulin and its important effects in later chapters. In the meantime, let's look at the bottom line.

Nearly everyone can achieve healthy low insulin levels and become insulin sensitive. A low-carbohydrate diet is the place to start, but some people may need to take more substantial measures (as we'll discuss in Chapter 6).

THE PLAN FOR LOWERING INSULIN

How do you go about lowering your insulin? The core strategy, based on science, is to lower the carbohydrate levels in your diet. The secondary consideration is to moderate your protein intake to appropriate levels, based on your muscle mass and exercise level, since excessive protein can also raise insulin levels. Finally, the bulk of your energy needs should be supplied by healthy, nutrient-dense fats. There are also many nondietary factors involved, such as getting enough sleep, exercising, and managing stress. All this forms the core of the Eat Rich, Live Long program, and we'll talk about it in more detail in Chapter 6.

People with insulin resistance can't burn fat effectively. Who are the people with the biggest insulin issues? See if you can pick out the group which you are in:

- **Slim, insulin sensitive:** Low blood insulin, super fat-burner, high life expectancy
- **Overweight, insulin sensitive:** Low blood insulin, moderate fat-burner, good life expectancy
- **Slim, insulin resistant:** High blood insulin, poor fat-burner, poor life expectancy
- **Overweight, insulin resistant:** High blood insulin, very poor fat-burner, very poor life expectancy
- **Type 2 diabetes (regardless of weight):** High blood insulin, dreadful fat-burner, dreadful life expectancy

Did you find your group? It's tricky if you have never measured your insulin. Did you notice that body weight is a weak indicator for judging your health outlook? What really matters is your insulin and blood glucose status. That's why many health authorities have been confused by the results of studies looking at body mass index and life expectancy. The trends and outcomes from these studies are all over the place, *because they're measuring the wrong thing.* Body mass index isn't the crucial factor; insulin is.

Before you embark on our plan to lower your insulin, it is important to know where you are starting from. This is not difficult to find out. The simplest way is to calculate what's called your HOMA value, which indicates your level of insulin resistance, using one of the many online calculators. (There's a good one at www.thebloodcode.com/homa-ir-calculator.) All you need for this is the measure of your fasting glucose and fasting insulin. These tests can be requested in any doctor's office. With those numbers in hand, you can plug your fasting glucose and insulin values into the calculator and get the result. If it is below 1.0, you have low insulin resistance. Between 1.0 and 1.5 is marginal and may require some corrective action. Approaching 2.0 and certainly above 2.0 indicates significant levels of insulin resistance. These must be tackled using our plan.

People with type 2 diabetes have major problems burning fat as a fuel—they have high blood glucose and high blood fat levels simultaneously. Over half of the US adult population is now classified as prediabetic or diabetic. Anyone caught in these categories has serious problems burning fat. That means the majority of American adults have a fat-burning problem, which is an absolute disaster for the health of our citizens.

If these folks have problems burning fat, does this mean they should eat less fat? No—that is not how it works. Insulin resistance (and the trouble with fat-burning it brings) starts with eating too much carbohydrate relative to dietary fat. Remember the worst mix a human can eat: lots of carb with plenty of fat.

For weight loss and longevity—by way of lower insulin status and insulin sensitivity—it is important to burn fat as your primary fuel, and that means significantly reducing the amount of carb you eat. Eating this way will also enable huge improvements in appetite control, since fat is so satiating. You

MARY'S STORY

At sixty-eight years old, Mary believed she was healthy and hardly needed a checkup. Sure, she had been overweight for twenty-five years, which was frustrating. But compared to her three siblings, who were all suffering from full-blown type 2 diabetes, she seemed healthy. She had always been careful with her diet and had exercised regularly for the past forty years. But "careful" had meant following the standard advice to eat a low-fat diet filled with whole grains and vegetables. And because no diet she'd tried had worked, she no longer believed in them and had thrown away her scale years ago.

Jeff's exam showed a serious level of prediabetes, so he prescribed a tailored low-carb diet of 70 percent of calories from fat, 20 percent from protein, and 10 percent from carb. It sounded strange to Mary, but she was willing to try it in order to avoid medications. She asked Jeff, "How do I eat that much fat when I've been trying to eliminate fat for forty years?" His advice: eat an avocado every day; eat more nuts, especially macadamias; and consume healthy fats, including coconut oil, olive oil, and butter. Later, she learned about adding more delicious fats and the wonderful health benefits of eliminating grains.

Within a few weeks, all Mary's friends were commenting on her transformation. Her clothes were becoming loose and her skin was glowing. After nine months of the new healthy-fat lifestyle, she had lost 40 pounds, her blood pressure was back to normal, and she had great cholesterol numbers. What's more, she no longer had arthritis pain, frequent urination, or low energy.

On a recent visit with Jeff, she asked, "How long should I be on this diet?" Jeff answered, "For the rest of your life." Mary was delighted. She is really enjoying her new lifestyle, which has freed her from obesity and serious health concerns and has given her renewed energy and vigor.

may even find that the increase in fat calories doesn't need to fully match the calories from carb lost from your diet. Pleasingly, your body fat can now become part of your fat-based fuel supply. This will particularly be the case after you have become "fat-adapted": after your body optimizes its fat-burning machinery and switches to preferring fat to glucose. This fat adaptation occurs in the first weeks of our plan and will be described in Part 2. When your body starts to rely primarily on fat for fuel instead of glucose, you'll be able to tap into your body fat stores in addition to dietary fat.

SAFE STORAGE IS EVERYTHING

Every time we eat, energy is stored in multiple different compartments in our bodies. That energy is then released steadily to fuel our activity when we are not eating. Think of your personal energy storage as a rechargeable battery in an electric car. When you eat, your batteries get charged up. Between meals, the batteries provide a steady release of energy to keep you alive. Let's briefly look at how carbohydrate and fat play into this process:

1. The glucose from food you eat is used for your body's immediate needs, and whatever remains is first stored in the *glycogen* battery. This glycogen reserve can hold around 2,000 calories' worth of glucose. These are short-term batteries—in the absence of food, they run out within a day or so. When glycogen is full, you will not be in a good state for the healthy burning of fat. *The healthiest state is one in which glycogen remains incompletely full.*

2. When the glycogen battery becomes full, excess glucose is converted into special fats that are released from the liver into the bloodstream. This process can drive up your "bad cholesterol" (LDL) and promote many other problems in the body. It is a very different phenomenon from the healthy processing of dietary fat. *The healthiest state is one in which glucose is not converted into these fats.*

3. The final storage depot is your body fat, or *adipose tissue.* The storage capacity here is huge, but most overweight people don't tap into it. *The healthiest state is one in which this battery is used almost exclusively.* To achieve this, you must stop drawing on glycogen (#1) and creating the special fats in your liver (#2).

Healthy dietary fats are the safest fuel in a well-formulated low-carb diet. They directly enable you to minimize your intake of glucose, and so achieve the optimization of 1 to 3 above.

In doing so, you can help keep your adipose tissue in good health and insulin sensitive.[11] When the cells of your adipose storage remain insulin-sensitive, they protect the rest of your body from metabolic dysregulation. In contrast, following a poor diet will allow your adipose tissue to become insulin resistant. When this happens, it is often the first step in the process that leads to your whole body becoming insulin resistant. In this way, much of modern chronic disease originates with unhealthy fat cells. (If you're interested in learning more about the importance of healthy fat cells, it's explored in more detail in Appendix D.)

For the majority of people, the worst diet to drive problems in adipose tissue is a high-carbohydrate diet—especially when it includes substantial dietary fat, and particularly if refined sugar and/or processed vegetable oils are added to the mix.

The best diet to achieve desirable insulin sensitivity is essentially the opposite of the silliness we've been sold. The best diet is low in carb and has good quantities of satiety-inducing healthy fats and protein. With the ratios right, your insulin is optimized. Much of the rest will follow. Obesity and chronic disease can be prevented and even largely reversed.

ARE YOU A SUGAR-BURNER OR A FAT-BURNER?

Your body's cells do not burn both glucose and fat at the same time. In fact, the core fat-burning mechanisms are intentionally shut down when glucose enters your system. Mammals always prioritize burning glucose when it is present—which makes sense, because glucose is toxic to cells when it is at elevated levels. Note that we only carry about 1.5 teaspoons of glucose in our entire blood supply. If it rises much beyond that, it will damage the body's organ systems. Fat, on the other hand, is easy for the body to store and reuse. But fat is not easy to tap into if carb is the main part of your meals.

The standard American diet relies primarily on carb—in fact, the government has told us for decades to make "healthy whole grains" the bulk of our calories. And most Americans are sugar-burners. What are the major implications of this higher-carb dietary strategy?

1. You experience blood sugar and insulin spikes.

   ▶ This downregulates the fat-burning machinery.
   ▶ For many, this can promote a speedier onset of post-meal hunger pangs.
   ▶ Over time, insulin spikes can lead to insulin resistance.
   ▶ With increasing insulin levels, the negative aspects of the diet become magnified.

2. You miss out on the benefits of nutrient-dense foods high in healthy fat and protein.

   ▶ For many, hunger pangs start sooner after meals that lack fat and protein.

   ▶ This promotes larger, hunger-driven meals and snacking behavior.

   ▶ A relative deficiency in fat-soluble nutrients can promote appetite to compensate for their lack.

Let's contrast the above with a diet that focuses on healthy fats and keeps carb intake low. The implications of this diet are as follows:

1. You will minimize blood sugar and insulin spikes.

   ▶ This upregulates your fat-burning machinery and reduces your dependency on sugar.

   ▶ It enhances smooth burning of body fat between meals, suppressing appetite and enabling you to skip meals without undue hunger.

   ▶ Over time, your insulin resistance levels will fall steadily, and with them your risk of chronic disease.

2. You will gain access to a whole range of nutrient-dense foods, which will enhance your health and vitality.

The above is only a brief summary of the advantages that come with a high-healthy-fat diet. We will be exploring them in more detail throughout the rest of the book.

In short, a higher-carb diet promotes a sugar-burning physiology, which directly impedes your fat-burning ability. This is the very last thing that you want, for either weight loss *or* longevity. But the worst thing about being a sugar-burner over the long term is that it drives up your risk of acquiring the most prevalent disease in our world today, which in turn underpins the risk for most diseases of modernity—heart disease, diabetes, Alzheimer's, and many cancers. We call this disease state metabolic insulin resistance syndrome (MIRS)—and the last thing you want to be on is the MIRS diet.

"**The more insulin resistant one was, the greater the negative impact of a high-carbohydrate diet.**"

—Dr. Gerald M. Reaven

CHAPTER 4

STOP THE TOXIC MIRS DIET

We have an explosion of health problems today. Obesity, type 2 diabetes, and a shocking array of afflictions associated with them are rampant. The dysfunctions of obesity and diabetes are so closely interlinked that the term *diabesity* has been coined, and the incidence of fatty liver disease—which is intimately connected to the foods we eat, just like obesity and type 2 diabetes—has increased massively; over a third of US citizens now have fatty liver, whereas in the 1960s, the condition was mostly confined to alcohol abusers.[1]

Since the 1970s, there have been reductions in the old causes of heart disease mortality. For example, we have greatly reduced rates of tobacco smoking. There has also been an explosion of medical therapy and surgical intervention to help reduce deaths from heart disease. And yet heart disease remains our number one killer, and its incidence is rising at frightening rates, outpacing our ability to manage it.[2] Extensive heart disease is just one price we pay for the failed nutritional dogmas—it's no coincidence that its rate rose as we reduced our natural fat intake considerably over the last few decades.[3]

We were told that all these problems were related to our consumption of natural fats. The evidence simply doesn't support that. Obesity and its related diseases, including heart disease, have skyrocketed since the 1970s; for dietary fat intake to be a key factor in this dysfunction, it should have risen, too. It did not. We followed official dietary advice and impressively reduced our intake of natural fats from red meat, fatty fowl, cheese, butter, and eggs, replacing them with industrially produced vegetable oils.

It is true that we have increased our caloric intake substantially over the past several decades, driven in a significant way by the appetite surge caused by a low-fat diet and trying to "eat less, move more." Yet we have not increased the number of calories we get from dietary fat. Overall, today we get about the same number of calories from fat as we did in the 1970s (though today we eat a lot more man-made fats). So where, then, did all the extra calories associated with the diabesity epidemic come from? They pretty much all came from *extra carbohydrate*.

HOW TO LOOK LIKE A SUMO WRESTLER

We are all familiar with sumo wrestlers, those leviathans of the sporting world. While there is muscle in there somewhere, definitely, an enormous amount of body fat covers the lean. This famous sport has been cultivated for more than 3,000 years. Sumo wrestlers know how to generate the required bloated bodies, that's for sure. They ingest a huge percentage of dietary carbohydrates, keeping fat relatively very low.[4] Sumo wrestlers stay healthy due to their grueling exercise regimen, but they tend to fall apart when their careers end.

METABOLIC MADNESS

Humans are clever. Generally, we find the best ways of doing things to get results, especially when money is involved. Fatty marbled meat has been desirable for centuries. So what key factor have we consistently used over the centuries to fatten cattle, pigs, and other animals rapidly, thereby marbling their meat? Grains—pure carbohydrate, pure glucose. Pigs are omnivores, with a physiology especially close to ours. Historically, the best method to fatten pigs was to feed them a combination of skim milk and grains.[5] In fact, farmers had to be careful not to feed them too much of this low-fat fare, lest the pigs become obese and metabolically damaged.

Or consider foie gras, created for centuries from fatty goose livers, made by force-feeding the poor geese grain, lots of grain—pure carbohydrate. People are no different: a healthy liver should *never* contain appreciable amounts of fat, but now half of adult Americans have that problem—because we eat so much carbohydrate.

Like other mammals, we humans are fattened primarily by carbohydrates. Any refining, such as mechanically refining grains or creating high-fructose corn syrup, supercharges the problem exponentially. (There's a great study on this effect explained on page 358.)

On top of the weight gain, with time, excessive carbohydrate intake drives metabolic dysregulation in most people: it causes excessive insulin secretion, which, over time, promotes insulin resistance, and other hormones that interact with insulin are affected and become dysfunctional as well. Overall, the body's hormonal systems that control appetite and weight gain become deranged—nothing works the way it was intended to—and we basically lose control of our weight and health.

This hormonal problem was given a name in the 1970s: metabolic syndrome. Later, it came to be known as syndrome X. High insulin levels and insulin resistance are now understood to drive metabolic syndrome, and it is sometimes referred to as insulin resistance syndrome. We refer to it as metabolic insulin resistance syndrome (MIRS) to highlight the fact there is no mystery about its origin, as "syndrome X" suggests—insulin dysregulation is at its very core. Calling it "metabolic syndrome" highlights that it is a metabolic problem but sidesteps its deeper nature. We believe that both elements of this crucial disease state—the fact that it's a metabolic problem and that it stems from problems with insulin regulation—should be acknowledged in the name. Especially given that this is the most common disease state in the world.

MIRS will scuttle your weight-loss efforts like nothing else. Unsurprisingly, rates of MIRS have exploded since the low-fat guidelines came into being.[6] The World Health Organization and many other bodies have slightly differing criteria for MIRS, but they all center on the same set of variables.[7] In sum, you have a serious MIRS problem if you suffer from three or more of the following conditions:

▶ Low HDL ("good cholesterol")

▶ High triglycerides (fats in your blood)

▶ Large waist size

▶ High blood pressure

▶ High blood sugar

No world authorities bother including LDL ("bad cholesterol"), because it has little relevance to disease for most people. We'll see why later. In contrast, the most powerful pair in the list are HDL and triglycerides. Having both low HDL and high triglycerides indicates that unhealthy hormonal signaling is afoot.

Note that insulin measures are not included in the list of criteria, either. Is this not bizarre, given that insulin is at the very core of MIRS? Unfortunately, for many decades it has been unpopular to measure insulin in population studies. It would raise many awkward questions around the cholesterol dogma and our current approach to managing chronic disease. Also, there are no saleable drugs that really tackle the problem of high insulin. (Medications for type 2 diabetes, such as metformin, treat high blood sugar primarily, rather than high insulin.) But there are *many* drugs that tackle things like high blood pressure, high triglycerides, and high blood sugar—all on the list of MIRS criteria. As a result, insulin as a screening measure for MIRS has been grossly neglected. This is one of the central reasons why our epidemic of obesity, diabetes, and heart disease has blossomed over the decades.

If you measured insulin metrics directly, you could diagnose MIRS in a heartbeat. Most doctors have not been educated on how it all works, however. They remain distracted by weak metrics like LDL, largely wasting their time.

Given the connection between insulin and MIRS, it's not surprising that MIRS is intimately connected to type 2 diabetes and obesity. However, it may come as more of a surprise that MIRS is a crucial factor in the heart disease epidemic. Heart disease remains the world's biggest killer in spite of enormous medical advances and a huge drop in smoking rates, and it shares metabolic root causes with the other MIRS diseases. We can see this by looking at people who develop heart disease at an early age. It's similar to how engineers approach a complex problem: they focus quickly on "early-in-life-cycle failures." These are the parts that fail much earlier than they should. When scrutinized, they can point to the problem's primary cause. So it is with the problem of heart disease. When we look at what causes people to develop heart disease at an early age, it tells us something important about heart disease itself.

An excellent recent scientific paper did this very analysis.[8] It is packed with all the risk factors that are most important for early-adulthood atherosclerosis. It hardly mentions LDL. When it does, it notes that there is a lack of evidence demonstrating that children with high LDL levels are more likely to later develop atherosclerosis. But it does call out as critical factors pretty much all of the phenomena that are intimately linked to MIRS: low HDL, high triglycerides, high blood pressure, high blood sugar, obesity/waist size. In fact, another study found that children between the ages of six and nineteen with metabolic syndrome (MIRS) had almost *fifteen times* the risk of heart disease in their future.

THE FRUCTOSE FACTOR

In the previous chapter, we discussed glucose as the fundamental element of carbohydrate. But we didn't discuss the other key carb molecule: fructose. Like glucose, fructose is a monosaccharide—a single sugar molecule—and it's a major part of our sugar consumption today.

In past millennia, human beings had access only to small amounts of fructose. Small amounts are perfectly okay for healthy humans, and fructose was historically available mainly from fiber-rich fruits, which were lower in sugar than they are today. Fructose was also accessible if our ancestors came across some honey, which is pretty much unrefined sugar with a few nutrients thrown in. Fructose was a relatively rare treat for our scruffy forebears; it was seasonal and access was sporadic. Things are very, very different now.

In the past hundred years, our consumption of fructose has exploded. Today we have high-sugar fruits that have been bred for sweetness, and we are encouraged to eat them every day, not just seasonally. Even worse are fruit juices and smoothies, which are actually promoted as healthy. Compared to ancestral whole fruits, these products expose you to much more fructose.

Table sugar is an equal mix of glucose and fructose molecules. This is a bad combination to consume in excess. In many processed foods, this compound has been mostly replaced by high-fructose corn syrup (HFCS): same badness, slightly different formula. (It is approximately 40 percent glucose and 60 percent fructose.) These compounds are present not only in sugary drinks and sweets but in just about every processed food product on the shelves: bread, cereal, weight-loss products, sauces, and much more.

How much refined sugar (both glucose and fructose) did humans ingest as the species evolved? The estimates are somewhere in the region of 1.5 teaspoons a day, mostly from occasionally available sources like honey. The World Health Organization now recommends no more than 6 teaspoons a day for adults and no more than 3 teaspoons for children—whether it comes from traditional refined sugar or HFCS makes little difference.[9] The average American currently consumes around 20 teaspoons of sugar per day, with teenagers ingesting more than adults.[10] It is therefore no surprise that teenagers' insulin levels are going through the roof: although fructose itself does not cause insulin excretion, it promotes insulin resistance through other pathways, which in turn drive higher insulin levels and the associated obesity.[11]

FRUCTOSE KILLS

The title of a 2014 study of fructose, well worth a quick read, illustrates just how bad fructose is for you: "Carbohydrate Intake and Non-Alcoholic Fatty Liver Disease: Fructose as a Weapon of Mass Destruction."[12]

The study team did not pull any punches with the title, and they have ample justification for it. As this review paper nicely lays out, fructose occupies a special place in the obesity and disease nightmare. Fructose may be okay in moderate quantities if you are slim and healthy—but it is the last thing that should pass your lips if you are not.

Glucose can be directly absorbed into most of your body's cells. In a healthy person, a relatively small amount is directed to the liver. Fructose, however—like alcohol—*must* be sent to the liver for processing. Once it gets there, fructose must be carefully managed in the liver, which has the ability to convert some of it into a form of glucose. For a huge number of people, however, it will generally be converted into fats or triglycerides. Some of those fats end up in the bloodstream, but some stay right in the liver, building up over time and leading to nonalcoholic fatty liver disease.

Excessive glucose can also lead to fatty liver; geese bred for foie gras are an elegant example of this problem. But a moderate glucose intake may be quite tolerable for many individuals—until appreciable fructose is added. That can tip the balance toward a dysfunctional buildup of liver fat. The mechanisms are many and include increases in post-meal triglyceride levels, visceral adiposity, and delivery of fats to the liver via its blood supply.[13] There are also many other pathways being clarified, including the promotion of uric acid production, which has many negative effects in the liver and throughout the body's organ systems.[14] The increase in triglycerides and cholesterol leads directly to lower levels of HDL cholesterol—one of the MIRS criteria. It also leads to increased levels of *small and dense* or *oxidized* LDL. While normal LDL may not present a problem, these forms of modified LDL can do so, leading to an increased risk of heart disease.

On top of all this, the liver wasn't designed to handle an abundance of fructose, and too much will accelerate metabolic issues, ruining both your weight-loss efforts and your health.

When we take in glucose and fructose together in high quantities (as in table sugar and HFCS), we experience an unfortunate double punch. The glucose ramps up insulin, which tends to direct the fructose toward conversion into fat—making *you* fat. The fructose-driven fat can also end up in your liver, pancreas, and other organs: another unfortunate way for your diet to fail.

A human experiment illustrates this effect on organ fat buildup (not to mention sugar's effects on other MIRS metrics).[15] The team selected sixty overweight people who were healthy and nondiabetic. They randomly assigned the people to four groups, and each group was given a different drink: a typical sugar-sweetened soft drink (SSSD), milk, diet soda (sweetened with artificial sweeteners rather than sugar), or water. The participants drank a liter (approximately 2 pints) of their assigned drink per day. Importantly, all groups remained isocalorific—there was no difference in calorie intake between the groups over the six months of the experiment. Remember, the sucrose used in the SSSD was composed of equal parts glucose and fructose.

While the other three groups showed no significant differences at the end of the experiment, the SSSD drinkers suffered:

▶ an approximately 25 percent increase in visceral fat (fat around the internal organs)

▶ an approximately 130 percent increase in liver fat

▶ a significant increase in blood pressure, triglycerides, and total cholesterol

Having fat around your internal organs is linked to all kinds of chronic disease, including—unsurprisingly, given what we know about MIRS—heart disease and type 2 diabetes.

Interestingly, building visceral fat is actually a key survival strategy for bears and other animals: the rich supply of fruit in the summer and fall allows them to consume copious quantities of fructose, leading to massive fat stores that let them survive the winter. But for modern human beings, winter never comes. We keep consuming "healthy" fruit all year. On top of this, sneaky sugar creeps in via most of the processed foods that we eat.

Fructose also triggers hunger in a way that even glucose does not. Insulin, which is released in response to glucose, plays its own role in managing the appetite system, and glucose sensors in the digestive system trigger a range of hormones involved in appetite and fat-storage management. In short, there are key regulatory mechanisms that sense the presence of glucose and help manage its effects on your appetite—when glucose is present, appetite is dialed down somewhat. Fructose is missing these key regulatory steps (possibly because it was less available in our ancestral past). Therefore, even when you consume large amounts of fructose, it does not adequately trigger your satiety system. You don't feel satisfied, and you want more and more.

STUDIES SHOW A HIGH-CARB DIET IS A MIRS DIET

There are countless scientific papers that highlight the problem of fructose.[16] The title of this one, for instance, neatly illustrates that it's fundamental to MIRS: "Fructose: A Key Factor in the Development of Metabolic Syndrome and Hypertension." Glucose, of course, with its insulin-spiking effects, also shares in the blame. Overall, this much is clear: a diet that's high in both is a diet that leads to MIRS.

In one recent and revealing study, researchers used a sugar-plus-fat diet to give rats four out of the five criteria for MIRS.[17] The fifth criteria was low HDL ("good cholesterol"), but it did not drop as much as it should have to properly model human MIRS. Adding even more fructose to the diet was great for accelerating the disease process, but HDL still wasn't dropping the way it does in humans, which was somewhat frustrating. The researchers wanted to find the *perfect* MIRS diet, one that would cause all five MIRS criteria to explode in the poor rats.

Then they had a revelation: A key ingredient in the human MIRS diet is *refined* wheat flour. Previously, all the rat experiments had been using *unrefined* wheat flour pellets. So the researchers cleverly decided to use refined flour instead. They struck HDL-destroying gold.

When the researchers added refined wheat flour to the high-fructose, high-fat diet, the rats' HDL dropped like a stone and they became diseased with MIRS much more rapidly than before. By replacing the standard fiber-rich wheat with refined wheat flour, the researchers achieved "hypertension [high blood pressure], hyperglycemia [high blood sugar], hyper-triglyceridemia [high triglycerides], and also HDL reduction … in only four weeks compared to the usual eight." The study was entitled "Fiber-Free White Flour with Fructose Offers a Better Model of Metabolic Syndrome."

Another study showing the importance of fructose on the road to MIRS is very interesting for three reasons: (1) it used quantities of fructose closer to what people may actually eat; (2) it used animals that are much, much closer to our human physiology than rats—rhesus monkeys; and (3) the experiment was allowed to run for a full year, which is long enough for any effects to manifest themselves.[18] The monkeys were fed a standard low-fat monkey chow, but in addition, every day each monkey was given approximately a pint of fruit-flavored drink that contained 15 percent fructose (a little over 2.5 ounces of fructose). After a year of consuming 2.5 ounces of fructose each day, what had happened to the monkeys? Every single one had developed MIRS, and four of the twenty-eight had developed full-blown type 2 diabetes. While unfortunately there was no control group to measure against, it would be staggeringly unlikely for twenty-eight rhesus monkeys on standard chow to go down with MIRS within a single year.

Researchers often call an unhealthy dietary regimen in a study a "high-fat diet," making sure that the blame for all the metabolic damage can be laid at fat's door. But these bad diets are invariably high in *sugar* as well as fat! The studies often fail to mention the sugar—but as you can see in the two studies just described, the *sugar* is really what propels the subjects into a terrible state of MIRS. Fat just goes along for the ride. It is important to note that in many studies, people with MIRS have seen stunning improvements with properly formulated high-fat, low-carb diets and ultra low carb ketogenic diets. In fact, the very worst enemy that MIRS has is a properly implemented high-fat, low-carb diet!

TOXIC OILS DRIVE THE MIRS DIET

Most orthodox diets push polyunsaturated vegetable oils. These are suggested to replace natural saturated fats. The 2015 *Dietary Guidelines for Americans* actually increased the recommended intake for polyunsaturated vegetable oils. Honestly, aren't we eating far too much of these compounds already?

Our obesity epidemic has mushroomed since we reduced natural dietary fat and began to eat more carbohydrates, but we also greatly increased our intake of polyunsaturated vegetable oils in the same period.

Over evolutionary history, humans ingested very low levels of polyunsaturated fats. These fats are indeed essential for human health. *But only very low intakes are required.* And only low levels were ingested for most of history. Our consumption of polyunsaturated fats has increased significantly in the past century, and this is unprecedented in human history. We now consume maybe twenty times more than the base requirement for health.

There are different types of polyunsaturated fats, but the main ones to note are the omega-3 and omega-6 varieties. Excessive intake of omega-6 fatty acids drives inflammation, and having the right ratio of omega-6 to omega-3—ideally, 1:1 to 3:1—is essential for good health. Omega-3 fatty acids come mainly from fish, animal foods, and certain plant foods. We have not increased our consumption of omega-3—in fact, consumption of foods containing omega-3 has actually decreased markedly. Omega-6, however, is a different story. Historically, it came mainly from animal foods and certain plant foods. But now it's found in huge quantities in refined vegetable oils, and we are drowning in them!

Soybean oil is the dominant source of polyunsaturated fats; it constitutes approximately half of all the vegetable oil consumed in the US. In fact, the estimated per capita consumption of soybean oil increased a thousandfold from 1909 to 1999. Largely as a result of this, omega-6 fats in our diets increased from 2.79 percent to 7.21 percent.[19] This is a huge change in human evolutionary terms.

What are the likely effects of these oils when taken in such excess? The emerging science says that they're highly negative. The effects range from increased systemic inflammation to significant weight gain to type 2 diabetes. There are very few properly executed studies in this area, however. As with the sugar situation, most of the research has been trying to frame health-promoting natural dietary fats. But one study from 2015 looked closely at the vegetable oil problem: "Soybean Oil Is More Obesogenic and Diabetogenic Than Coconut Oil and Fructose in Mouse: Potential Role for the Liver."[20]

Although it was conducted in mice, this study was well executed and the mechanisms were carefully explained. The title itself is revealing. The detailed conclusions were shocking. Basically, polyunsaturated soybean oil drove the development of type 2 diabetes and weight gain. Coconut oil, which is high in saturated fat, was relatively benign in comparison, even when the researchers added fructose to it. The combination of polyunsaturated oil and fructose, however, was a disaster. And this nasty combination has gone through the roof in the past century. Most processed foods are laden with both polyunsaturated oils and sugar—modern breads alone are a perfect example of the problem. Many more studies and animal experiments that illustrate the dangers of excessive vegetable oils are emerging. Tragically, these studies have been done only in the past few years—decades after this work should have been done.[21]

The industrial process that produces these polyunsaturated oils causes the fats to become damaged and essentially unfit for human consumption.[22] If you saw the multistep industrial process used to create these oils, you would not touch them. High temperatures, high pressures, petrochemical solvents, bleaching, and more! This rancid concoction goes through a deodorizing step near the end of the factory line, and it desperately needs it. The workers in the factory need to wear respirators while making this "food." (You can get an idea of the process by watching a YouTube video on the FatHeadMovie channel, www.youtube.com/watch?v=omjWmLG0EAs.) Yet we are told to replace natural, genuinely healthy fats with these chemical compounds.

A complete review of the impact of excessive vegetable oils on human health is included in Appendix E. After you read it, we are sure you'll do the right thing. Remove polyunsaturated oils and processed foods from your diet. You will get plenty of polyunsaturated fats from our healthy whole-foods diet plan.

In essence, the most important thing about any diet is the extent to which it prevents or reduces the effects of MIRS in your body. The best dietary strategies to achieve this are ones that minimize the consumption of refined carbohydrates, sugars, and vegetable oils. Of course, once you eliminate these foods, you will need to replace these missing calories with healthier alternatives. And that is where healthy fats come to the rescue!

DAVID'S STORY

David Bobbett is an Irish business leader who came close to being one of millions who die from heart attacks—long before they are diagnosed with insulin problems. He had catastrophic levels of heart disease, but none of his blood tests revealed the reality.

In 2012, David appeared to be an unusually healthy fifty-two-year-old man, running several days a week to maintain his slim and fit physique. The father of six children, he had many reasons to ensure his personal longevity. David had been passing his executive medical exams with flying colors. All his blood tests were good, and his cardiac treadmill tests put him in the top fitness bracket for his age.

But he accepted and believed in the high-carb nutritional guidelines. He was therefore careful to avoid fats, and he fueled himself mostly on carbs. This serious mistake was speeding him toward an early grave.

Most heart attacks are linked to hyperinsulinemia and insulin resistance. These issues don't always show up in common blood tests, especially for physically fit people. And David, like most people, never had his insulin checked—doctors simply don't test people for elevated insulin. So with all the positive test results he got, David had been given an illusion of good health.

But for many years, David's arteries had been secretly burning. He came very close to losing it all, but he got a really lucky break: he happened to get a CT scan of his heart, which gave him a coronary artery calcium (CAC) score, the very last word on how much heart disease is burning inside you. We'll talk more about this crucial scan in Chapter 11, but essentially, it shows where arteries have recruited calcium to shore up the most damaged parts of the arterial wall. Genuinely healthy people of his age can have a score of zero calcium, which experts call a "fifteen-year warranty." David's score of 907 put him in the worst 1 percent of heart disease severity for his age. His arteries were those of an eighty-seven-year-old. Three-quarters of people with his score go on to have a serious heart attack within ten years.

After the shocking results of the CAC scan, David's doctors finally measured his blood glucose and insulin levels following a meal. They were catastrophically high. He was a secret diabetic—one of countless millions. The most underdiagnosed disease in the world was rapidly destroying his arteries.

After a period of intense personal research, David realized two things. The first was that the CAC scan is an incredibly powerful technology that is grossly underused at present. To address this, he funded a documentary movie about it called *The Widowmaker* to help others get the wake-up call that had saved his life. The second thing he learned was that he, like most of us, had been misinformed about the dietary drivers of heart disease and other chronic issues. He rapidly lowered his carb intake to begin healing his heart and took many other measures to repair his body and become truly healthy. We will share all of them with you so that you can do likewise.

The happy ending to David's story is that he succeeded in slowing the progression of his disease to safe levels. His later CAC scans demonstrated that his risk level had plummeted. He maintains exquisite control over his blood glucose through applying all of the rules in our plan—without using any diabetic medications. He is thriving on his new regimen and is now focused on giving something back. Because he had the rare opportunity to discover his disease and to save himself, he now dedicates substantial resources to ensuring that others can have the same opportunity. He founded the Irish Heart Disease Awareness (IHDA) charity to let people know heart disease is both measureable and preventable. In his own words, this is "simply the right thing to do."

(We highly recommend watching the fascinating movie *The Widowmaker* at vimeo.com/ondemand/thewidowmakermovie2015.)

" It's highly likely that carbohydrates, and not fat, cause inflammation. "

—Dr. Colin Champ

CHAPTER 5

LOW-CARB, HIGH-FAT FOR THE WIN

So if a diet that's high in carb and high in fat is the worst possible diet, what's the *best* possible diet? It's one that's low in carb and high in healthy natural fats.

There are huge benefits to a low-carb, high-healthy-fat diet. There are so many that to claim them all can come across as unrealistic. But claim them all we will, because they are all genuine. A properly formulated low-carb, high-healthy-fat diet:

► is hugely effective in resolving prediabetes and diabetes

► enables and enhances appetite control to achieve desired weight loss

► optimizes the absorption of the crucial fat-soluble vitamins A, D, E, and K

► enhances immune system function and promotes resistance to infection

► minimizes systemic inflammation

► enhances rapid recovery after sustained vigorous exercise

► allows us to enjoy the power of fasting for slimness, longevity, mental acuity, and increased productivity

► lowers the risk of heart disease

► slows aging effects and enables vitality, energy, and youthfulness

► enhances libido

► promotes healthy skin, hair, nails, and many other outward signs of health

All this is possible because reducing carb and eating more healthy fats lowers insulin levels. As we talked about in Chapter 3, keeping insulin levels low is the most important thing that you can do to lose weight, reduce your risk of heart disease, and increase your longevity.

ADAPTATION IS THE KEY

Your body is a hybrid machine that can burn glucose (carb) or fat, depending on what's available—but it does not like to burn both at the same time. Rather, it switches between the two modes. When we sleep at night, we are essentially fasting and therefore switch to fat-burning mode. So in a sense, everybody fasts intermittently.

But while everyone can switch to burning fat, some people are experts at it. These people are truly fat-adapted—their bodies run spectacularly well on fat, and they hardly use their glucose-burning capability at all. This is a very healthy, low-inflammation way to run the body's systems.

Fat adaptation is the process that leads to a person becoming a highly efficient fat-burner. Fully fat-adapted people are well able to safely manage a big load of dietary fat—as long as it's not eaten with a lot of carb. They are also able to smoothly access body fat for fuel whenever there's a need.

We have around 20,000 to 40,000 calories of energy stored on our body. Fat-adapted people can tap into this fuel readily when power is required. They are spared jittery low-blood-sugar hunger—those annoying pangs that drive the non-adapted back to the cookie jar.

The easiest and best way to become a fat-burner is to eat a well-formulated low-carb, high-fat diet. A week or two into our low-carb plan and you will be burning fat like never before. You can become a master in this art, and this in turn will enable you to become a master at fasting for health and slimness. The beauty is that regular periods of fasting will also enhance your fat-burning ability. It is a truly virtuous cycle.

One reason that exercise is good for you relates to this very phenomenon. Sustained or vigorous exercise benefits your fat-adaptation development. It can also drain your glycogen stores enough to switch on your fat-burning mechanisms.

LOW-CARB, HIGH-FAT SURE BEATS STARVING YOURSELF!

In Chapter 13, we will look in more detail at studies that prove the benefits of a low-carb, high-fat diet. For the moment, let's look quickly at one of the most important studies, which shows just how much a high-fat diet can improve your risk factors for heart disease.

This study looked at a range of people affected by MIRS.[1] The participants were randomly assigned to four groups. One group was put on a low-fat, very high carb diet, one on a moderate-fat, high-carb diet, one on a high-fat, low-carb diet, and one on a high-fat, low-carb diet that emphasized saturated fat. All the participants followed their diet for three weeks without reducing their calories.

The result? The high-fat, low-carb diet that emphasized saturated fat yielded incredible improvements in blood markers that indicate risk of heart disease. (We'll talk more about those markers in Chapter 11.) The other high-fat diet also gave great results.

After three weeks, the participants stayed on the same diet but reduced their calories by 1,000 calories per day. They followed this drastic starvation plan for nine weeks.

All the groups saw improvements after nine weeks. But what's really amazing is that after nine weeks, the participants following highest-carb diets saw only *half* the improvement that the highest-fat group saw after three weeks *without any calorie restriction at all.*

In other words, following the classic low-fat diet and starving yourself is only half as effective as following a healthy high-fat diet and eating normally.

WHAT EXACTLY IS A "HEALTHY FAT"?

The simplest definition of "healthy fat" is "fat that can be found in natural, ancestral foods." These can be from animal or plant sources. There is no credible evidence that natural fats are anything other than nutritious fuel for humans. In the absence of credible evidence, it is absurd to blame the foods humans ate while evolving for today's health epidemics.

But keep in mind that the healthful nature of fats depends in part on what you eat along with them. If you consume them alongside refined carbohydrate, all bets are off. A diet that's high in both fats *and* carbs is the worst possible diet and will lead straight to MIRS.

Healthy high-fat diets depend on carb moderation for their benefits to accrue. They also depend on using genuinely healthy fats rather than industrially created ones. Here's a quick overview of healthy fats:

▶ The healthiest fats are those found in fish. The fattier the fish, the better. Examples include wild salmon, mackerel, and sardines.

▶ Plant sources of fat are many and varied. Nuts, avocados, olives, coconuts, and the like contain a range of beneficial fats to provide nutritious and satiating energy for our bodies.

▶ Fats from land animals are also overwhelmingly good to eat in a well-formulated low-carb diet. Contrary to what we've been led to believe, animal fats are not made up exclusively of the much-vilified saturated fat. For example, lard from pigs contains more monounsaturated fat (the same kind found in olive oil) than saturated fat.[2]

You should not run short on variety when seeking out sources of nutritious fat energy. We'll provide much more detail, along with delicious recipes, in Part 2. And Chapter 13 explains the deeper science supporting the healthy use of fat.

On the polyunsaturated front, you should optimize your omega-3 intake and moderate your omega-6 intake. You can achieve most of the required omega-6 reduction by greatly restricting processed foods—the phrase "just eat real food" always applies. Replace all vegetable oils (canola, soybean, cottonseed, sunflower, safflower, etc.) with olive oil, coconut oil, and other cold-pressed oils, which are extracted directly from real foods.

You will not believe the appetite control that is possible once you have adapted to a diet rich in healthy fats. This change must be made properly, however, and that's what Part 2 is all about.

ARE THERE EXCEPTIONS TO THE HEALTHY-FAT RULE?

While most people respond optimally to the full range of ancestral fatty foods, there may be a minority who require a customized approach. The most established example is people who have the ApoE4 genotype, which is associated with higher cholesterol and a slightly higher rate of coronary heart disease. In people with ApoE4 who have sustained lasting metabolic damage from high-carb diets, consuming excessive meat or even cheeses may spike insulin and glucose levels. As a result, they achieve much greater benefits through targeting fish, eggs, avocado, and other non-meat sources of fat. Low-cost genetic tests for ApoE4 are readily available (for instance, from 23andMe.com). For more on how you can optimize your health if you have ApoE4, see page 343.

DIFFERENT LOW-CARB, HIGH-FAT STRATEGIES

Even in the low-carb world, there are several different views on what the optimal ratio of macronutrients might be. To summarize, there are three main lower-carb approaches:

▶ Paleo: medium carb, moderate to high protein, moderate fat

▶ Low-carb, high-fat (LCHF): low carb, moderate protein, high fat

▶ Keto: very low carb, moderate protein, very high fat

The Paleo diet is based on the belief that we should eat as our ancient ancestors did, before the advent of modern foods. Therefore, it prohibits foods that were not eaten more than ten thousand years ago, including breads, refined grains, and dairy products like milk and cheese. In terms of macronutrient ratios, Paleo is generally 50 percent fat, 20 percent protein, and 30 percent carbohydrate. In contrast, a standard low-carb, high-fat diet is approximately 60 percent fat, 20 percent protein, and 20 percent carbohydrate.

Keto is a special case of low-carb. *Keto* is short for *ketogenic diet,* so named because burning fat produces unique molecules called ketones, which are used for energy. On keto, the body enters a state of *nutritional ketosis,* in which it is fueled by fat. Keto is essentially a very low carb regimen, with a very high percentage of energy coming from dietary fats—or your own body fat. Achieving a state of nutritional ketosis can result in major health and weight-loss benefits, even when compared to a classic low-carb approach. In a sense, keto is the ultimate fat-burning diet. We will explain it further in Chapter 13. In the meantime, we'll highlight that the keto macronutrient mix is approximately 70 percent or more fat, 20 percent protein, and less than 10 percent carb. The accomplished nutritional researchers Jeff Volek and Steve Phinney have produced a useful diagram to capture the primary macronutrient approaches, Figure 5.1.

We favor LCHF as the best strategy in today's world because it has proven overwhelmingly beneficial for resolving MIRS; although Paleo is also a much healthier diet than the standard American diet, it doesn't have the benefits provided by reducing carb further and increasing fat. Keto, as a more extreme

Figure 5.1. Different macronutrient ratios for different dietary strategies. Used with permission from Jeff Volek and Steve Phinney, Beyond Obesity LLC.

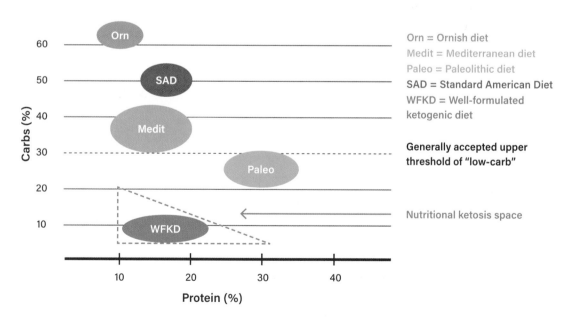

Dietary Protein and Carbs by Diet Type

Orn = Ornish diet
Medit = Mediterranean diet
Paleo = Paleolithic diet
SAD = Standard American Diet
WFKD = Well-formulated
ketogenic diet

Generally accepted upper threshold of "low-carb"

Nutritional ketosis space

version of LCHF that pushes carb even lower and fat even higher, certainly has these benefits, but the ratio of macronutrients may be more difficult to achieve consistently. That said, many will benefit further from pushing into the keto space, especially people with long-established MIRS damage and seriously diabetic physiology. We personally follow LCHF, but we regularly shift into keto for enhanced low-carb benefits. In most cases we enter keto by skipping meals or more widely spacing them, which results in much of our calorie intake coming from body fat. (We'll talk more about this strategy in Chapters 6 and 8—in particular, see page 113.) Essentially, we are living on the low-carb/keto spectrum, moving back and forward to hone our health.

SUCCESS STRATEGIES

Most people will benefit hugely from a dietary approach that turns the classic weight-loss advice on its head. It's not too surprising, as the classic low-fat approach has failed catastrophically and continues to cause harm. Here are the core approaches that boost your chances of losing weight, regaining your health, and living a long time, which we'll discuss in more detail in Part 2:

► Greatly reduce carbohydrate in your diet, especially refined carbohydrate of all types

► Greatly reduce fructose, so no processed foods and very few high-sugar fruits

► Greatly reduce omega-6 polyunsaturated fats, so no processed foods or vegetable oils

► Ensure adequate intake of high-quality, satiety-inducing protein

► Acquire the bulk of your energy from nutrient-dense natural, healthy fats

A range of other factors are also important to tackle and resolve, and different types of people need different targeted strategies. An insulin-resistant slim person will follow a different path than an insulin-sensitive obese person. In Part 2, we will show you how to determine *your* type and take the correct path to success.

Part 2 also explains how to implement a personal plan for weight loss and longevity and ensure maximum success. That said, we believe that having a good understanding of how everything works is an important factor in long-term success. Therefore, we believe it is important that you read and understand Part 3 as you get going on your plan. It includes important details about the science that supports our strategies and explains how insulin, carbohydrate, fat, and protein all impact metabolic processes and overall health.

We will also detail hugely important diagnostic measures, like the pivotal CAC score from a simple CT scan of the heart and cholesterol ratios that predict heart disease far better than the much-hyped LDL. There will also be a detailed summary of all the most important vitamins and supplements—being short on these can really scupper your weight loss and longevity goals. Understanding all these factors will help you to understand why the Eat Rich, Live Long plan works so well!

WARREN AND JOSHUA'S STORY

The low-carb, high-fat approach is not just for overweight older people with insulin issues. We mentioned in Chapter 4 that young people today are riddled with insulin resistance and MIRS. Two of Jeff's recent patients are a great example.

Warren and Joshua are teenage brothers who were sent to see Jeff by their mother, who had recently taken an interest in healthier nutrition and had learned about the low-carb diet. She was concerned about the boys' health as they were steadily gaining weight.

Since recently completing high school, Warren and Joshua have been working hard to support themselves financially. As with many teens, food, activity, and health were the last things on their minds. They ate on the run without regard for nutrition and admittedly ate mostly carb-heavy and processed foods. Their activity level was moderate and mainly job-related—they were on their feet most of the day at work.

Both boys had about 30 pounds to lose; as is typical, weight issues ran in their family. Their fasting blood work, which included LDL levels, did not reveal any issues. However, they were severe-ly hyperinsulinemic: their insulin levels were off the chart. They were seething with MIRS, but they were too young for the problem to show up in standard glucose measurements.

The brothers were on their way to becoming full-blown diabetics in the coming decades, and because post-meal glucose and insulin measurements are hardly ever considered by health professionals, it might not have been caught until serious damage was done.

The boys are already seeing results from taking a lower-carb approach to their diet. They are also focusing on more-nutritious food choices and are committed to being more active. Their weight is dropping and their health is rebounding.

Warren and Josh's story is typical of many young adults. Proper screening, along with providing the right tools and education, will help even the youngest people. And lowering carb intake is a linchpin of recovery from MIRS.

2

THE EAT RICH, LIVE LONG PRESCRIPTION

" For the master, surrender means there are no experts. There are only learners. "

—George Leonard

" Winning is the science of being totally prepared. "

—George Allen

CHAPTER 6

YOUR WEIGHT-LOSS MASTER CLASS

In Part 1, we talked about *why:* why we've been taught to follow a low-fat diet and "eat less, move more" and why these are actually terrible strategies for weight loss and overall health, why lowering insulin is the linchpin to managing weight and reducing chronic disease, and why a low-carb, high-fat diet promotes health.

Now we'll look at *how*. This chapter will share with you our fundamental strategies for weight-loss success, optimal health, and longevity. Our ancestors, while plagued by infectious disease and other problems that modern medicine effectively addresses, managed to avoid both obesity and chronic diseases—which are, of course, closely related to diet, and which are poorly handled by modern medicine. We cannot re-create our ancestors' exact environment, nor should we try to do so. We do, however, need to replicate the great advantages that they had in diet and lifestyle—but using an approach that will be effective for modern people.

We'll start with some important high-level approaches, including mindset and macronutrient goals. We will then focus in detail on ten key action steps that will deliver both slimness and optimum health.

MANAGING MINDSET

We want to discuss psychology a bit before you embark on your low-carb, high-fat journey. This will help you immensely as you apply our prescription for weight loss and longevity.

The truth is, it's not easy to overcome an indoctrination that started in your earliest years, and we have all been indoctrinated in bad nutritional science. It has been drummed into us for most of our lives. All of our scientific leaders parroted the same distorted half-truths about the benefits of a low-fat diet and "healthy" carbs. Our subconscious will not easily surrender these deep-seated instructions and fears. No book or scientific logic can eradicate them fully. The programming is simply too profound. Our minds have enormous difficulty accepting that our best and brightest leaders have been wrong for decades. But wrong they were.

And so you will face a challenge; we don't deny it. You will have to wrestle with the oldest force in human history: your subconscious. In the first weeks, you will feel this force holding you back. You will have to overcome the artificial fear of natural fats. You will have to overcome the powerful dogma that exalted the "complex carbohydrates" at the base of the food pyramid. You will have to remind yourself that these carbohydrates are mostly just glucose (sugar) with some nutrients and fiber—which are easy to get from far, far healthier foods.

Do not underestimate the power of this high-carb propaganda. It is a psychological poison that you must clear from your subconscious—the rock on which our modern disease epidemics have been built.

Keeping this threat in your mind will enable you to defeat it. You will overcome the brainwashing, just like the millions who have already done so.

Do not worry. You will succeed. We know you will. But underestimating the subconscious enemy is the biggest threat to your success.

Do not let the legacy of bad science undermine your efforts.

A NEW LIFE STARTS HERE

Many people experience apprehension when starting a new phase in life. There is the fear of the unknown and the fear of failure. There is also the fear of what may be left behind, what we may miss in the new life. This is natural, but you will overcome it. Luckily, in the Eat Rich, Live Long plan, the upsides massively outweigh any challenges—the benefits are enormous and the sacrifices few.

We want you to hit the ground running in your first week on the plan with the best measures, but we don't want to overburden you with mountains of instruction. Jeff's patients succeeded best by focusing on changing their diet first and then, once they'd adapted to that, tackling other important lifestyle issues, such as stress and sleep—and we are certain that you will, too. It's just a matter of prioritizing key dietary elements in the first week, and then bringing in more tools when you have found your feet.

Prepare to transform both your personal appearance and your vitality! You will be free from trying to reduce your calories. You will be free from gnawing cereal like a rodent or chewing fibrous feed like a horse. You will spurn the processed junk and fake foods of our misguided society. At best they gave you a cheap thrill—a momentary pleasure that soon turned to hunger and emptiness. Their main effect was to make you fatter and sicker.

You will instead eat rich ancestral foods that give you vitality, health, and slimness. You will realize how delicious they are compared to the carbs and vegetable oil that we've been sold. This transformation in your diet will lead to great improvements in your appearance. People will be noticing within weeks and commenting on your newfound radiance and slimmer body. They will want to know how you are doing it. You can tell them, if you like, that you are simply applying good science. You will be thrilled to leave the junk science behind—and you will feel better than you ever have.

It is important to pick the right time to start your new life. Avoid starting at a particularly stressful time or when major life events are coming up in the near future. It's best to pick a stable period when you have a couple of weeks with no major events occurring. Perhaps it could be a quiet period in work, or even when you are on vacation. Make sure to give the first week, in particular, the attention it deserves.

Clear the bad food out of your pantry and fridge and replace it with the foods highlighted throughout this chapter. You don't need to be obsessive, but you do need to be reasonably thorough. Clear out the old and welcome in the new.

CROSSING THE BRIDGE TO FAT-BURNING

Now we reach the essential part of the program: converting your body from a sugar-burning machine to a fat-burning one.

As we discussed in Chapter 3, the body's fat-burning mechanisms are shut down when significant amounts of glucose enter your system. This means it's very difficult for your body to burn fat (including your own body fat) when you're consuming high amounts of carbohydrate—in other words, when you're a sugar-burner.

Most people who are overweight are trapped in sugar-burning mode. Their bodies have become dependent on a steady supply of carbs. Escaping this trap is something to be fiercely proud of. When you consume high amounts of fat and, simultaneously, very little carb, your body transforms into a fat-burner. Millions of new fat-burning enzymes will be rapidly manufactured during this wonderful and miraculous transition.

Think of this transition as a bridge. You start out on one side as a sugar-burner, but by following the ten steps of the Eat Rich, Live Long plan (coming up on page 72), you'll make the journey across the bridge. Life as a fat-burner awaits you on the other side.

One of the most important factors in your transition to fat-burning is the quantity of carbohydrate you ingest. The ideal quantity varies for different people, but for everyone, we recommend looking at net carbs, not total carbs. The net carb content of a food is the total carb minus the grams of indigestible fibrous carb. For example, 1 ounce of Brazil nuts has 3.4 grams total carbs, but 2.1 grams of that is indigestible fiber. Therefore, the net carbs for an ounce of Brazil nuts is only 1.3 grams. In contrast, cashews are high in carbs. One ounce of cashews has 9.3 grams of total carbs, and 8.4 grams of this is net carbs. It would be a great idea for you to print out the carb cheat sheet available at thefatemperor.com/carb-cheat-sheet and stick it on the fridge.

We espouse the 40/80/120 rule for carb intake. It can be explained as follows:

▶ If you have established insulin resistance, prediabetes (consistently high blood glucose), or type 2 diabetes, the net carb intake needs to be less than 40 grams daily. You will be living on the keto end of the low-carb spectrum (see page 298). You may be able to relax this rule once you meet your insulin-sensitivity targets. (Note that the easiest way to estimate your insulin sensitivity is using the HOMA index, as explained on page 39.)

▶ If you're insulin-sensitive, your net carb intake should be around 80 grams daily. Insulin sensitivity is a sign that you're relatively healthy and can live in the low-carb, high-fat part of the spectrum.

▶ For the vast majority of people, net carb intake should never exceed 120 grams per day. There is no useful benefit and many potential problems with higher carb intake. The one exception may be athletes who are striving for peak energy bursts. (We'll talk more about athletes on page 345.)

If you have prediabetes or type 2 diabetes, you have established metabolic issues and are highly carb intolerant—that is, your blood sugar and insulin levels are out of whack and aren't managing your intake of carb correctly. You may have found that you're dependent on a steady stream of carbs just to feel okay from hour to hour. It's like being a smoker who needs a steady stream of cigarettes to avoid the jitters.

A smoker who quits smoking gains freedom from the physical addiction within a few days, but he or she may still have a leftover psychological yearning for the poison. So it is with carb addiction for people with established metabolic disorders such as insulin resistance, prediabetes, or type 2 diabetes. If this describes you, it is imperative that you break the addiction cycle and become a fat-burner as soon as possible. When you do, only the psychological urge will remain. This is simply a subconscious memory of the days when carb injections were needed. This sneaky memory is easy to control when you are prepared for it.

In contrast, if you are relatively insulin sensitive, you do not need to be so rigorous on the carb front. For you, around 80 grams of carb per day is very workable.

The insulin-sensitive overweight are a particularly interesting group. Often they find it difficult to lose the excess weight. They may experience a weight-loss plateau, even on a low-carb diet. They often do not gain much extra benefit from going ultra low carb, either. If this describes you, meal spacing is much more important (see page 113). Switching to fat-burning mode will make this step easy to apply.

MASTER THE BASICS TO BECOME A MASTER

Ivor has occupied the role of "technical master" in a huge high-tech multi-national corporation. Engineers are by their nature highly technical people. But only a small percent of engineers achieve master level. Ivor achieved it through excellence in complex technical problem-solving. It required decades of practice to hone this art.

There is no "technical master" role in medicine as such. Nonetheless, Jeff is certainly a master in weight loss and preventative health. Again, he honed his art through decades of practice. The stories throughout this book about his patients and the success they've had in improving their health stand as testament to it.

We followed very separate paths to achieving mastery in the area of health and nutrition. We were both fueled by a burning desire to understand the scientific principles involved and have spent countless hours researching and decoding them. Successfully applying the science to craft a truly health-promoting diet has been our reward.

You can become the master of your weight control. No question about it. You just need to understand the rules and apply them all correctly. Below, we list the rules you need to hammer in your first week. Ivor did this and lost more than 30 pounds in eight weeks. Jeff lost almost 40 pounds in the same length of time. We transformed our blood test results for the better without adding any significant exercise to our regimens. Countless numbers of Jeff's patients have achieved the same, and millions are now doing the same thing under the guidance of low-carb doctors around the world.

ACTION STEPS FOR CONTROLLING YOUR WEIGHT AND IMPROVING YOUR HEALTH

The following list of steps does not cover everything—no list can in such a complex, multifactorial challenge as weight control. But it will address most problems for most people. If applied, these steps will deliver success. If applied optimally, they can deliver spectacular success.

Here's the master list. After identifying these steps, we'll explore each one in more detail in the rest of this chapter.

1. Eliminate refined carbohydrates and sugars from your diet. They are a biochemical battering ram. They act like locks, trapping you in an overweight state and keeping you there.

2. Eliminate refined vegetable oils from your diet. No one interested in either weight loss or longevity should be eating these oils. They are easy to replace. Olive oil, coconut oil, and other healthy oils are readily available.

3. Greatly restrict processed food. This will help hugely with #1 and #2. Processed foods are invariably loaded with refined carbs and disgusting oils.

4. Eat only nutrient-dense and slow-burning carbohydrates, which can promote gut and general health (we'll talk more about this later), and keep carb intake low. Your initial target should be approximately 15 to 20 percent of your total calories.

5. Eat nutrient-dense sources of protein. Always consume high-quality protein—make that protein count. Your target should be approximately 0.4 to 0.6 gram per pound of lean body mass if you are not athletic—more if you're more active.

6. Get most of your calories from fats that come from nutrient-rich foods. These fats should supply 60 to 65 percent of your total daily calories. *Do not ingest fats with abandon.* Simply replace the carbs you're cutting out with healthy fats. Your healthy fat intake should be from real-food sources. Eat according to genuine hunger signals only—no bingeing!

7. Eat only three main meals a day—ideally two, if you can manage it. You can make this a wonderful habit for life. You will learn to relish each meal. Your body will positively hum with this regimen.

8. Ensure that you consume adequate vitamins and minerals (as outlined in Chapter 15). This is important—nutrient deficiencies can trigger hunger. Also ensure that you have an adequate intake of water—several pints per day.

9. Be mindful of your lifestyle and environment. Poor sleep, stress, and lack of healthy sun exposure will hammer your weight-loss efforts. Do not neglect these environmental influences.

10. Partake in healthy exercise. Resistance exercise is best.

An overweight person following these ten rules will transform him- or herself and his or her health status. The first few in the list are somewhat obvious. They will benefit anyone who wants a quick fix. But all are needed for sustained and healthy weight loss. If you pick and choose only a few rules from the list, all bets are off.

Let's now take a closer look at these ten weight-loss action steps.

1. ELIMINATE REFINED CARBS AND SUGARS

Refined carbohydrates have to be dumped. This rule is an easy one. Following it means that dropping breads and pastries is a given. Most commercial breads are a concoction of finely ground carb, sugars, and oils. And modern wheat is a disaster for most humans in any case, refined or otherwise. Don't worry—we will provide bread alternatives for sandwich lovers.

Mechanically grinding carbs—that is, refining them—turns them into a super-fattening fuel and a driver of obesity and diabetes. Refined carbs cause very detrimental hormone responses in your digestive tract. Specifically, they cause your levels of the hormone GIP to flare up. GIP is a primary trigger for insulin release, and insulin spikes to rally to the rescue of your elevated blood sugar.

If you eat some fatty food along with this carb, you will suffer even more. Highly digestible carb turns healthy fat into a liability: insulin spikes shut down fat oxidation, preventing healthy metabolism of the dietary fat. In this way, the combination of refined carb and fat is a biochemical disaster that has been instrumental in condemning our population to epidemic obesity. Maintain fat as the healthy fuel it should be—by keeping your insulin low and safe!

Do not eat processed carbohydrate. Period.

Processed carbohydrate leads to a form of addiction over time. When you're a sugar-burner, your body senses deprivation soon after a carb-filled meal. What is happening is that blood glucose rises fast just after the meal and drops excessively in the hours following it. This leads to a low blood glucose level, in a body that depends on glucose—hence the feeling of deprivation.

So what happens if you reduce your intake of processed carb but sneak some refined carbs or sugar occasionally? Well, think about what happens when ex-smokers sneak a few cigarettes. You know the sorry story—they're back to buying packs and cartons in no time. The smoking cessation analogy can be extended further. Once you dump refined carbs, their addictive power will quickly fall away. A sense of freedom and well-being will kick in. As with cigarette cessation, your appetite for refined carbs will exist only in your mind after a few weeks—the physical addiction will be gone. By understanding that the desire for refined carbs is now only a memory, you can resolve the problem for good. (Interestingly, this very type of understanding formed the basis for the most successful smoking-cessation strategy of all time, Allen Carr's *Easy Way to Stop Smoking*.)

2. ELIMINATE REFINED VEGETABLE OILS

Refined vegetable oils have to be dumped along with refined carbs. Vegetable oils are extracted from seeds in a multistep chemical process. Vegetable oils were originally used as machine lubricants. Then someone got the bright idea of feeding them to humans. As we discussed in detail on page 53, refined vegetable oils are toxic for people. Various animal studies have shown that excessive omega-6 fatty acids, abundant in vegetable oils, drive obesity more than natural monounsaturated or saturated fats, abundant in animal sources.[1] It is unlikely that you will consume excessive omega-6 quantities while eating a whole-foods diet, especially the one that we prescribe. The science suggests that vegetable oils are contributing the vast majority of the omega-6 problem in our world today. Vegetable oils are more fit for use in a lawnmower than in your body.

Cold-pressed olive oil, coconut oil, and other natural oils are unquestionably the best choice. The "eat real food" rule applies here—seek out real food from the era before obesity took over the world.

3. GREATLY RESTRICT PROCESSED FOOD

Not all food processing is bad. Much of the food that we eat has *some* level of processing. For example, the following real-food-based items undergo some processing:

▸ High-quality cured meats and sausages with no grains or added oils

▸ Ready-to-eat meals made from primarily real-food items

▸ Premade soups that are low-carb and contain primarily real-food ingredients

We aren't saying that you need to avoid these, though we do recommend limiting them. They're convenient, and sometimes in order to avoid truly unhealthy processed food, you'll find yourself reaching for these. As long as it's not frequent, that's okay—it's more important to avoid the really bad processed food. The problem is that when processed foods are part of your diet, you are simply not in control. You cannot monitor their contents constantly to make sure they're real-food-based and don't have refined grains, vegetable oils, and added sugar, and label-studying habits fade. The safest option is to do what we do: simply eliminate processed foods from your diet. Form a new real-food habit and stick to it.

But the most important thing is to completely eliminate bad processed food. Let's clarify what we mean by that.

These foods include:

▶ Most breads, which are made from finely ground grains, vegetable oils, added sugar, and many other bad things

▶ Most packaged foods—cereals, soups, and so on—which contain powdered grains, vegetable oils, and sugars

▶ Nearly all "healthy" snack bars—they are normally made from powdered grains, vegetable oils, and sugars, and they are almost always too sugary

All these will disrupt your body's hormonal weight control system, cause increased hunger, and trigger weight gain—along with health problems.

4. CORRECT YOUR CARBS

Your goal should be to reduce your carb intake to approximately 15 to 20 percent of your total calories.

The other part of this step is to target the carbs that can help you. These have no refining to make them dangerous, and they have plenty of fiber on board for satiety and insulin moderation. These are also the carbs that can improve your gut microbiome. A healthy gut microbiome in turn helps with many things, including insulin sensitivity. The Eat Rich, Live Long plan is not about eliminating carbs. It is about eliminating *junk* carbs while optimizing potentially useful carbs.

Focus on nutrient-dense carbs that are generally slower to digest. Slow-digesting carbs do not spike blood sugar and insulin as much, and they stimulate hormones that help pancreatic function and moderate appetite. Center your carb allocation on above-ground non-starchy vegetables, like spinach, broccoli, and cauliflower. In moderation, some tubers like sweet potatoes can also be okay—boiled rather than baked lowers insulin response.

CALCULATING YOUR MACRONUTRIENTS

While you do not need to be obsessive about ratios of fat, carb, and protein, you do need to have an overall idea of how to monitor them. We will give a simplified summary here.

Carbohydrate and protein both have 4 calories per gram, while fat has 9 calories per gram. Let's say you eat a meal that has 100 grams of net carb (this doesn't include fiber—see pages 69 to 70), 100 grams of protein, and 100 grams of fat. This equals 400 calories of carb, 400 calories of protein, and 900 calories of fat, for a total of 1,700 calories. Your macronutrient ratio for that meal would be 23.5 percent carb, 23.5 percent protein, and 53 percent fat.

You can look up the nutrient details—including total carb and fiber, so you can calculate net carb—for any food online.

High-fiber carbs provide material that can promote the growth of beneficial bacteria in your gut—your microbiome. The science of the microbiome has been advancing rapidly in recent years. Your microbiome can have a large influence on your insulin sensitivity and weight gain tendencies; some less-beneficial bacteria can directly trigger insulin and promote insulin resistance.[2]

For higher-carb treats, dark chocolate is a good bet—80 percent cacao or higher is ideal. If you are skipping a meal or feeling hunger pangs, dark chocolate hits the spot with minimal damage. It contains multiple antioxidant compounds and a range of important minerals, such as magnesium, manganese, and copper, and if it's 80 percent cacao or more, the sugar content won't be too high. Berries with cream is another relatively low-sugar treat—you get the benefits of antioxidants, nutrients, and fiber with a minimal sugar load.

5. EAT NUTRIENT-DENSE SOURCES OF PROTEIN

This step is pivotal: consuming quality protein is imperative. Protein provides key amino acids your body needs. Consuming these wonderful molecules means that your body won't trigger hunger in an attempt to pursue them. There are additional satiety effects from optimum protein intake. Do not fall down on the quality protein imperative. Whenever you eat, always think protein.

At the same time, we do not believe in consuming excessive protein, as high intakes can be converted into glucose, trigger inappropriate insulin release, and promote related growth pathways. Growth is fine for a young person, but once you are middle-aged, driving growth pathways can be problematic. We will talk about protein in more detail in Chapter 14.

A healthy protein intake can help with weight-loss efforts through established mechanisms; here are the top two:

▶ The thermogenic effect of protein—some energy from the food is lost as heat during digestion rather than being used. These losses are much higher for protein than for the other macronutrients—you might get 85 calories of usable energy from 100 calories of protein, whereas you might get 95 calories of usable energy from 100 calories of fat.

▶ Protein absorbed in the digestive tract activates hunger-suppressing hormones like peptide YY, GLP-1, and others.

To illustrate, a recent trial was specifically designed to assess long-term weight maintenance following weight-loss efforts.[3] Researchers randomly split the subjects into two groups and put them on a very low calorie diet for four weeks. Both groups lost the same amount of weight, 5 to 10 percent on average. Then their diets were returned to the normal amount of calories and their protein intake was adjusted: one group had their protein intake set to 18 percent, while the other group was set at 15 percent. Even with this very small protein tweak, the 18 percent group regained significantly less weight than the 15 percent one. The 18 percent group also showed a decrease in waist size, while the 15 percent group showed an increase. Finally, analysis showed that the "satiety before breakfast" score was higher in the 18 percent group, which speaks to the appetite-suppressing effects of protein.

Getting adequate protein can also help stimulate muscle growth. When combined with physical activity, this can enhance lean muscle mass. Muscle is the primary place where glucose and fat are burned. Increasing your lean muscle mass improves insulin sensitivity by enhancing glucose disposal. When combined with a healthy low-carb diet, it will also accelerate your fat-burning ability.[4]

It's important not just to get enough protein but also to always target *high-quality* protein—protein that provides more of what we need. We favor ancestral animal products for the most essential amino acids, which we have to get through the diet—we can't make these on our own. Finally, animal foods are particularly nutrient-dense when compared to most plant foods. The best examples of desirable animal foods are wild-caught fish, sardines, pastured eggs, organ meats, shellfish, and fatty cuts of other grass-fed meats. That said, high-quality protein can also be consumed through a carefully formulated vegetarian diet (see page 307).

CALCULATING YOUR LEAN BODY MASS

It is quite easy to estimate how much lean body mass you have, but you do need to know your body fat percentage. This can be estimated using a simple caliper at your doctor's office or gym, or you can pick one up for around $10. Once you know your body fat percentage, multiply it by your weight in pounds, and subtract the result from your weight. This gives you your lean body mass. For example, if you are 200 pounds and have 25 percent body fat, then your lean body mass is 200 − (25 percent of 200) = 150 pounds.

Remember that for nonathletic people, the goal should be to consume 0.4 to 0.6 gram per pound of lean body mass. More can be added according to your activity level. In terms of the macronutrient ratios, we recommend getting about 20 percent of your calories from protein.

6. GET MOST OF YOUR CALORIES FROM FAT

Embrace delicious and nutritious fat-filled foods. Hear the voices of your ancestors cheer you with their approval! Your hunger and your health will be transformed. You will feel your body hum again. Both the weight and the years will fall away.

Aim to get most of your energy from nutrient-rich fats—your target should be to get 60 to 65 percent of your total daily calories from them (see page 76 for how to calculate this).

A diet high in healthy fats provides nutritious fuel, but no diet enables you to gorge with abandon. You can eat rich, but that doesn't mean you can be a glutton. Eating rich is about enjoying the delicious fatty and protein-rich foods of our ancestry. It is not about overeating them. Simply let the healthier fat replace the now-reduced carb intake. For example, if you were eating 1,200 calories from carb and cut that down to 400 calories, increase your intake of healthy fats by 800 calories.

A primary advantage of diets high in healthy fat is their appetite-control edge: you simply won't feel hungry. But you need to make this advantage count. Focus on nutritious real-food sources of fat and protein, like fatty fish, eggs, meat, avocado, and other high-fat plant foods. The best real-food sources of healthy fat generally come with high-quality protein on board. They will also be delicious and satisfying once you wean yourself off the demon carb—double win. The ultimate example of a perfect food is an egg from a pastured hen—it is a fantastic nutrient-dense balance of fat and protein that's very low in carb. Lower-protein sources of healthy fats are olive oil, coconut oil, and butter (which has more nutrients than the other two). All of these can be used in sauces and dressings, as well as in main dishes. However, it is generally preferable to get healthy fats from whole foods rather than oils.

7. EAT ONLY THREE MEALS A DAY

We evolved by alternating feast and famine. It is encoded in our genes. Respect this rich history. Balance any indulgent blowouts with appropriate restraints. Master the power of fasting.

Spacing your meals well is so important. Eat only three main meals a day, maximum—two is even better.

Remember that you are crossing the bridge to become a fat-burning machine. You must strive to make that bridge a short one. Get to the safe side quickly. Leaving long gaps between meals forces your body to set itself up for smooth fat-burning. Eating meals too often will stretch the bridge and get in the way of this process. It will frustratingly keep you away from the fat-burning practice your body needs to optimize quickly in the early stages of the plan, to make things easy for you going forward. If you really need a snack, a small dish that combines fat and protein is the emergency option—but only in the first few days, and only if really necessary.

The idea of regularly going for stretches of twelve hours or more without eating is called intermittent fasting, but we prefer to think of it as simply "meal skipping." We've been using it as part of our weight-maintenance toolkit for years. It is not a chore—in fact, it is quite liberating. We never restrict our calories as such or weigh portion sizes. Why should we? Did our slim and healthy ancestors have to count calories?

Our high-fat diets have turned us into excellent fat-burners. It can be quite satisfying to know you're burning your own body fat, and we would never go back to the habit of eating meals at assigned times—it's so restrictive. Eating by the bell provokes our weight-gain hormones with unhelpful regularity, as many studies on weight-challenged people have verified.[5] The time at which you eat your meals can also have an effect, and we do not recommend eating within three to four hours of bedtime.[6] But the most important point is to keep the number of meals low, leaving large gaps between them to minimize hormonal disruption. (We'll talk more about meal spacing on page 113.)

You, too, can make meal skipping a superb habit for life. It will bring your hunger signals under *your* control. This is because when you've transformed yourself into a fat-burner, your body will become far more fluent at using your body fat for energy. With this source of energy unlocked, hunger becomes a much, much weaker force—one that you can easily control. This is a wonderful way to live, and it will deliver increased mental acuity and personal performance levels, too.

Separating meals widely:

▶ promotes insulin sensitivity and excellent regulation of other weight-related hormones

▶ resolves stubborn residual insulin resistance in prediabetic and/or overweight people

▶ improves and enhances your hunger-control abilities

▶ hands you back the controls of your body

▶ improves your concentration and mental acuity after you achieve fat-burner status

We cannot stress enough how powerful a tool this is. With a diet high in healthy fats, your body can become a fasting machine. Hunger becomes a weak and highly manageable force, and your appetite is under your control.

8. CONSUME ADEQUATE VITAMINS AND MINERALS

As you cross the bridge to becoming a fat-burner, your body will be undergoing wonderful changes. But these changes will bring new requirements for particular nutrients. We'll talk much more about vitamins and minerals in Chapter 15, but for now, know that the most important minerals to pay attention to are sodium, magnesium, and potassium. (See pages 101 to 102 for more on these.) If you neglect these, the bridge will lengthen; deficiencies have been known to prevent people from reaching the other side. And hunger can be triggered by nutrient and mineral deficiency, as our body tries to prompt us to eat more to get more of them.

Also, make sure you're getting enough water—several pints a day.

9. BE MINDFUL OF ENVIRONMENTAL FACTORS

Weight control is not only about what you put in your mouth. Other aspects of your life and environment can have a huge influence on your success as well.

Chronic stress severely disrupts the hormonal system that regulates weight control by causing the release of stress hormones, including cortisol. The resulting imbalances create a pattern that disturbs the glucose/insulin system, increasing both insulin and insulin resistance. The release of these hormones is a normal evolutionary response to stress that's designed to mobilize glucose and free fatty acids to fuel a fight or your escape from danger. An interesting study measured the free fatty acids in a race car driver's bloodstream just before a big race. They were through the roof.[7] Having high glucose and high fats in the bloodstream is helpful in the short term but a disaster in the long term—particularly for insulin sensitivity and weight-loss efforts. This point is best illustrated by the metabolic disaster that is type 2 diabetes. This disease is essentially defined by elevated insulin, insulin resistance, blood glucose, and blood fats—all occurring simultaneously. We are not designed to have this combination, and it puts severe stress on our vascular and organ systems.

Having poor sleep patterns will also hurt your chances of weight-loss success. Many studies have explored the effects of inadequate sleep on insulin sensitivity.[8] Reducing sleep to four to five hours a night for even a week can have a surprisingly large harmful effect: insulin sensitivity and your ability to control blood glucose levels can drop by 20 to 40 percent. As you can imagine, this will not help with your weight-loss efforts, even if you are on a relatively good diet.

Healthy sun exposure brings many benefits, though there is much controversy in this arena. The main problem is that excessive sun exposure can increase the risk for the nonmelanoma skin cancers. What is often not appreciated is that studies have shown that on average, people who get these "cosmetic" skin cancers live longer than those who don't. Also unappreciated are the huge range of benefits of sun exposure.[9] Sun and light deprivation will also hamper your weight-loss efforts and promote obesity by disrupting your circadian rhythm and melatonin production.[10]

We always get as much healthy sun exposure as possible—without getting a sunburn, of course, since that is where the risks lie. Balance is the key. The exact amount you need each day will vary depending on skin type, latitude, time of day, amount of skin exposed, and other factors. The overall goal is to achieve a blood vitamin D level greater than 30 ng/ml; in the summer in the US, this will require approximately 30 minutes of sun exposure. Because of all the variables, we simply get as much healthy sun exposure as possible (again, without sunburn!).

10. PARTAKE IN HEALTHY EXERCISE

We have a rule of thumb when it comes to weight loss, the 80/20 rule. Weight-loss success is at least 80 percent determined by what you put in your mouth—both the types of food you eat and how you manage appetite so you can avoid overeating (which itself depends largely on what type of foods you eat).

Only 20 percent of weight-loss success is determined by exercise. In other words, you can get 80 percent of the weight-loss success you're seeking while only doing the basic movements of life—walking to the store, climbing stairs, doing housework, and so on. The slim and supremely healthy people of Kitava, an island in Papua New Guinea, do not exercise intensively, but they have half the insulin levels of even the most active people in Sweden.[11] They achieve this excellence mainly through other elements from our list of rules. (See page 363 for more on the Kitavans.)

Without a doubt, there are many health benefits from working out: it increases your lean muscle mass, releases endorphins for a feel-good boost, and even boosts mental clarity and alertness.[12] Just don't depend heavily on exercise for major weight-loss benefits. Exercise can, for instance, allow people to eat more bad food without ballooning. Is this a good thing? Not really. The bad food will cause damage regardless. You cannot outrun a bad diet. In the long term, it will take you down.

But exercise has a quite different result if you are on a healthy low-carb plan like ours. The right exercise regimen will then enhance your transition to a fat-burning physiology. It will promote muscle gain and improve your metabolic health. It can drain your glucose stores (glycogen), prompting your body to burn more fat, and switch on your fat-burning turbines. Particularly when combined with a low-carb lifestyle, exercise will speed your transition to becoming a fat-burner. Therefore, it can be a very useful tool, and we highly recommend it.

The key point with exercise, though, is that it should not be used in a way that will simply generate more appetite. You should be fueling exercise mostly from your body fat stores. By doing so, you can avoid excessive hunger in the period following the activity. The flow of fat that was switched on to fuel your efforts will overshoot in the period afterwards. You will continue to be smoothly fed from your fat.

In general, resistance exercise (also called weight training or strength training) is best for fat-burning and growing muscle. Examples of this exercise type include push-ups, squats, and chin-ups. When doing these you should always "push to failure"— until you can do no more. Your body senses that the muscles have been pushed to the limit and triggers the many processes required to create more muscle. These processes are all highly beneficial for your health and give great muscle-building payback with only a few short training sessions per week.[13] We will talk more about exercise and even provide an easy and effective routine on page 119.

Finally, we remind you again not to be fooled by the "eat less, move more" ruse. Exercise has usually been promoted via the "calories in, calories out" logic—the idea that if you increase the number of calories you burn by exercising more, you'll lose weight. This is a clever lie that seems to most benefit the food and fitness industries. (See Chapter 3 for a more in-depth discussion of the problems with the "eat less, move more" theory of weight loss.)

Managing these nondietary factors—exercise and environment—can be difficult. We understand this, so don't worry—there are workarounds and tricks available. If you focus on steps 1 through 8 in the first week, that's okay. The benefits from the first eight steps will enable you to better tackle these last two later on. So hold tight and focus. We will tease out steps 9 and 10 in a little while, after you have the first week under your (now-shrinking) belt.

APPLYING THE RULES: INDIVIDUALIZED MAGIC

While all ten of these rules apply to everyone, different types of people need to focus on different rules. To keep it simple, there are mainly two types of people—the insulin resistant and the insulin sensitive. (See page 39 on how to gauge your level of insulin resistance using the HOMA index.)

▶ **Insulin resistant:** If you're insulin resistant, you will benefit from applying rules 4 and 6 quite hard: cutting carb intake down and focusing on slow-burning carbohydrates, and getting most of your calories from healthy fats. Make sure you push to very low carb levels—fewer than 40 grams daily.

▶ **Insulin sensitive:** If you're insulin sensitive, you'll need to focus more on rule 7: eat no more than three meals a day, preferably two. You can consume more carbs; around 80 to 100 grams per day is okay. But it's still important to follow all the rules in order to switch from burning primarily sugar to burning primarily fat. And once you're a fat-burner, skipping meals regularly will help you burn body fat for fuel.

KNOW YOUR NUMBERS!

Avoid all foods that spike your blood sugar levels. No good comes from bumping up your blood glucose. In fact, it is the last thing you need in the first week—or ever. Luckily, you can find out exactly how your food choices affect your blood glucose levels. This can help you identify and eliminate your problem foods, so you can fine-tune your regimen over time.

WHAT ABOUT FASTING GLUCOSE?

In addition to checking your post-meal blood glucose, keep an eye on your fasting glucose—your blood glucose level first thing in the morning, following an overnight fast. It should generally be below 100 mg/dL. Repeated readings above this indicate a problem, and at that point you should ask your doctor to test your fasting insulin to see if there is a genuine problem afoot.

You'll need a blood glucose meter to check your post-meal glucose. The price of these meters has plummeted in recent years due to the exploding diabetes epidemic. Get yourself a dependable model and a pack of disposable test strips. We use the Freestyle Optium from Abbott, which has the added advantage of measuring ketone levels, too. (You'll remember that ketones are produced when your body burns fat, so measuring your ketone levels is a good way to find out if your body has become a fat-burner.)

Occasionally check your blood glucose before and approximately one hour after a meal. If your blood glucose increases by more than 30 mg/dL after a meal, you'll know that something you ate is a problem for you. Some people have problems with dairy. Others are sensitive to certain meats or a higher protein intake. A blood glucose meter gives you instant feedback on what to avoid in the future.

Early on, we used blood glucose meters to chart our course. They were extremely valuable and provided excellent insights. We rarely use them anymore because now we know how our bodies react to various foods. So it will be for you; as your real-food expertise grows, the need for this tool will fall away. Phasing out your meter use will be a sign of your significant progress toward slimness and excellent health.

THE DAWN PHENOMENON

The "dawn phenomenon" is the occurrence of higher blood glucose in the morning, before eating, and it's particularly prevalent in people who have a strong history of diabetes or insulin resistance. It is the result of your body creating excess glucose based on hormonal signals that occur in the waking hours. (That's right—as we talked about back in Chapter 2, the body can synthesize its own glucose, so you really never need to eat carb.) You might conceivably experience this phenomenon even as your overall blood glucose and insulin resistance (measured by your HOMA figure, page 39) is improving over time. The best way to tackle the dawn phenomenon is through fasting strategies. Fasting for 20 to 24 hours occasionally has proven to be of great help in stubborn insulin-resistance cases.

OTHER BLOOD TESTS

We won't burden you with too much stuff around blood tests. That said, it would be great to get a baseline in certain areas before you start the Eat Rich, Live Long plan. The reason is twofold. First, everyone should know their values for these basic measures of health. Second, it is very useful to have a reference or baseline before you embark on the plan, so any changes that occur once you've started the plan can be explored properly. Here are the tests we would recommend, should you be willing to get them:

- ▶ Fasting blood glucose and fasting insulin
- ▶ A1C (average blood glucose over several months)
- ▶ Standard lipid panel (triglyceride, total cholesterol, HDL, and LDL)
- ▶ Vitamin D levels (the detailed name is the 25(OH)D test)
- ▶ Liver panel with GGT, AST, and ALT. When the levels of these liver enzymes are high, it indicates inflammation—low levels of GGT, in particular, are very important.
- ▶ Serum ferritin (iron loading in the blood) and homocystein levels (a significant heart disease risk factor when high indicates low B-vitamin intake and other issues)

If you wish to track your progress closely, we recommend the following more-advanced tests. These are very detailed assessments of your insulin status and cholesterol quality. We will explain the implications of these in Chapters 10 and 11.

- ▶ Oral glucose tolerance test with insulin assay (or simply a two-hour post-glucose insulin, which gives similar information but is much easier to acquire)
- ▶ Advanced lipoprotein profile with ApoB, ApoA1, and sdLDL. These measure the number and size of your cholesterol-carrying particles and will be discussed in more detail in Chapter 11.

THE ULTIMATE TEST OF YOUR CURRENT HEALTH

The other crucial test that will benefit any middle-aged man or woman is a CAC scan, which is a CT scan of the heart that measures coronary artery calcification (CAC). It shows where your body has tried to repair damaged arteries by depositing calcium in the arterial walls, so it reveals how much heart disease you have and also how much inflammatory damage you have sustained over the years. It's more powerful in assessing health than any measurement of risk factors. The CAC scan can really help bring clarity where the risk factors can confuse. This is particularly true if you track how your CAC score changes over time. Because it sees the actual evidence of inflammatory disease impact in your body, it essentially gives you the bottom line on your health status. It does not just show the extent of coronary heart disease—it really reflects the damage from the broad root causes of modern chronic disease. Therefore, it can be very useful for anyone tracking their progress toward achieving optimal health.

To take advantage of this, ideally you would have a CAC scan before embarking on the Eat Rich, Live Long plan. The CAC score from this scan would become your baseline status. Subsequent scan results would then tell a more compelling story than any blood tests. It gives incredibly useful information about your genuine health status and risk for chronic disease. For instance, if you have a score of zero in middle age, your risk of all-cause mortality is extremely low. A zero score is being called "a warranty for humans."[14] Striving to keep this zero score into old age is the ultimate strategy for health and longevity. Nothing else comes close, because the CAC scan sees how the disease itself progresses.

If you get a score higher than zero, all is not lost by any means. The key is to now stop your score from rising significantly over the years. You can achieve this by applying the ten action steps like a pro. Interestingly, many studies conclude that an individual's CAC score inevitably rises over the years. They assume that the score increase cannot really be stopped—it is just a fact of life. But they are wrong in this assumption—there have been documented cases of regression seen through nutritional interventions.[15] Jeff has also seen regression in his patients (you can read about one patient's story on page 272), and many more people are declaring their CAC regression in online forums. But we are only at the very start of this new revolution. The orthodox researchers have no knowledge of our ten steps and their synergistic effect on disease progression, and the people in their studies are certainly not applying the steps. So of course their disease and CAC scores progress unchecked—until they experience the sickness and early death that result from this tragic lack of understanding.

The key is to keep your CAC score from increasing more than 15 percent per year. Ideally, it will increase by only 5 percent per year or less. You do not need to reverse your score; the vast majority of the longevity benefits will come from keeping the progression at a low level.[16] When this is achieved, you will have put yourself way ahead of the average person with coronary heart disease, whose disease is progressing rapidly and doesn't even know it. Applying the ten steps and checking your progress with CAC will put you way ahead of this pack.

You don't need to get a CAC scan very often at all. If you have a low score (0 to 10) and are following the Eat Rich, Live Long plan, you might check in five to seven years later. If you have a very high score (higher than 400), then it would be prudent to check back within two years to verify that progression has been brought under control. In this way, you can complement the results of regular blood tests. You can also put isolated high readings of, say, LDL cholesterol into perspective, since the level itself can be misleading. The CAC score, which reflects actual disease progression, trumps risk factors and can put them into context. There are countless excellent scientific papers demonstrating the incredible power of the CAC score, with the best ones summarizing many sources.[17]

The next chapter will focus on what to do in your first week on the Eat Rich, Live Long plan. We know that you will make a great effort during this crucial week. Feel good about propelling yourself toward successful weight loss—and greatly improved health and longevity.

LARRY AND KAY LYNNE'S STORY

Larry and Kay Lynne were both obese and in ill health when a family tragedy prompted them to question everything. A much-loved family member became profoundly ill and incapacitated with a disease known to be driven by obesity. At the time, their daughter was only two years old. They began to fear that she would soon be left alone in the world, so Larry decided to take action. He had a science background and decided to use it to analyze nutrition and health. Larry's academic training gave him a perspective on nutrition that encompassed evolutionary biology, history, and culture. The only thing that made sense to Larry was that conventional nutrition advice had to be wrong—especially because chronic, preventable diseases had become epidemic over the past fifty years.

Larry engrossed himself in the metabolic theory of obesity, which powerfully resonated with him. The metabolic theory places the blame for obesity on the hormonal dysregulation mechanisms that we discussed previously. Larry began to decode for himself what we are revealing in this book. He started to link his grandmother's early death from type 2 diabetes, his uncle's death from Alzheimer's, and his own ill health and constant hunger to the same root cause: insulin resistance.

Larry immediately started cutting out bread, pasta, potato chips, candy, and ice cream. But if fat was a problem, as he'd been taught, then what could he replace them with? At this point, he did a Google search that he will never forget: "Why do we think dietary fat is bad?" This brought up the name Ancel Keys and his highly flawed Six Countries Study and Seven Countries Study (see page 23). Larry realized that these were, shockingly, the basis for conventional dietary advice. He discovered that properly designed studies instead showed that a low-carb, high-fat diet would deliver salvation.

Larry switched completely over to a healthy low-carb regimen. He found that he loved many of the mainstay foods of LCHF, so he adopted it wholeheartedly. Within a couple of weeks, he felt better than he had in decades. He also noticed a dramatic reduction in his appetite. Larry never counted calories or went hungry—those were two rules he had that he would not deviate from. But as he healed his insulin resistance, a voluntary reduction in calories occurred and Larry finally could access his stored body fat. Larry ended up losing 125 pounds—100 pounds in the first year.

Seven months later, Kay Lynne became his partner in good nutritional science. Kay Lynne ended up losing 70 pounds. They both resolved numerous lifelong health issues: for Larry, lifelong asthma, IBS, allergies, anxiety, sleep apnea, and brain fog; for Kay Lynne, joint pain, panic attacks, anxiety, depression, and skin conditions. Their young daughter also thrived on a real-food LCHF diet, going from the third percentile in height to the twenty-fifth percentile.

Larry and Kay Lynne beat insulin resistance and obesity with LCHF. They are now slim, insulin sensitive, and ruggedly healthy. They no longer fear leaving their daughter behind at an unfairly young age.

CHAPTER 7

THE EAT RICH, LIVE LONG PLAN:
DAYS 1 THROUGH 7

> " Whatever you can do, or dream you
> can do, begin it. Boldness has genius,
> power, and magic in it. "
>
> —Goethe

The first week on the Eat Rich, Live Long program is very important to get right. It is when the right habits are laid down, and some focus and dedication are required to do this properly. Weight loss and longevity are multifactorial challenges. Playing around with one or two factors while ignoring the others is a recipe for failure. Therefore, in your first week, you must hit the big factors hard and hit them together.

But we do not want to overcomplicate your first week, so we suggest that during this time, you make fixing your food your primary focus. The more you can add in steps 7 through 10, the better, but don't worry too much about them right now. We'll talk more about maximizing those steps when we talk about days 8 through 21. Right now, for days 1 through 7, let's focus on food.

FOODS THAT WILL KEEP YOU ON TRACK

For the sake of simplicity, we've created a list of the foods that will keep you on track during your first week. Make a photocopy of this list and keep it handy so you can easily refer to it.

THE FOOD-QUALITY CONSIDERATION

In the US, animals bred for meat are often raised under questionable circumstances. The quality of their feed, living conditions, and the use of antibiotics, hormones, and other chemicals raise many questions. These practices no doubt have a negative effect on the quality of the products made from the animals; how much this will impact human health is a controversial topic. Without question, we highly recommend targeting pastured, grass-fed, and organic sources. Likewise, we recommend choosing wild-caught fish and prioritizing smaller fish, which acquire lower levels of toxins from their environment.

Most plant-based foods have also been impacted by modern agricultural methods. Intensive horticulture, genetically modified organisms (GMOs), and widespread use of chemical fertilizers and pesticides mean that similar questions of quality arise when choosing plant-based products. Selecting organic, non-GMO produce can help minimize any potential risks.

It can be difficult (and expensive) to always choose the best-quality foods. Consuming a low-carb, real-food diet provides the main benefit and is the primary goal, even if some cheaper, lower-quality choices sneak into your grocery basket.

DO EAT

Wild-caught seafood is the ideal "meat" for great health. Seek out fatty fish in particular: mackerel, sardines, salmon, hake, tuna. Shellfish are also delicious and bring many nutrients, like iodine, to the party.

Natural and unprocessed grass-fed or pastured meats, such as lamb, duck, pork, beef, turkey, and chicken (legs are better than breasts, and leave the skin on!), offal, etc. Always go for the fattiest cuts.

Pastured eggs: Eggs, eggs, eggs—any way you like them. They are a true superfood in every way!

Full-fat dairy, including heavy cream, butter, ghee, full- and high-fat cheeses, and full-fat yogurt. Dairy is a great source of natural fats. While some people need to be careful not to overdo it with dairy, most benefit greatly when it replaces carb in the diet. However, cheeses are incredibly delicious and easier to overeat than some other fatty foods—so if you are stuck on a weight-loss plateau, maybe taper back the cheese.

Vegetables, including above-ground leafy greens and cruciferous vegetables like broccoli and Brussels sprouts

Healthy natural fats, including butter, beef tallow, lard, avocado oil, macadamia nut oil, coconut oil, and more

Nuts, including Brazil nuts, walnuts, almonds, macadamias, and walnuts

Certain non-grain-based flours, such as coconut flour, almond flour, and other nut flours

Some sweet foods, including coconut, dark chocolate (greater than 80 percent cacao, preferably greater than 85 percent), berry fruits (occasionally), and high-fat, low-sugar desserts. Artificial sweeteners, ideally xylitol or stevia, are okay in minimal quantity, though there is evidence that excessive use of sweeteners will affect your weight-loss efforts. The goal is to reduce or eliminate sugary and sweet items, including artificial sweeteners, over the long term. Our recipe section goes easy on you for the first three weeks and allows for a fair amount of the "less bad" sweeteners. However, salty, savory, and fatty treats are the safer way to indulge over the long term.

Alcohol that's low in carb/sugar: red wine, spirits (moderation is advised)

This is a very simplified list. We are constantly asked to "just tell me what I can eat—keep it simple, please." When you're busy and just trying to tackle a problem, too much information and too many options can be overwhelming. So for this first week in particular, we've taken a commonsense approach that focuses on the bottom line. There is enough change going on without grappling with an encyclopedia of allowed foods.

FOODS THAT FOIL YOUR PLAN

Here is the list of the foods to avoid. Make a photocopy of this list and keep it at hand. Don't worry about the occasional item that you are not too sure of. There are plenty of foods on the "do eat" list to keep you alive for one week! The truth is that the foods on that list kept our species alive and healthy for all of history.

We remind you that you are running across the bridge to fat-burning during this week. Imagine that the bridge itself is burning. For many people, it's not too comfortable to dawdle on. You really want to get across it quickly to where wonderful health and vitality awaits. Obsessing about the details won't speed you along. Rather, you must focus on the core: eating healthy fats and eliminating unhealthy carb. Don't complicate your crossing. Most of all, you need to stay well clear of the foods in the following list.

DON'T EAT

Starches such as breads, crackers, pasta, potatoes, grits, rice, porridge, popcorn, etc.

Sweets, including sugar, honey, agave, milk chocolate (dark chocolate is okay—see page 76), fruit juices, pastries, cookies, pies, cakes, etc. Limit dried fruits to only occasional exceptions—these can be sugar bombs!

Grains such as breakfast cereals/muesli, wheat, corn, couscous, oats, rye— avoid pretty much all grains

Bad meat products, including low-fat processed meats, low-quality luncheon meats, and sausages with grain fillers. The fact that we use the word *products* is a big clue. (Contrast these with healthier but still processed meats like Parma ham, high-quality beef jerky without additives, and unadulterated lardons have had minimal processing or additives, which can all be consumed in moderation.)

Problematic dairy, including low-fat or skim milk and low-fat cheeses. The great thing about dairy is it's a good source of healthy fats, which makes low-fat versions an absurdity. We note, too, that excessive cheese consumption has been associated with insulin-spiking in the sensitive minority of people (e.g., ApoE4 people with history of diabetes—see page 343). Checking your blood glucose after a meal (see page 84) can be very useful in figuring out if you are in the sensitive minority.

Toxic fats, including all the industrially processed oils: soybean, sunflower, canola, peanut, rapeseed, grapeseed, safflower, sesame, flaxseed (cold-pressed is okay), cottonseed, etc.

High-sugar fruits, including grapes, mangos, pomegranates, cherries, bananas, and melons. Low-sugar fruits like strawberries and blueberries are okay.

Legumes—moderate the intake of peanuts, lentils, and beans

Sweet alcohol with a high carb/sugar content: beers, ciders, sweet wines

BREAD, THE DIET DESTROYER

What single complaint do we hear more than any other from people who have accepted the science that a low-carb, high-fat diet is healthy but are faltering with its practical aspects? It involves something known as a sandwich. It turns out the biggest problem faced is a lack of bread.

We don't want you to feel deprived in the first week. So we had better get this one out of the way right now. Cheap, convenient junk food didn't just arrive in the past century. It really came about several thousand years ago when humans began to cultivate grains. Through clever processing of these grains, our ancestors created various breads. For a long time, these contained some nutrition and were useful for meeting energy needs. They became staple products all over the world. In the past century, however, they have led to a growing problem.

The selective breeding of grains has greatly increased their level of anti-nutrients—molecules that prevent the body from absorbing nutrients. It has also depleted their level of nutrients (what little they had in the first place). On top of this essential lack of nutrients, breads today are made from refined flour and have added sugar. With the majority of American adults now insulin resistant, breads have become a massive liability.

Breads are appetite enhancers. They spike insulin, disrupt the gut, and tweak the brain's pleasure center in disastrous ways. Breads quietly signal us at a deep level. They whisper one message: "Eat me … You need more …"

And sadly, breads have become central to our eating routine, particularly at lunch. In addition to loaves of bread, we now have wraps, bagels, crackers, rolls, pizzas, and more needed to hold our lunches together. If you take these carb bombs away, the very structure of our lunch routine implodes. So we are left with a dilemma. We must reject all breads to enable weight loss, metabolic health, and longevity. There is really no choice in the matter when desiring health and slimness. But what to eat instead?

Luckily there many solutions to this tricky problem. Below are some of them:

► Take the contents of that sandwich you were going to make for your work lunch. Put them in a small lidded container. Add a small bottle of balsamic vinaigrette or other tasty dressing, along with a knife and fork—without bread, you'll need them.

► Really need the "hold it between two slices" experience? Take a few minutes to make some safe slices for yourself. Shred 1 small cauliflower and mix it in a large bowl with 3 eggs and 2 ounces (60 g) grated Parmesan. You can add chiles, chives, or other herbs to taste. Spread into bread slice–shaped patties in a hot greased pan and cook until firm, flipping halfway to cook both sides. In this way, you can make a batch of delicious "bread" (about 6 to 8 slices). While most delicious when eaten straight away in a hot sandwich, they can be stored in a plastic bag after cooling. Leave the bag slightly open to keep them from getting moist. If not used within a day, they can be stored in the fridge for 2–3 days.

► Make a batch of "oopsie bread." It is quick to make and in its most basic form uses just a handful of ingredients, though many taste tweaks are possible with the addition of seasonings such as dried herbs. It's perfect for sandwiches or hamburger buns, and it doubles as a crust for low-carb pizza. It's not surprising that oopsie bread is such a popular bread substitute in the low-carb movement. Here is a great version from Diet Doctor: www.dietdoctor.com/recipes/oopsie-bread.

► You can also bake a dizzying array of safe breads using almond flour, coconut flour, and other non-grain-based flours. They are delicious, and the internet is filled with recipes for these low-carb breads.

Sadly, there are as yet no good substitutes for bread on the supermarket shelves. We believe there will be in the coming years, as the world wakes up to what humans really need. So for the moment, you need to look after yourself. It is not hard to do. Bread is one of the worst things that can sneak its way into an otherwise healthy diet. Please don't let this Trojan horse food undermine your weight-loss and longevity efforts.

Just say no.

SNACKING: EMERGENCY OPTIONS

We cannot overstress the importance of widely spacing meals (action step 7). You must give your digestive hormones extended breaks between meals. Otherwise, the bridge to smooth fat-burning will lengthen painfully. You do not need a barrier to success like this placed right in your path.

We understand that there will be pressure points during the first week of your journey. We have been there. For instance, you may be doing very well after lunch, holding off on eating anything until your evening meal, when with a couple of hours to go, you find yourself in your workplace with a problem: a deep-seated hunger growing in you.

The key is to be prepared for these moments. You need to have safe fuels available if and when they strike. It is better to have a healthy snack that won't spike your insulin than to reach out and eat something nasty. Also, targeting very low carb snacks means there is minimal lengthening of the bridge to fat-burning. Often, you will need only a small shot of energy to get you through the moment of weakness. Where this emergency shot comes from is crucial. The real problem occurs if you approach a vending machine or snack counter. In these places, only foods of failure exist. You will be like a newly former smoker taking a cigarette from a guy in a bar. Once the junk is ingested, many days of great achievement are undone.

All you need to do to avoid this is keep the best emergency foods nearby. These snacks should be practical, high in fat and/or protein, and very low in carb. Here are the ones we recommend for emergencies.

If no refrigeration is available:

- ▶ Dark chocolate (80 to 85 percent cacao or greater)
- ▶ Nuts (macadamia nuts, Brazil nuts, hazelnuts, pistachios, walnuts, pecans, etc.)
- ▶ Canned fish (tuna, sardines, etc.)
- ▶ High-quality cured meats or dry sausage without grains or added oils

If refrigeration is available:

- ▶ Bone broth (and other low-carb, low-calorie broths)
- ▶ Cheeses (whatever full-fat variety is your favorite)
- ▶ Mix of olives, feta cheese, and lardons

If you don't have any healthy snacks available when you feel hunger hit, there are other stopgaps you can try to get you through:

- ▶ Drink a large glass of water
- ▶ Take a short walk in fresh air—take deep breaths and think of the proper meal of real food that awaits only an hour or two away. You will savor it all the more having waited for it.

Note that with time and adaptation, you will very rarely feel the need to snack. Freedom awaits you.

Let's now check in on what the early days will look like in your new life.

DAYS 1 THROUGH 7: A SAMPLE WEEK OF MEALS

We do not want to tell you every bite that should go in your mouth during the first week. With all the information you've read so far in this book about how the body responds to different foods, you're already way ahead of the game—you know how food affects the body and what makes a particular food a good or bad choice. That said, it may be useful to see a sample week's worth of meals. Later in the week you can start to bring in rules 7 to 10—if you feel you are ready for it, wider meal separation is key.

Remember to keep healthy snacks within reach for tough situations. Avoid indulging if possible—but use these as a lifeline when you need them rather than resorting to carb-loaded junk. And don't forget to keep a water bottle handy. Always try to drink several pints of water a day, mainly away from your mealtimes. The reason is twofold: drinking water can help manage appetite between meals, and drinking large amounts of water with meals can impact some people's digestion process.

The meal plans for days 1–7, below, and for days 8–21 (pages 120 to 127) were designed to give you a ratio of macros for each day consisting of roughly 60 percent fat, 20 percent protein, and 20 percent carbohydrates. Both plans feature recipes from Chapter 9 as well as basic, simple-to-prepare meals. But please don't feel wedded to these meal plans; you can choose any of the recipes from Chapter 9—just keep in mind the balance of macros for each day. Later, as your appetite becomes better controlled, portion sizes will naturally get smaller and you'll need less fat to feel full. You can also get meal ideas from excellent low-carb websites such as Diet Doctor (dietdoctor.com), which is managed by our friend and colleague Dr. Andreas Eenfeldt.

Although this meal plan does include snacks, avoid them as much as possible. These are meant to replace unhealthy carby snacks if you feel significant pressure to eat between meals. But the longer you go without eating, the shorter your bridge to fat-burning will be!

Unless otherwise noted, all the Chapter 9 recipes in the meal plans serve four people. All recipes that serve more than four people can be frozen for later and/or are used as leftovers later in the week, saving you prep time. The brief descriptions of basic meals are given in per-person quantities, so you will need to scale them up as needed. If you're feeding just yourself and are concerned about having too many leftovers, make a half batch of the recipes referenced from Chapter 9. (*Note:* Salt and pepper are not included in the simple meal descriptions; we assume you will season the meals to your taste. Feel free to add fresh or dried herbs to the simple meals to further personalize them.)

DAY 1

BREAKFAST	Three eggs, any style, with 2 to 3 slices cooked bacon *(Serving per person)*
LUNCH	A salad of crisp lettuce topped with cold or warm cooked chicken, 2 tablespoons Caesar dressing (page 166), 1 tablespoon Parmesan shavings, and 1½ tablespoons cooked bacon bits or lardons *(Serving per person)*
DINNER	1 batch Almond & Parmesan–Crusted Baked Salmon (page 192)
STOPGAP SNACK OR TREAT	1 batch No-Bake Cocoa Peanut Butter Protein Balls (page 175) *(This recipe makes 12 servings but keeps for a month in the freezer. Leftovers may be used on days 4 and 5 of this plan.)*

DAY 2

1 batch Bacon, Gruyère & Red Pepper Egg Muffins (page 138) *(This recipe makes 8 servings; leftovers may be used on day 6 of this plan.)*	BREAKFAST
Taco salad: A bed of chopped or torn lettuce topped with 4 ounces (115 g) ground beef (grass-fed, 80% lean), browned and seasoned with taco seasoning, along with ½ cup diced onions, ½ cup diced bell peppers, 1 cup diced tomatoes, 1 cup shredded full-fat cheese, and about a tablespoon each of sliced scallions and sliced olives. You can dress this salad with sour cream and squeeze a half lime over it for further flavor. *(Serving per person)*	LUNCH
1 batch Squid "Pasta" with Pan-Seared Cod, Chorizo & Spinach (page 204)	DINNER
1 batch No-Churn Avocado & Salted Pistachio Ice Cream (page 212) *(This recipe makes 8 servings; leftovers may be used on day 4 or day 5 of this plan.)*	STOPGAP SNACK OR TREAT

DAY 3

1 batch High-Protein Breakfast Smoothie of choice (page 152) A handful of mixed nuts, such as Brazil nuts, walnuts, and almonds *(Serving per person)*	BREAKFAST
1 batch Crispy Boneless Chicken Wings with Buffalo Ranch Dip (page 178)	LUNCH
Hamburger patties: In a large bowl, mix together 1½ pounds ground beef (grass-fed, 80% lean), 1 large egg, 3 ounces (80 g) shredded cheese, 1 tablespoon olive oil, 1 tablespoon (15 g) butter, parsley, salt, and ground black pepper. Shape the mixture into 8 patties and cook on a grill or stovetop. *(4 servings of 2 patties each)* 1 pound green cabbage, shredded, sautéed in 3 ounces (85 g) butter until softened to desired texture	DINNER
Small handful of favorite nuts or a few squares of dark chocolate (80 percent or higher cacao) *(Serving per person)*	STOPGAP SNACK OR TREAT

DAY 4

BREAKFAST	Three-egg omelet filled with 2 ounces (60 g) fresh (soft) goat cheese and chopped fresh herbs, such as chives, parsley, and tarragon or basil *(Serving per person)*
LUNCH	1 batch Creamy Chicken-Mushroom Soup (page 156) *(This recipe makes 6 servings, but you can divide it into 4 servings for slightly larger portions.)*
DINNER	1 batch One-Pan Thai Coconut Chicken & Vegetable Bake (page 198) *(This recipe makes 6 servings; freeze any leftover portions for later.)*
STOPGAP SNACK OR TREAT	½ cup (75 g) fresh blueberries drizzled with heavy cream or *leftover* No-Bake Cocoa Peanut Butter Protein Balls or *leftover* No-Churn Avocado & Salted Pistachio Ice Cream *(Serving per person)*

DAY 5

BREAKFAST	Pesto and sun-dried tomato scrambled eggs: Scramble three eggs in a pan greased with olive oil over moderate heat; when the eggs begin to set, stir in 1 tablespoon pesto, 3 chopped sun-dried tomatoes, and ⅓ cup shredded full-fat cheddar cheese *(Serving per person)*
LUNCH	Baked portobello mushroom caps stuffed with crabmeat and goat cheese: Season a large destemmed portobello mushroom cap with salt and pepper. Bake, cavity-side down, in a preheated 400°F (205°C) oven for 10 minutes to soften. Turn the cap over and fill with 5 ounces (150 g) crabmeat and 3 ounces (90 g) fresh (soft) goat cheese. Return to the oven and bake until the cheese and crabmeat are heated, about 6 minutes. *(Serving per person)*
DINNER	1 batch Incredible Keto Pizza (page 160)
STOPGAP SNACK OR TREAT	1 batch Double Chocolate Pudding (page 206) or *leftover* No-Bake Cocoa Peanut Butter Protein Balls or *leftover* No-Churn Avocado & Salted Pistachio Ice Cream

DAY 6	

Leftover Bacon, Gruyère & Red Pepper Egg Muffins	**BREAKFAST** (optional; see sidebar)
Tuna salad made with 2-Minute Homemade Mayonnaise (page 132), diced celery, and a squeeze of fresh lemon juice *(1 cup per person)*	**LUNCH**
1 batch Slow Cooker Beef Stew (page 195) *(This recipe makes 6 servings; freeze any leftover portions for later.)*	**DINNER**
A few squares of dark chocolate (80 percent or higher cacao)	**STOPGAP SNACK OR TREAT**

DAY 6 OPTION

See if can you bypass breakfast altogether. Have a stopgap snack available if skipping the morning meal isn't working out for you—there are some great low-carb snack recipes on pages 170 to 178. If it does work, make sure that you visualize your body fat slowly burning to feed you throughout the morning. Sense your growing fat adaptation as you accelerate your ability to burn fat. Feel and be proud of the benefits that come from self-reliance. Most importantly, look forward to that tasty lunch with great anticipation! We and many others find that extending your overnight fast by skipping breakfast is the best strategy for meal spacing, but you can opt for skipping lunch instead. If you wish to try this option, then it is best to have a substantial breakfast, ideally one that's egg-based.

DAY 7	
BREAKFAST	Two-egg omelet filled with ½ cup (80 g) diced or chopped vegetables, sautéed, and ¼ cup (35 g) shredded full-fat cheese or 2 ounces (60 g) cooked meat *(Serving per person)*
LUNCH	Ham salad made with 2-Minute Homemade Mayonnaise (page 132), diced olives, avocado, and cheese, with sliced tomatoes and pickles on the side (1 cup per person)
DINNER	1 batch Seared Liver with Bacon & Wild Mushrooms (page 200)
STOPGAP SNACK OR TREAT	1 batch Cucumber & Raspberry Mojito Mocktail (page 220) *(This recipe makes 2 servings; increase as needed. Note: If following the meal plan, make this mocktail recipe virgin, as written.)*

WHAT TO DRINK

For this first week, here are the beverages we recommend:

▶ Water

▶ Wine in moderation (dry red varieties are preferable due to lower sugar content)

▶ Tea (no sugar, little whole milk)

▶ Coffee (no sugar—enrich with heavy cream if you like)

You can use a low-carb sweetener in tea or coffee if you feel you really must, but ideally you will wean yourself off these and go sweetener-free.

You can also drink, in moderation, low-carb drinks sweetened with reasonably safe to consume low-carb sweetener.

Do not consume the following drinks:

▶ Soft drinks

▶ Fruit juices

▶ Sweetened beverages

▶ Lattes or cappuccinos (too much milk—cream is much better for you)

DAYS 1 THROUGH 7: SUPPLEMENTS

You are switching to a healthy low-carb lifestyle. This means crossing the bridge to fat adaptation, as we have said. But some other things will also be happening in your body as you leave bad food behind. One of these is an enhanced requirement for certain nutrients. Here we will cover what you need for a successful first week.

POTASSIUM

With this diet you will be reducing glycogen (glucose) stores in your body. This can cause a drop in potassium in the short term, though over time potassium levels will stabilize. The natural foods you're now eating should provide a lot of the potassium you need, but it may not be enough for everyone. In recent years the daily potassium intake guidelines have been increased to a minimum of nearly 5,000 milligrams per day. You want to make sure that you are *at least* getting this amount. Therefore we advise taking a potassium supplement to make sure you're covered.

We recommend a half teaspoon of potassium chloride ("lite salt") mixed in with food or drinks during the day. This is a mixture of potassium and sodium, so it will help with both requirements. Keep in mind that the best way to get your potassium is from real foods. Some of the best sources are avocados (about 1,000 mg), nuts (100 to 300 mg per ounce), dark leafy greens (840 mg per cup, cooked), salmon (about 800 mg per filet), and mushrooms (100 to 200 mg per cup).

SODIUM

As your insulin levels drop because you're consuming less glucose, you'll shed fluids and, with them, salt. That means a healthy low-carb diet actually increases the body's demand for salt, so sodium becomes a really good thing to add to your regimen.

It's possible that many people who eat a lot of processed foods may be consuming too much sodium. But even then, the problems with high sodium have been grossly exaggerated in the past decades. A recent book by Dr. James DiNicolantonio exposed the truly dreadful scientific methods that were used to vilify the crucial nutrient that is natural salt.[1] Salt may indeed be a problem for a small proportion of people (salt-sensitive hypertensives), but for most people, lack of it is a bigger problem. That's especially true for people who are fixing their health with low-carb diets. People on low-carb diets who aren't getting enough sodium may experience fatigue, light-headedness, headaches, and constipation.

Getting adequate sodium is an imperative. Adding 2 to 3 grams of sodium a day is advisable. This can be most easily achieved by adding salt to soups, broths, drinks, and savory dishes. Specialized salt products such as pink Himalayan salt, Aztec salt, and sea salt are often rich in valuable minerals. It is an excellent idea to always have these at hand and use them liberally.

MAGNESIUM

Regardless of diet, the majority of people get way too little magnesium. Low magnesium can lead to fatigue, neurological issues, muscle cramps, and more. A low-carb diet can accentuate the need for magnesium. This is because lower insulin initially causes loss of fluids and, with it, electrolytes, and also because many of the high-carb foods you'll be avoiding have significant amounts of magnesium, and you need to ensure you're still getting enough. This would not have been so much of a problem for our ancestors. But today magnesium in the soil is depleted, which means there's less magnesium in our food, too. You should still get reasonable amounts of magnesium from avocados, full-fat yogurt, and low-carb nuts like Brazil nuts and almonds. Dark chocolate will give you a boost, too.

That said, we highly recommend taking a magnesium supplement. We use magnesium citrate powder, which is cheap and can be purchased in bulk online. You can sprinkle it onto savory dishes with no real impact on flavor. Note that it can have a laxative effect until you get used to it. For this reason, spread your intake throughout the day, so you don't get too large a dose at once, and ingest it with or just after a meal. Approximately 300 mg of magnesium in supplement form should suffice, assuming you are also getting reasonable quantities from your healthy food intake.

OMEGA-3 FATTY ACIDS

Start taking an omega-3 fish oil supplement straightaway. By following the action steps, you will eliminate the dreadful omega-6-filled vegetable oils from your diet, so you will be well on your way to fixing your ratio of omega-6 to omega-3. In the standard American diet, that ratio is around 20:1, but ideally it should be between 1:1 and 3:1. Taking supplemental omega-3 will also help with your triglyceride level, neurological health, and many other things. With your new healthy low-carb diet you should be consuming more omega-3. However, a supplement of 2 grams extra per day is a great addition. The best capsule sources can be expensive. We actually go for the tried-and-true traditional solutions. We simply take a half tablespoon of high-quality cod liver oil each day. We favor the "high strength" version from Seven Seas because it contains enhanced concentrations of EPA and DHA, the two key types of omega-3. In this way cod liver oil can give you what you need at close to a tenth of the price of capsule supplements. You may not be crazy about the taste, so quickly down the tablespoon after a meal and wash it down with a glass of water.

OTHER SUPPLEMENTS

We don't want to weigh you down with too many supplements in the first week. The only other ones we'd recommend are vitamin D and iodine. Vitamin D insufficiency is connected to so many health problems that you need to tackle it straightaway. Although it is better to access vitamin D from healthy sun exposure or healthy foods, the reality is that supplementation is a great enabler. If you have a blood test that indicates healthy vitamin D levels (ideally over 30 ng/mL), then there is not much need. If your results are below this or you don't know what your vitamin D level is, a good place to start is with 3,000 to 4,000 IU per day. We will revisit this in Chapter 15.

In this first week, you're embarking on a journey that will change your cholesterol numbers for the better. But iodine deficiency and associated thyroid function issues are also intimately connected to triglyceride and cholesterol problems. You do not want to start fixing your cholesterol and leave a related factor swinging loose by becoming deficient in iodine. In any case, most American adults are not receiving enough iodine in their diets and cannot even reach the low targets in the recommended intake guidelines. Best to start fixing this right away by taking an iodine supplement. There is a lot of debate around how much should be taken, from a few hundred micrograms (mcg) to many thousands. Excess iodine intake can present a problem for some individuals, so we compromise at 500–1000 mcg per day. Sea kelp tablets are a good supplement for bioabsorbable iodine.

GINA'S STORY

Gina made the switch to a healthy low-carb lifestyle after a "final straw" experience. She had a long history of irritable bowel syndrome (IBS), but she never realized that these issues are often driven by high-carb diets.

On a road trip to a wedding, Gina felt a bad attack coming on. Her stomach was gurgling, and she was about to have an issue in the middle of nowhere. Sitting fearfully in the passenger seat, she started looking at cures for IBS using her phone. She luckily came across a blog that showed people were having amazing success with low-carb lifestyles. She decided to become a low-carb eater.

Prior to that day, weight was always a struggle for Gina. Her primary care physician pushed lots of fruits and vegetables, along with whole grains and lean meats. Her typical diet would be bananas, low-fat Greek yogurt, whole-grain pasta, lean chicken, whole-wheat bread, turkey, oatmeal, and the like. For nearly two years, she followed her meal plan precisely, worked out a few hours each week, and managed to lose small amounts of weight. Then the poor results with this high-carb dietary strategy caused her to let the truly rigorous adherence slip.

In fairness, Gina continued to avoid cookies, cakes, ice cream, and candies. She continued to stick with the whole-grain, low-fat lifestyle in principle, never realizing that she was on the road to diabetes with this fare. And she steadily gained weight until she was quite obese. At 38, she was now the heaviest she had ever been, while largely following her doctor's nutritional guidance. Not once did her doctor suggest removing carbs from her diet.

Since eating low-carb, high-fat, Gina has lost around 70 pounds in less than a year. She has gone down a few dress sizes and her energy has skyrocketed. Her IBS issues have disappeared. Her cholesterol, blood pressure, and other metrics are now excellent. She is no longer on the road to diabetes. She is delighted with her new body weight and massively improved sense of wellness. And she achieved all of this by following our key rules.

CHAPTER 8

THE EAT RICH, LIVE LONG PLAN:
DAYS 8 THROUGH 21

> " We are what we repeatedly do.
> Excellence, then, is not an act but a habit. "
>
> —Will Durant

The next two weeks on the Eat Rich, Live Long program will establish your new, healthier habits. While in the first week you focused primarily on getting the food right, now it's time to add some more strategies to achieve optimal results over the longer term. Most notably, this means focusing on steps 7 through 10. As a reminder, these are: widely spacing meals, getting enough vitamins and minerals, managing environment factors, and exercising. As with the first week, some focus and dedication are required to do all this properly, but rest assured, covering all the steps is the recipe for success.

But first, let's check in on how the first seven days went.

FIRST AND FOREMOST: CHECK IN ON YOUR FIRST SEVEN DAYS!

At the end of the week, you should be feeling much better than you did before. Your belt should be looser, your mind should be clearer, and your mood should be more stable. You should be facing the next fourteen days with determination and gusto.

But what do you do if you are also experiencing some challenges?

We then need to check in on potential pitfalls. First, make sure that you are following the action steps on pages 72 to 73 correctly. If you're not, then address any gaps. Finally, you may need to adjust your plan according to your specific needs.

Here is a list of potential roadblocks and their remedies. (We'll talk about some other challenges that can happen over time in Chapter 16.)

▶ **"Low-carb flu."** When you're crossing the bridge to fat-burning, you may experience some symptoms as your body makes the transition away from sugar-burning. These symptoms can include headache, lethargy, nausea, confusion, brain fog, and general irritability. Usually these can be traced back to dehydration or sodium deficiency. Review the supplements section for the first week again (page 101). Boost your intake of salt and make sure you're drinking plenty of water. Chicken or beef bone broth—or even a bouillon cube that contains salt dissolved in water—can be a huge help. As an emergency measure, you can add a small amount of healthy carbs back into your diet—for example, add some sweet potato with one of your meals. We do not recommend this, however, as it may only delay the switch to fat-burning.

▶ **Muscle twitches and aches.** If you're experiencing muscle cramps, restless legs, achiness, and the like, it may be related to a nutrient deficiency. Boost your intake of salt and make sure you're drinking plenty of water—these are the most likely culprits in the first week. Muscle symptoms may also be a sign that you're low in magnesium, however. Take a good supplement (see page 102) and do not go low on this miraculous element.

▶ **Constipation.** Although most people experience improvements in this department, constipation can occur. Yet again, dehydration may be the culprit. You may also need to tweak up the vegetable intake, while being careful to avoid those problematic grains. Magnesium citrate can also come to the rescue. It is an extraordinary bowel-mover, to the point that many people have to be careful with it. Taking the maximum daily dose of 1,000 milligrams will make constipation impossible to maintain!

▶ **Heart palpitations, blood pressure fluctuations, and other cardiovascular concerns.** The solution to these issues is similar to the other ones—drink plenty of water and eat plenty of salt. But it is important to check with your doctor in advance before making any significant lifestyle changes. You need to be sure you are aware of any underlying heart issues, and if you do have a heart concern, talk to your doctor about this diet before making the switch and again if you experience any heart-related symptoms on the diet. You need to also be careful if you are currently on medication for diabetes or high blood pressure. The sudden switch to a genuinely healthy diet may mean that the conditions these medications are meant to treat are no longer there, as blood pressure and blood glucose drop naturally. If you're taking medications designed to have these effects, they may result in particularly low blood glucose or blood pressure. You can discuss this with your physician as necessary, although it would be ideal if he/she is well-informed on the low-carb science.

► **Hair loss.** Mild hair loss can occur during any significant diet change, and so it is with switching to a low-carb regimen. The phenomenon is a temporary one. During the first few months following the switch you may notice more hairs coming away when you brush. After a few more months new hair follicles will replace the old, and the experience will fade. Essentially, the sudden switch causes a global replacement of the hair. Usually this replacement process is occurring randomly across your scalp and is not so noticeable.

PERSONALIZING YOUR PLAN

Back in Chapter 3, we identified four main kinds of people based on insulin status and body weight. Each type of person will benefit from tailored advice for the next fourteen days. On the next page is an overview diagram to illustrate the primary types and where they should focus.

THE INSULIN-RESISTANT OVERWEIGHT PERSON

This is the most common type among American adults nowadays. Let's take a look at where you are now, after your first week on a low-carb, high-fat diet.

During the first week, there was a prompt fall in your insulin and glucose levels. This alone has begun to dismantle the insulin/glucose roller coaster in which you were trapped. Our recommended very low net carb intake (less than 40 grams per day) accelerates this crucial process. Likewise, your body's stores of glycogen (glucose) finally have begun to deplete. Glycogen carries a lot of water, so you'll have experienced weight loss due to this factor alone as your body drops water weight. But toward the end of the week, you'll also have seen the beginnings of body fat loss. You're starting to feel that belt loosening.

Personalizing Your Plan

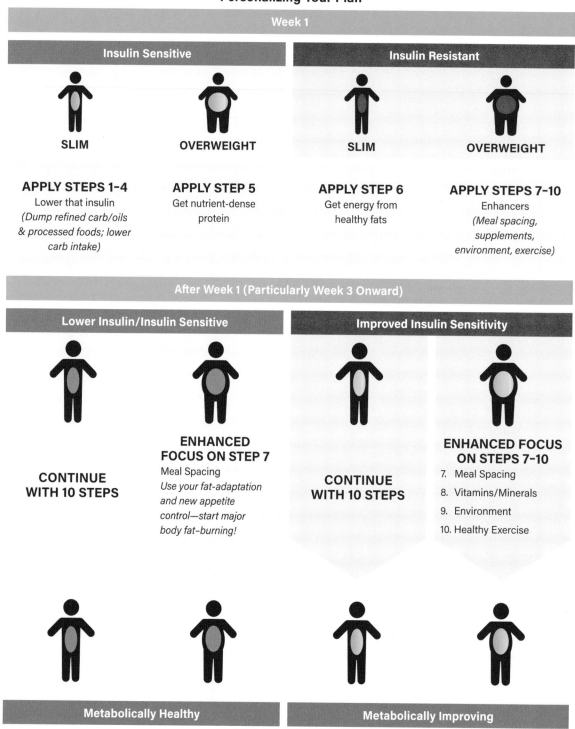

Week 1

Insulin Sensitive

SLIM

APPLY STEPS 1–4
Lower that insulin
(Dump refined carb/oils
& processed foods; lower
carb intake)

OVERWEIGHT

APPLY STEP 5
Get nutrient-dense
protein

Insulin Resistant

SLIM

APPLY STEP 6
Get energy from
healthy fats

OVERWEIGHT

APPLY STEPS 7–10
Enhancers
(Meal spacing,
supplements,
environment, exercise)

After Week 1 (Particularly Week 3 Onward)

Lower Insulin/Insulin Sensitive

**CONTINUE
WITH 10 STEPS**

**ENHANCED
FOCUS ON STEP 7**
Meal Spacing
*Use your fat-adaptation
and new appetite
control—start major
body fat–burning!*

Improved Insulin Sensitivity

**CONTINUE
WITH 10 STEPS**

**ENHANCED FOCUS
ON STEPS 7–10**
7. Meal Spacing
8. Vitamins/Minerals
9. Environment
10. Healthy Exercise

Metabolically Healthy

Metabolically Improving

The fall in insulin is also opening the door to your new fat-burning physiology. You are getting most of your energy from healthy fats now. Your body is beginning to switch over its machinery to burn this fat more efficiently.

Your insulin and glucose levels have begun to drop, particularly your postmeal levels. Likewise, the most important cholesterol numbers have started to improve—the ratios of triglycerides to HDL cholesterol and total cholesterol to HDL (we'll talk about these much more in Chapter 11). If you have been tracking your blood pressure, you should see those numbers beginning to drop also. All these and more indicators of health status are improving. Your body has started to repair itself. It is becoming ready for a much healthier future.

All this is great news, but people with very high insulin and associated insulin resistance may experience a double-edged sword in the first week. On the one hand, they tend to have the most extreme improvements in health status. But they may also have more challenges. This is where continued focus on all ten of our steps is very important. Resolving profound insulin issues requires more than simply restricting carb intake–protein and healthy fat intake matter, too, along with meal spacing, environmental factors, and exercise. The action steps must all be tackled to eradicate this near-universal driver of poor health and obesity.

If you're insulin resistant and overweight, here's what you should be focusing on over the next fourteen days:

▶ Address any challenges that you may have experienced in the first week.

▶ Continue following the prescription for meals and supplements from days 1 through 7, but go beyond the diet. Start really working all ten action steps.

▶ If things are going well and you are comfortable, begin to focus particularly on action step 7, meal spacing / fasting.

Remember that following the other action steps will enable you to apply step 7 effectively. You cannot apply meal spacing effectively when enslaved in the high-carb hunger trap. You must break the cycle and develop some degree of fat-burning capability in order to practice healthy fasting habits. These habits in turn will enhance your fat-burning metabolism. They will actually end up enabling themselves.

After some level of fat-adaptation is achieved, you can deploy meal spacing as a powerful intervention. Make this a primary goal over the coming fourteen days!

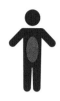

THE INSULIN-RESISTANT NORMAL-WEIGHT PERSON

This kind of person is often called "thin outside, fat inside" (TOFI). It is a common category—these people experience a huge number of surprise heart attacks. They share most of the health risks associated with the insulin-resistant overweight, but they seem relatively healthy—until one day a heart attack comes out of the blue. They may not need to lose much weight, but for longevity and genuine good health, they need a low-carb, high-fat diet just as much as overweight folks.

If you are insulin resistant but not overweight, your experience after the first seven days is probably similar to that of the insulin-resistant overweight type, though you've probably lost less weight. Most importantly, a similar fall in your insulin and glucose levels has taken place. Our recommended very low net carb intake (less than 40 grams per day) has kick-started your exit from insulin dysregulation. Your body's stores of glycogen have finally begun to deplete. The body fat loss will be coming particularly from the fat in your belly region. An insulin-resistant person will likely have significant visceral adipose tissue—fat in and around their internal organs. This is the fat you really need to tackle, as it can affect overall health. You should be beginning to feel some belt-loosening effects as this occurs.

The fall in insulin levels is promoting your fat-burning physiology, which is crucial for your longevity. It will also inoculate you against significant weight gain as you age.

Your insulin and glucose levels have begun to drop, particularly your post-meal levels. Likewise, the most important cholesterol numbers have started to improve. Many TOFI people have "unexplained" high blood pressure, mostly driven by high levels of insulin and insulin resistance. So your blood pressure should have begun to drop naturally, too. All these and more indicators of your health status will improve. Your body has started to repair itself. It is getting ready for a much healthier future.

Continued focus on all ten of action steps is still important. That said, if you're insulin-resistant but not overweight, you'll have experienced a rapid improvement in well-being by the end of the first week.

Here's what your primary focus should be on over the next fourteen days:

▶ Be sure to address any challenges you may have experienced (see page 106).

▶ Continue following the prescription for meals and supplements from days 1 through 7, but go beyond the diet. Start really pushing all ten of those action steps.

- While weight loss may not be needed, step 7 should be a focus to help you further accelerate the switch to a fat-burning physiology.
- Action steps 8 through 10 will really help accelerate progress to true insulin sensitivity and the ultimate goal: habitually low insulin levels.

THE INSULIN-SENSITIVE OVERWEIGHT PERSON

The path forward for people in this category can be a little tricky. If you are one of these people, you may not have experienced a dramatic weight transformation in the first week. You certainly should have noticed significant changes, but perhaps less so than the insulin-resistant folks.

Our recommendation to you was a low to moderate net carb intake (40 to 80 grams per day, with a maximum of 120 grams). During the first week, you likely saw a moderate drop in your insulin and glucose levels. The extent of the change will of course depend on how healthy or low-carb your previous diet was. Let's look at the most likely outcome from the first week in more detail.

Your body's stores of glycogen have begun to deplete. Toward the end of the week, there was also body fat loss. Your belt should be easing somewhat from its previous tightness.

During the first week, you too started crossing the bridge to fat-burning—just like your insulin-resistant colleagues. With most of your energy now coming from healthy fats, you will be much better prepared for the actions required during the next fourteen days. Your key focus in the next fourteen days will be to leverage your growing ability to burn your own body fat. You are keeping the carbs down—this is good. But dietary fat is providing the energy you need to simply stay where you are in terms of body weight.

Your body is now carrying reserves of what is essentially healthy fat. Your fat cells are not insulin resistant and are functioning very well—which will support your overall health. Metabolically, you are in reasonably good shape, but there is no internal driver to burn stored body fat. Therefore, you must intentionally create a driver to achieve this. You are one of the few types of people who should keep an eye on caloric intake. Our guideline would be to aim for less than 1,800 calories per day, which will help you burn your body fat for fuel. This is, of course, a rough estimate for an average adult—and your primary focus should always be on following the ten action steps.

In terms of blood tests, your insulin and glucose numbers should have been reasonable before starting the first week. That said, your post-meal levels might not have looked quite so good but are now improving. While your ratio of triglycerides to HDL cholesterol was likely okay, your post-meal triglyceride levels were likely higher than optimal. These metrics should now have improved. Although it's less likely that blood pressure is a problem for you, it should have dropped a little by the end of the week.

So things are improving, and indeed weight loss may be progressing satisfactorily. But for the insulin-sensitive person, it may not progress as rapidly as desired. So let's focus now on what you need to do for it. Here's what your primary focus should be on over the next fourteen days.

- ▶ Continue following the prescription for meals and supplements from days 1 through 7, but go beyond the diet. Start really pushing all ten of those action steps.

- ▶ For insulin-sensitive weight loss in particular, you must focus heavily on action step 7 (meal spacing / fasting). This will become increasingly easier as your fat-burning and appetite-control mechanisms become established.

- ▶ Keep an eye on calorie intake. As mentioned, we recommend staying below 1,800 calories per day as you apply the action steps to lose weight. Depending on your ability and comfort with meal skipping, you may go much lower than this. Check out Simon's story on page 116 to see how it's done.

- ▶ Remember that applying the other action steps correctly will enable you to develop effective fasting habits. You must develop some degree of fat-burning capability first. Otherwise, it will be difficult to practice healthy fasting habits. This is not simply about calorie restriction, either. Meal skipping is about cycling fasting periods on a regular basis and depends on your ability to smoothly burn your own body fat for energy. This strategy of cyclical fasting will in turn enhance your fat-burning capabilities. This is the virtuous cycle that an insulin-sensitive person really needs to foster.

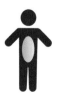

THE INSULIN-SENSITIVE NORMAL-WEIGHT PERSON

Okay, you're the lucky type who was already in good shape before adopting the Eat Rich, Live Long plan. That said, you may not remain in such good shape as you age. By following our prescription, you can continue to hold on to your health in the coming decades. You can also prevent the middle-aged spread that has become near inevitable.

Although you do not have much weight to lose, after the first week of the plan your belt should be beginning to ease. Your blood glucose and insulin were already at good levels, but your insulin is starting to drop even more. Your triglyceride/HDL ratio should have been pretty good, but now you're tuning them to even better values. Your average glycogen levels are dropping, too, and you are on your way to optimal fat-burning. Keep focusing on the ten action steps to stay in great shape.

Let's visit in more detail the action steps to start prioritizing in the coming weeks. Practicing these will indeed make perfect. They will become your tools for life. The first six steps will pretty much continue to be applied as before. In the next fourteen days, however, action steps 7 through 10 need some extra focus. You now have a growing muscle in the fat-burning department. Get ready to flex it.

ACTION STEP 7: MEAL SPACING

It's time to start putting your body fat to work. It won't get off its butt all by itself—you need to encourage it, and going for longer periods without eating will get your body to burn some of that stored fat. Let's look at some meal-spacing realities.

There are two primary states you can be in: fed or fasted. Here's the bottom line on each.

The Fed State: This applies both while you are eating and for a period of several hours after eating. Insulin is elevated and body fat either is being added or, at best, is immobilized. When you are in the fed state, there is no net burning of body fat—quite the opposite, in fact. The best way to trap yourself in an overweight state is simply to ensure that you eat too often. Making your meals high-carb ones will seal the deal.

And eating too often while also attempting to reduce your calories is a fool's game. Frequent eating will maintain the fed state and hamper your progression to a fat-burning mode, and eating many calorie-restricted meals with high carb content is not sustainable for most. Hunger will eventually cause you to fail.

The Fasted State: This state begins a few hours after a meal. Insulin is lowered and body fat is leveraged to fuel your body—you're now beginning to achieve a net loss of body fat. (This only occurs, however, when the body's stores of glycogen are depleted—that is why it's beneficial that glycogen stores start to drop on a low-carb, high-fat diet.) That's why the best way to shift stubborn weight is to ensure that long gaps between meals are the norm, so you stay in a fasted state longer. Make these well-spaced meals low-carb ones to seal the weight-loss deal.

Calories do matter at some level, especially for insulin-sensitive overweight people. But our approach is far more effective than general calorie restriction because it takes advantage of how the body and brain work—it does not rely on monotonous self-denial. That's neither effective nor sustainable over the long term. Most calorie-restriction diets fail, but our science-based strategy will not; you won't get hungry, and you'll reduce your calories naturally, through eating the right foods.

It is important to take advantage of the fat-burning machinery you've started to create during your first seven days. We believe it is crucial to strike while the iron is hot. If you experienced significant challenges during your first week, then consider continuing to focus on steps 1 through 6 and holding off working on meal spacing for another week or so while you apply the solutions discussed at the start of this chapter. Otherwise, you'll benefit from doubling down on your efforts now and following that magical step 7.

We and countless other meal-spacing followers have found that you can learn to really *enjoy* fasting. Crazy, perhaps? Not at all. It only seems crazy if you've swallowed the "eat regularly" brainwashing of the past forty years. When you understand the enormous health benefits of fasting, it becomes a pleasure to bypass breakfast. You also realize that you are performing a metabolic workout during fasted periods, making your body provide fuel. You are effectively advancing your health and fitness—without going near a gym.

There are marked increases in mental acuity during the fasted state also. When you experience these increases, you will become highly motivated to fast. For instance, we always prepare for challenging events—like stressful meetings, public speaking engagements, or difficult negotiations—by dropping meals in advance. Fasting creates a heightened sense of awareness and sharpened frame of mind. Therefore we make a point of not eating in the first part of the day before the event. We go in fasted and thus achieve peak performance. Of course, we gain this edge only because we are fat-adapted—our bodies have their fat-burning machinery in place so we can burn our own body fat smoothly, just as our ancestors could. It would not work so well for a sugar-burner, who would just slump after a few hours without a carb fix.

Fasting gives you an edge if you are a capable fat-burner. It is an edge that you will grow to desire and even depend on. And you will be honing your health as you use this advantage.

TIPS FOR WORKING ACTION STEP 7

The easiest way to start using this tool is simply to drop one meal on a couple of days each week. It is important to enjoy your two meals as normal, eating until you're satisfied. In fact, you should relish them—the eating experience will now be enhanced.

To keep it simple, there are two primary approaches to meal spacing—either skip breakfast or skip lunch. We prefer to skip breakfast. We have, at most, a coffee with a couple of tablespoons of heavy cream instead.

This breakfast-skipping strategy works well for several reasons:

► You have fasted right through the night and fat-burning is already underway. So you can keep it going quite easily for the win.

► On a real-food regimen, there are often minimal feelings of hunger, especially in the mornings. Take advantage of this—don't waste the edge it affords.

► It eliminates the hassle of preparing food on a busy morning. This gives you back valuable time, to help you start your day with gusto.

► You can look forward to "breaking the fast" around lunchtime with colleagues or friends. What's more, you can really relish this meal when it comes. You can savor it as you should.

Sometimes we change things around by having breakfast and skipping lunch instead. This can be a good strategy for those who really feel that they need their breakfast in the morning. If you go this route, make sure you eat until you're fully satiated at breakfast—an egg-based breakfast is ideal. The following are some more tips for success:

► Make your breakfast substantial, with plenty of fat and protein. A perfect breakfast on a lunch-skipping day would be several eggs with fatty bacon, topped off with coffee with heavy cream.

► Have access to a backup real-food snack (see page 95). Use this only if you really feel it's necessary.

► Plan a particularly delicious meal for the evening. Relish it as a reward for your meal-spacing achievement.

SIMON'S STORY

Simon began loosely following a low-carb diet in the year 2000, based on his extensive research. This enabled him to reduce his insulin resistance, become much healthier, and lose some weight in the process. But even after this health success, his weight continued to fluctuate. In 2014, he was quite overweight and hurt his back in an accident. He then experimented with a protein-sparing modified fast (PSMF) followed by a strict ketogenic regimen (see page 298). PSMF involves dropping dietary fat intake and simultaneously skipping meals. This enables your body to be fueled with fat that primarily comes from your body's own stores. Although the diet does not have a high percentage of fat, the calories your body uses are still coming predominantly from fat.

The clever combination of PSMF and keto enabled Simon to lose 50 pounds in a year. His blood tests now showed that he had achieved insulin sensitivity. When his weight loss plateaued, he made some final tweaks to the winning PSMF/keto formula: he simply nudged up the protein, which enabled him to skip even more meals without hunger. He went on to lose *another* 50 pounds in the following three months. So after twenty years of experimentation, he had applied the magical formula of PSMF/keto to finally achieve an ideal weight.

He achieved this because the ketogenic regimen made him a fat-burner, not a sugar-burner, and skipping meals allowed him to burn body fat rather than dietary fat. Measured by calorie intake, his weight-loss diet was 30 percent carb, 25 percent fat, and 45 percent protein. The fat intake was lower to account for the significant amount of body fat he was now burning. It is crucial to remember that this plan works for him because (1) his prior low-carb, high-fat lifestyle had already tackled much of his insulin resistance, and (2) his ketogenic diet enabled him to burn body fat smoothly, without hunger.

You may think that this PSMF diet is not ketogenic, as the fat calories look low in percentage terms. But as Dr. Stephen Phinney explains, "With a weight-loss ketogenic diet, you eat less fat on your plate because you're burning the fat that comes from your inside." You may be consuming fewer calories from fat, but when you add in the body fat being burned, then you actually are getting most of your energy from fat. The real caloric percentages of Simon's fuel actually look like this: 10 percent carb, 70 percent fat, and 20 percent protein. Simon was expertly maintaining a keto diet—but much of the fat content was coming from his ample body fat stores!

Simon's insulin sensitivity enabled him to easily slip into ketosis. He could gain weight easily, but he could also lose weight easily given the right environment. He did it by applying step 7—eat no more than three meals a day, ideally two—in a most expert fashion.

ACTION STEP 8: ENHANCE YOUR ENVIRONMENT TO PROPEL YOUR PERFORMANCE

With the first week under your (shrinking) belt, it is time to apply some helpful steps. Step 8 is so important for long-term success. We include three key factors in this step. Falling short in any of these can have very negative effects on your long-term success.

Sleep cycle and quality. Achieving quality sleep is very important. Ideally, you should be getting at least seven hours of quality sleep per night.

The science of sleep has exploded in the past ten years. Poor sleep drives up cortisol levels, disrupting your insulin signaling and glucose metabolism. It also messes with many other hormones involved in neurological signaling, promoting poor decision-making (including making food choices).[1] Moreover, it increases the levels of the hunger hormone ghrelin and slows your metabolism. Countless people have undermined their weight-loss plans through poor sleep hygiene—don't let it make your journey much harder!

Stress management. Chronic stress makes weight loss much harder to achieve and sustain. It also significantly undermines long-term health. A certain amount of stress is inevitable in the modern world, but how you deal with it is the variable that you can control. We like to use brisk exercise in the fresh air to control stress—a regular short run or vigorous hill-climbing type of activity is ideal. Other methods of managing stress include the practice of mindfulness and various forms of meditation. Find the stress-management practice that works best for you and make time for it in your life.

Sunlight exposure. It can be difficult to get adequate sunlight each day—working hours and many other commitments that keep us indoors conspire against us. But you will benefit hugely from accessing good natural light for at least thirty minutes in the morning after awakening—not through windows but out in the fresh air. We also recommend getting healthy sun exposure on your skin in the middle of the day when possible (without burning, of course—know your limits).

The many benefits of healthy sun exposure include weight control, vitamin D, and much more. We have been sold a twisted and one-sided story of the sun as villain. This has been a huge disservice to the health and well-being of the Western world.

ACTION STEP 9: DON'T FALL SHORT ON VITAMINS AND MINERALS

We will cover all the core supplements in detail in Chapter 15. For now, here is the list of supplements from Chapter 7 as a reminder of those that you'll want to focus on now. These are very important, and being deficient in them can have significant consequences. Continue to access them through food or supplementation during the coming fourteen days:

▶ Potassium

▶ Sodium

▶ Magnesium

▶ Omega-3 fatty acids

▶ Vitamin D

▶ Iodine (possibly from iodine-rich foods rather than supplements)

ACTION STEP 10: GET THE RIGHT KINDS OF EXERCISE

As has been demonstrated repeatedly in many studies, exercise is not an effective tool for long-term weight loss—unless, however, you use it to enhance fat-adaptation. Then it can be a really helpful adjunct to your weight-loss efforts. You can use exercise to help you become a fat-burning machine.

Exercise can contribute in many ways to your fat-burning capabilities. It has all the following benefits:

▶ Depletes the body's glycogen stores and lowers blood glucose

▶ Lowers insulin levels and enhances insulin sensitivity

▶ Enhances the fat-burning machinery of muscles via mitochondrial changes

▶ Liberates fatty acids from adipose tissue so they can be burned as fuel

▶ Encourages cells to renew themselves

These effects are wonderful and will accelerate your adaptation toward efficient and automatic fat-burning. Long, brisk walks in the fresh air are the easiest option for many people. Ideally they will be conducted over hilly ground to enhance the beneficial effects.

The best exercise for enhancing muscle function and insulin sensitivity, though, is resistance training, sometimes called weight training. This does not mean you need to use expensive equipment or join a gym. Neither of us frequents a gym at all—we just do basic strength training at home using, at most, a pull-up bar and some dumbbells.

Below is a sample routine suggested by our MD pal Ted Naiman, an expert in the field and host of the website BurnFatNotSugar.com. We think this is an absolutely super approach. You can easily do this routine in your living room. You can even watch television or listen to a podcast throughout. What's more, the routine takes only fifteen to twenty minutes.

▶ Virtual jump-rope (5 minutes)—you can use an actual rope, but you don't really need one

▶ Push-ups

▶ Sit-ups

▶ Chin-ups (using a basic pull-up bar attached to a doorway)

▶ Wall squats (squat down with your back lightly pressed against a wall, rise to standing, repeat)

The key for each exercise type is to continue it until you cannot manage another rep (this is known as "maxing out" or "pushing to failure"). This means the last rep of each exercise should be very difficult to complete. That's all. When you have pushed to failure for all the exercises, you have a choice of starting again at the top, but you'll get great benefits just by doing one full set.

You only have to do this simple routine a few times a week to accrue truly amazing benefits. Again, no gym or equipment is required.

You will gain the greatest benefits by exercising in a fasted state, long after a meal. We find that a great time is just before you sit down to your evening meal. There are two key advantages to this timing:

▶ You should already be in a somewhat glycogen-depleted state. This will enable you to deplete your glycogen even further before your next meal. An ideal state will thereby be reached—excellent for your insulin sensitivity and the optimal processing of the energy from your meal.

▶ This timing will further enhance your body's tendency to use fat as a fuel over the long term.

If you follow these simple exercise guidelines, you will put yourself way ahead of the vast majority of folks. After only a couple of weeks, you will feel an enormous difference, especially when combining these exercises with the other elements of the Eat Rich, Live Long plan.

Of course, there is also the option to do some aerobic exercise out on the road or in the park. If you are up for the aerobics, we favor relatively short jogging sessions of twenty to thirty minutes. Ideally, these will incorporate an element of interval training as well. This just means that at regular intervals during your jog, you break into a short, hard sprint of around 100 yards. Doing these sprints every three minutes or so will enhance the value of your routine.

We hope that you will apply the exercise rule during these fourteen days and beyond. It will greatly enhance your path to slimness and longevity.

DAYS 8 THROUGH 21: TWO WEEKS OF MEALS

Now let's look at a good meal plan for your next two weeks.

If you have followed our instructions, you should be pretty fat-adapted by this point. Therefore, you should try some meal skipping in the second week of this plan, as per action step 7. You can extend your overnight fast by skipping breakfast (or just have a coffee with heavy cream instead). Alternatively, you could skip lunch and really savor a delicious evening meal. The snacks have been omitted from this meal plan because it's time to focus on meal spacing, but keep some healthy stopgap snacks (see page 95 and pages 170 to 178) within reach for tough situations, including a failed meal-skipping event. Don't forget to keep a water bottle handy, either. Try to drink several pints of water a day, mainly away from your mealtimes.

If you need a reminder of how many people the meal plans are designed to feed, jump over to the introduction to "Days 1 Through 7: A Sample Week of Meals" on page 95, where the logistics of using the meal plans are discussed.

DAY 8	
BREAKFAST	1 batch High-Protein Breakfast Smoothie of your choice (page 152)
LUNCH	Asian lettuce wraps: Two large Boston lettuce cups filled with 4 ounces (90 g) ground pork or diced bacon cooked with ¼ cup (60 g) diced onions, ¼ cup (20 g) sliced mushrooms, ½ teaspoon minced garlic, 1 teaspoon minced fresh ginger, and 2 teaspoons soy sauce. (Serving per person)
DINNER	1 batch Zucchini, Ricotta & Parmesan Lasagna (page 186) (This recipe makes 10 servings; leftovers are used on day 12 of this plan.)

DAY 9	
1 batch Overnight Blueberry & Chia Breakfast Pudding (page 146) *(This recipe makes 6 servings; make a smaller batch, if required, to suit your needs.)*	BREAKFAST
1 batch Macadamia-Crusted Halibut with Orange-Sesame Salad (page 182)	LUNCH
1 batch Pesto-Mozzarella Chicken with Caprese Salad (page 188)	DINNER

DAY 10	
Three eggs, any style, with 2 slices cooked bacon *(Serving per person)*	BREAKFAST
8 slices beefsteak tomato, each topped with a slice of fresh buffalo mozzarella, fresh basil, and arugula with scattered walnuts and/or other nuts (not peanuts). Drizzle with virgin olive oil and balsamic vinegar as desired. *(Serving per person)*	LUNCH
1 batch Slow Cooker Chicken in Creamy Bacon Sauce (page 202)	DINNER

DAY 11

BREAKFAST	1 batch Butter "Cappuccino" (page 218) *(This recipe makes 2 servings.)*
LUNCH	1 batch Asian-Style Shrimp & Vegetable Wraps with Peanut-Cilantro Slaw (page 162)
DINNER	1 batch Juicy Turkey Swedish Meatballs (page 184)

DAY 12

BREAKFAST	1 batch Vanilla-Almond Granola (page 144) *(This recipe makes 20 servings but keeps for a month. If you're concerned about the quantity, make a half batch. Leftovers are used on day 14 of this plan.)*
LUNCH	1 batch Chicken Tikka Skewers with Cilantro-Lime Dipping Sauce (page 174) *(This recipe makes 6 servings; freeze any leftover portions of chicken for later.)*
DINNER	*Leftover* Zucchini, Ricotta & Parmesan Lasagna

DAY 13	
Three-egg omelet filled with 2 ounces (60 g) fresh (soft) goat cheese and chopped fresh herbs, such as chives, parsley, and tarragon or basil *(Serving per person)*	BREAKFAST
1 batch Pan-Roasted Chicken, Avocado, Apricot & Prosciutto Salad (page 164)	LUNCH
1 batch Squid "Pasta" with Pan-Seared Cod, Chorizo & Spinach (page 204)	DINNER

DAY 14	
Leftover Vanilla-Almond Granola	BREAKFAST
2 ounces (60 g) smoked salmon with chopped fresh dill, capers, a large spoonful of crème fraîche, and diced red onion; serve with a crisp salad dressed with oil and vinegar *(Serving per person)*	LUNCH
1 batch Bunless Burgers with Halloumi Fries (page 168)	DINNER

DAY 15

BREAKFAST	1 batch Zucchini, Sausage & Melted Cheese Casserole (page 142) *(This recipe makes 8 servings; leftovers are used on day 19 of this plan.)*
LUNCH	BLT stuffed avocado: Fill two hollowed avocado halves with chopped lettuce, 2 slices cooked and chopped bacon, diced tomatoes, and a dollop of 2-Minute Homemade Mayonnaise (page 132); serve with a low-carb side salad. *(Serving per person)*
DINNER	1 batch Philly Cheesesteak Lettuce Wraps (page 158)

DAY 16

BREAKFAST	Two hard-boiled eggs with 2 ounces (60 g) full-fat cheese *(Serving per person)*
LUNCH	1 batch Indulgent Chocolate Milkshake (page 221) *(This recipe makes 2 servings.)*
DINNER	1 batch Indian-Style Coconut Butter Chicken (page 180)

DAY 17	
½ batch Cheddar & Almond Flour Biscuits (page 148)	BREAKFAST
1 batch Pesto-Mozzarella Chicken with Caprese Salad (page 188)	LUNCH
1 batch Pork Loin Schnitzel with Tomato Pesto & Mozzarella (page 190)	DINNER

DAY 18	
1 batch Butter "Cappuccino" (page 218) *(This recipe makes 2 servings.)*	BREAKFAST
1 batch Caesar Salad with Seared Salmon & Parmesan Crisps (page 166)	LUNCH
1 batch Slow Cooker Chicken in Creamy Bacon Sauce (page 202)	DINNER

DAY 19

BREAKFAST	*Leftover* Zucchini, Sausage & Melted Cheese Casserole
LUNCH	1 batch Macadamia-Crusted Halibut with Orange-Sesame Salad (page 182)
DINNER	1 batch Caesar Salad with Seared Salmon & Parmesan Crisps (page 166)

DAY 20

BREAKFAST	1 batch Cheesy Cauliflower "Grits" with Garlicky Portobello Mushrooms (page 150)
LUNCH	1 batch Creamy Tomato-Basil Soup (page 157) with side salad *(This soup recipe makes 6 servings; leftovers will keep for up to 4 days.)*
DINNER	1 batch Shrimp Fried Cauliflower "Rice" (page 194)

DAY 21	
Meal-skipping option (see below) or 1 batch Butter "Cappuccino" (page 218) *(This recipe makes 2 servings.)*	BREAKFAST
1 batch Pesto & Tomato "Flatbreads" with Chicken Parmesan Crust (page 154)	LUNCH
1 batch Provolone & Ham–Stuffed Pork Tenderloin (page 196) *(This recipe makes 6 servings; freeze any leftover portions for later.)*	DINNER

MEAL-SKIPPING OPTION THROUGHOUT DAYS 8 THROUGH 21

As your body becomes more accustomed to burning fat, see if you can skip breakfast regularly or have a cup or two of bone broth instead. Have a stopgap snack available (see page 95) if it's not working out for you. If it does work, congratulations! As you extend your natural overnight fast, your ability to burn fat is being accelerated and you're burning body fat for fuel. Take pride in how your body is becoming healthier, and look forward to a delicious lunch!

CHAPTER 9
RECIPES

The recipes that contain sweetener were created with Sola, a granulated low-carb sweetener that measures exactly like sugar. See page 352 for more information.

MOZZARELLA PASTRY DOUGH

PREP TIME: 10 minutes

COOKING TIME: 5 minutes

MAKES 8 servings (enough for 1 large pie or quiche)

Did you think pastry was off-limits on a low-carb plan? So did we, until we discovered mozzarella pastry dough: a combination of mozzarella cheese, almond flour, and eggs that, when baked, tastes amazingly close to the real thing. This versatile pastry dough can be used to replace traditional pastry in any recipe; the mozzarella flavor is so mild that you can add low-carb sweetener and use it in your favorite sweet dishes, too.

1½ cups (165 g) almond flour

¼ teaspoon fine sea salt

2 teaspoons baking powder

1½ sticks (¾ cup/165 g) unsalted butter

3 cups (335 g) shredded low-moisture mozzarella cheese

2 large eggs

1. Place the almond flour, salt, and baking powder in a mixing bowl and whisk thoroughly.

2. Place the butter and mozzarella cheese in a large saucepan over low heat. Stirring constantly, melt the butter and cheese (they may look separated at this point, but they will combine nicely when mixed with the other ingredients).

3. Pour the melted cheese and butter mixture in the bowl of a stand mixer fitted with the paddle attachment. With the mixer on low speed, add the almond flour mixture and the eggs and turn the speed up to high. Continue to mix for 1 to 2 minutes until you have a smooth, soft dough. Alternatively, this can be done using an electric hand mixer or by hand, but a stand mixer works best.

4. Allow the dough to cool slightly, then use in any recipe to replace flour-based pastry.

CHEF'S TIPS

▶ Roll the dough out on clean work surface. If you find the dough is sticking, lightly dust the work surface with almond flour.

▶ This pastry dough is easier to roll out when warm, so work quickly. If it becomes too stiff to roll out, heat the dough in the microwave for 20 seconds on high power to make it pliable again.

▶ If using for a sweet recipe, such as the Blueberry Custard Tart on page 208, a touch of sweetener is nice, but not required. If using, add up to 3 tablespoons of the granulated low-carb sweetener of your choice to the almond flour mixture in Step 1.

NUTRITION FACTS (PER SERVING)

CALORIES	FAT	PROTEIN	NET CARBS	CARBS
416	36g	17g	4g	6g
	78%	16%	4%	

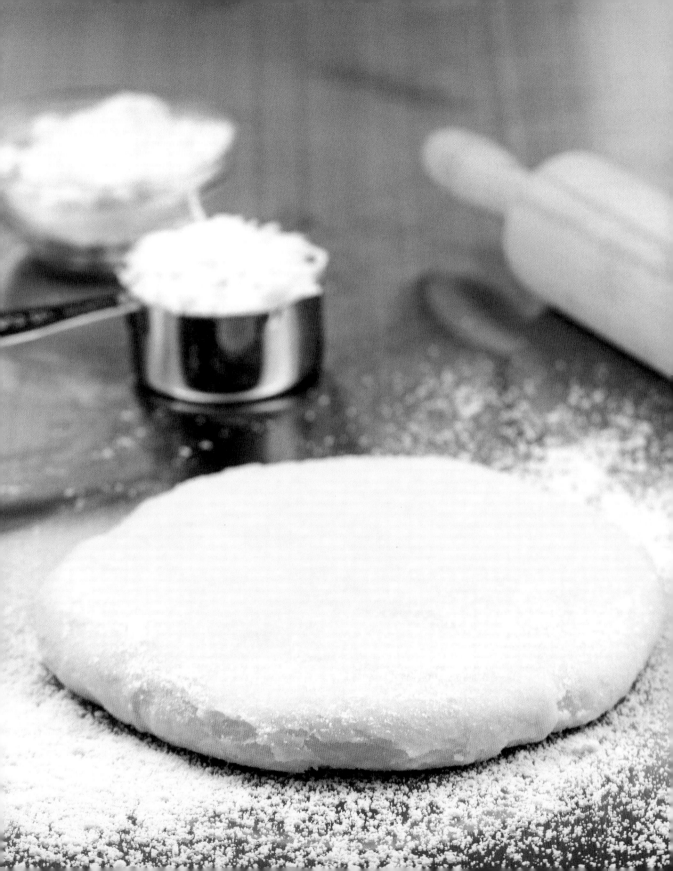

2-MINUTE HOMEMADE MAYONNAISE

PREP TIME: 2 minutes

MAKES 16 servings (1 tablespoon per serving)

This recipe takes less than two minutes to prepare and requires virtually no cooking skills. If you find yourself short on mayonnaise and are looking to avoid store-bought mayo made with canola or soybean oil, then this is the recipe for you.

Simply place all ingredients into a large mug and use an immersion blender to whip the mixture into a smooth creamy mayonnaise in a matter of seconds. This mayonnaise can be made with your favorite healthy oil. We recommend a mild-tasting oil such as avocado oil, macadamia oil (though this one is expensive!), or light olive oil. You should avoid using extra-virgin olive oil—it will give the mayonnaise a strong flavor.

1 large whole egg (see Tip)

½ teaspoon fine sea salt

½ teaspoon ground mustard

2 tablespoons fresh lemon juice or white wine vinegar

1 cup (240 ml) avocado oil, macadamia oil, or light olive oil

1. Place all ingredients into a large mug or widemouthed mason jar, big enough for an immersion blender to do its work. (The blender needs to be able to reach all the way to the bottom of the mug.)

2. Place the immersion blender into the mug and pulse while moving the blender up and down. Within seconds you'll have a smooth, creamy mayonnaise.

3. Remove the mayonnaise from the mug and store in an airtight container in the refrigerator for up to 1 week.

CHEF'S TIP

▶ The fresher the egg here, the better. Fresh eggs—one week old at most—have superior binding properties and help to ensure the mayonnaise emulsifies.

NUTRITION FACTS (PER SERVING)

CALORIES	FAT	PROTEIN	NET CARBS	CARBS
126	14g	0g	0g	0g
	100%	0%	0%	

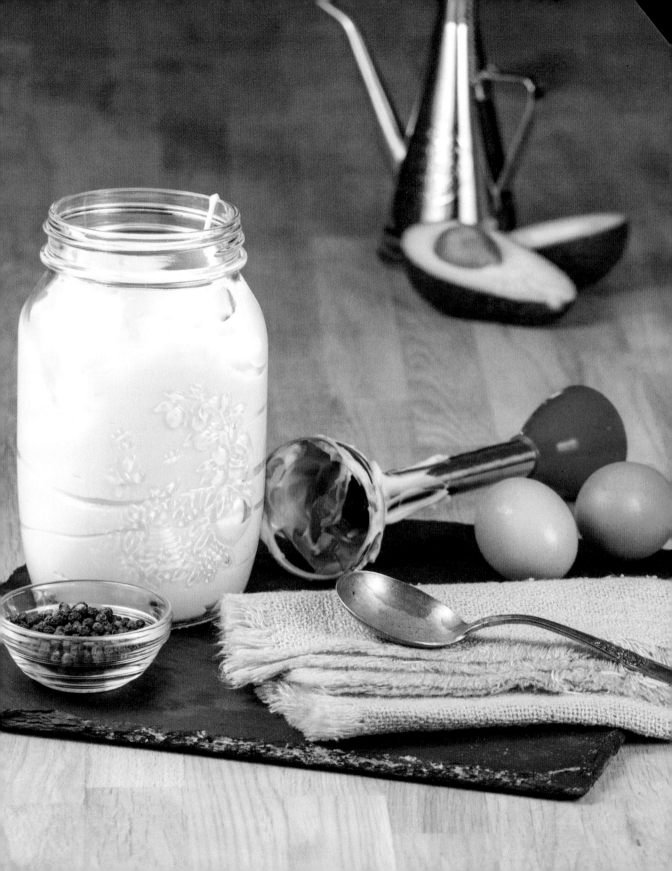

LOW-CARB ALMOND BREAD

PREP TIME: 10 minutes
COOKING TIME: 35 minutes
MAKES 1 loaf (16 slices, 1 slice per serving)

This chewy, mildly sweet bread is almost reminiscent of a carby off-limits yeast bread; it can be toasted for sandwiches and used in any recipe calling for a slice of traditional glutinous bread. You can top it with just about anything you like; we topped the loaf in the photograph opposite with 1 teaspoon sesame seeds and 1 teaspoon flax seeds. Other ideas are listed below. Use the leftover egg yolks to make Blueberry Custard Tart (page 208) or Double Chocolate Pudding (page 206).

2 cups (180 g) almond flour

½ teaspoon fine sea salt

4 ounces (110 g) low-moisture mozzarella cheese or mild full-fat cheddar cheese, shredded

2 teaspoons baking powder

10 large egg whites

½ stick (¼ cup/55 g) unsalted butter, melted but not hot

SUGGESTED TOPPINGS

Flax seeds

Poppy seeds

Pumpkin seeds

Sesame seeds

Sunflower seeds

Dried herbs of choice

Grated Parmesan cheese

1. Preheat the oven to 325°F (163°C). Line a 9 by 5-inch (23 by 12.75-cm) loaf pan with parchment paper, leaving about 1 inch (2.5 cm) of paper overhanging.

2. Place the almond flour, salt, cheese, and baking powder in a mixing bowl and mix until well combined.

3. In a separate bowl, whip the egg whites until stiff (using a stand mixer, electric beaters, or a hand whisk). Add the cooled melted butter to the whipped egg whites, then very gently fold in the almond flour mixture, keeping as much air in the whipped egg whites as possible.

4. Transfer the batter to the loaf pan and sprinkle about 2 teaspoons of the topping(s) of your choice on top. Place the pan on a middle rack in the oven.

5. Bake until the loaf has risen by about one-third and is golden brown, about 35 minutes. Remove from the oven and allow to cool in the pan for 10 minutes, then remove the loaf from the pan and allow to cool completely on a wire cooling rack before slicing.

6. Store in an airtight container in the refrigerator for up to 4 days.

NUTRITION FACTS (PER SERVING)

CALORIES	FAT	PROTEIN	NET CARBS	CARBS
150	12g	8g	2g	4g
	72%	21%	5%	

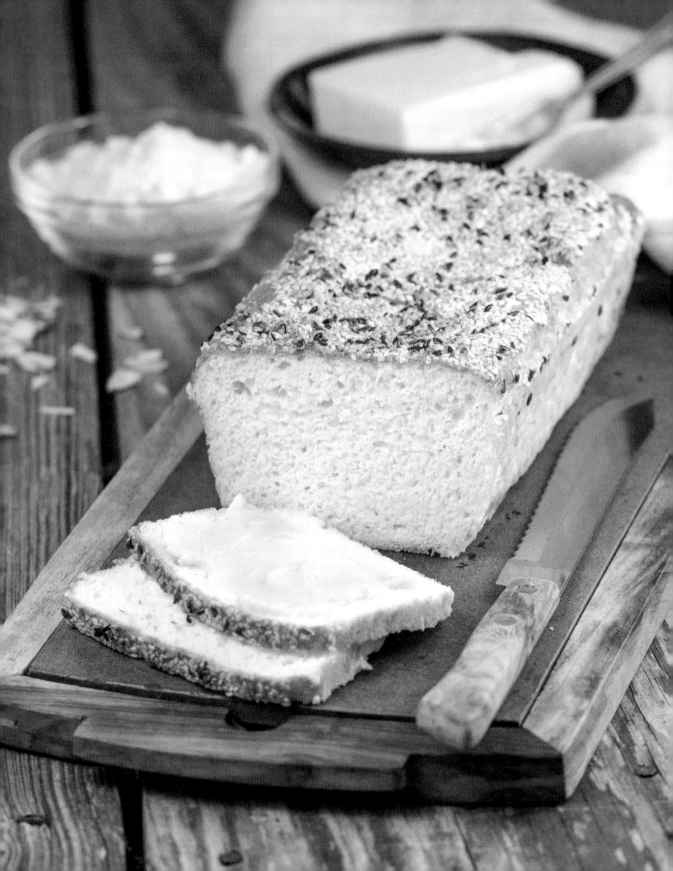

SIMPLE CAULIFLOWER "RICE"

PREP TIME: 10 minutes
COOKING TIME: 5 to 10 minutes
MAKES 4 servings

This rice substitute is one of my favorite starch replacers; the finished dish doesn't have an overpowering cauliflower flavor (as one might expect), and it has a great texture that makes it ideal for pairing with a wide range of meals. This is a basic recipe that can be used as a starting point for a wide range of flavored rice dishes.

1 medium cauliflower (about 1½ lbs/675 g)

2 tablespoons olive oil

Fine sea salt and freshly ground black pepper

1. To rice the cauliflower, remove the leaves and stalk from the cauliflower and roughly chop into florets. Place the cauliflower into a food processor with the S-blade in place. Process the cauliflower in short pulses until it is chopped up into pieces the size of grains of rice. Alternatively, you can use the grater blade for your food processor to grate the florets. If you do not have a food processor, you can also use the large holes on a box cheese grater to shred the cauliflower into rice-size pieces.

2. Place the cauliflower into a large saucepan and drizzle with the oil. Cover the pan and gently steam over low heat for 5 to 10 minutes, stirring regularly and keeping the lid on until the "rice" is tender. Remove the saucepan from the heat, season to taste with salt and pepper, and serve immediately.

3. Store leftovers in an airtight container in the refrigerator for up to 4 days. Reheat in the microwave for 2 minutes in a microwave-safe bowl covered with plastic wrap.

ON OLIVE OIL

We use two types of olive oil in the kitchen: extra-virgin olive oil and refined olive oil. The latter is often simply called "olive oil" and a description of its cooking applications is sometimes included on the label, such as "for sautéing and grilling." Extra-virgin olive oil should never be used in cooking; instead, use it for cold applications only, such as when drizzling olive oil over plated dishes, as a finishing oil, or in recipes such as gazpacho or vinaigrettes. When using olive oil in cooking, always reach for what's called simply "olive oil."

CHEF'S TIPS

► Don't add any water to the cauliflower; there is enough naturally occurring water in the cauliflower to help steam the rice.

► Remove the rice from the heat when it is just barely tender; don't overcook it, as it can become mushy. Cauliflower rice will have a slightly firmer texture than regular rice.

► Raw cauliflower can be riced ahead of time and stored in the refrigerator in an airtight container for up to 4 days until ready to cook.

NUTRITION FACTS (PER SERVING)

CALORIES	FAT	PROTEIN	NET CARBS	CARBS
103	7g 61%	3g 12%	4g 16%	7g

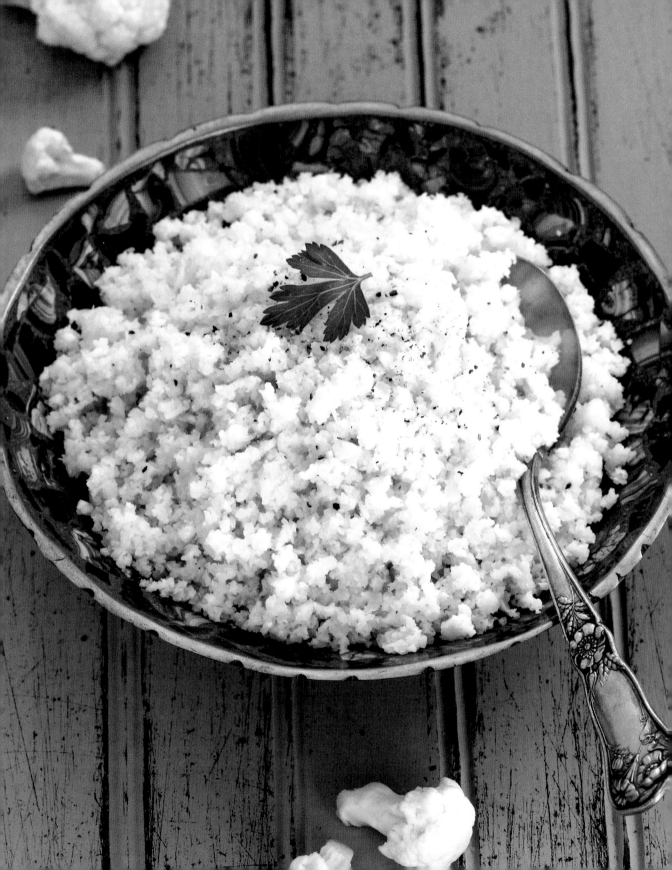

BACON, GRUYÈRE & RED PEPPER
EGG MUFFINS

PREP TIME: 10 minutes

COOKING TIME: 25 minutes

MAKES 8 muffins (1 per serving)

These delicious, protein-packed savory muffins are great for on-the-go breakfasts. You can make a big batch on Sunday and heat them up quickly on busy mornings. Fresh eggs are blended with cream and Gruyère cheese to create a rich, quichelike texture. This recipe is easily customizable; add any of your favorite ingredients to the muffin pan before putting in the egg mixture for endless flavor variations.

A nonstick silicone muffin pan is best for easy removal and cleanup. If you are using a metal muffin pan, be sure to grease it well with butter or another healthy cooking fat.

6 slices bacon, cooked and finely chopped

3 ounces (85 g) jarred roasted red peppers, diced

½ cup (120 ml) heavy cream

4 large eggs

8 ounces (220 g) Gruyère cheese, shredded, divided

Fine sea salt and freshly ground black pepper

Finely chopped fresh parsley, for garnish (optional)

1. Preheat the oven to 350°F (177°C).

2. Divide the chopped bacon and diced red peppers evenly among 8 cups of a standard-size 12-cup nonstick muffin pan.

3. Place the cream, eggs, half of the cheese, and a generous pinch each of salt and pepper in a blender and blend until smooth, 1 to 2 minutes. Divide the mixture evenly among the muffin cups, pouring it over the red pepper and bacon and filling each cup about three-quarters full.

4. Place the muffin pan in a baking dish and pour 1 inch (2.5 cm) of boiling water into the dish, around the muffin pan. Sprinkle the remaining cheese over the tops of the muffins and bake for 25 minutes.

5. Remove the pan from the oven and let the muffins cool in the pan. To serve, gently tap the egg muffins out of the muffin pan. Garnish with a sprinkle of parsley, if desired. Eat the muffins right away or store in the refrigerator and reheat individually as desired. Or eat them cold if you want! Store in an airtight container in the refrigerator for up to 4 days.

NUTRITION FACTS (PER SERVING)

CALORIES	FAT	PROTEIN	NET CARBS	CARBS
188	16g	10g	1g	1g
	77%	21%	2%	

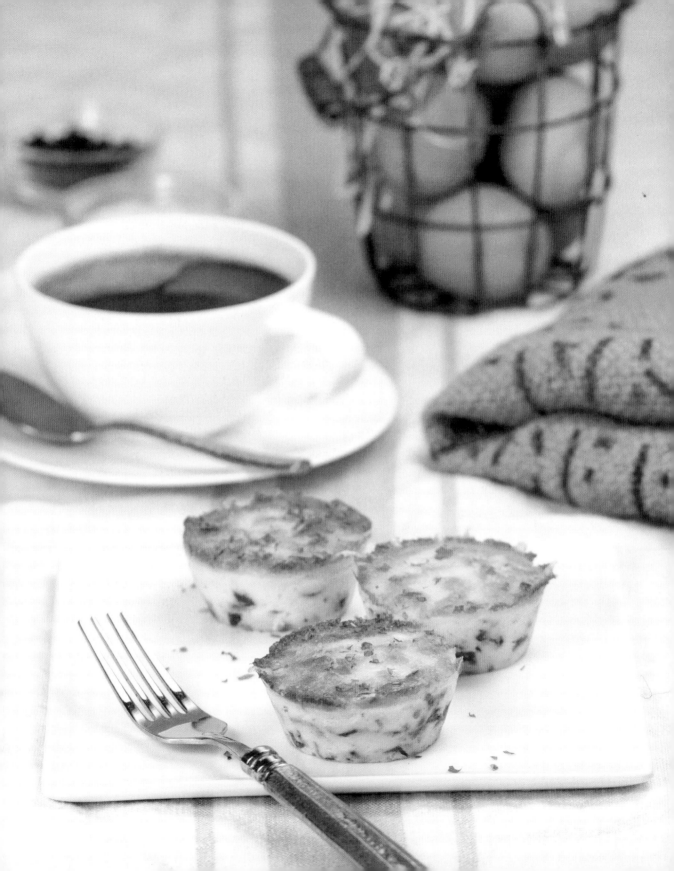

BACON-WRAPPED ROASTED SQUASH
EGG MUFFIN CUPS

PREP TIME: 10 minutes

COOKING TIME: 15 minutes

MAKES 8 muffins (1 per serving)

These delicious egg muffin cups can be a grab-and-go breakfast or part of a to-go lunch. They can be reheated quickly or enjoyed at room temperature. Use this recipe with your own favorite fillings for thousands of possible variations (see a handful of our suggested combinations below).

A nonstick silicone muffin pan will simplify the removal of the muffin cups from the pan, as well as the cleanup. If you are using a metal muffin pan, use cupcake liners for easy cleanup.

8 slices bacon, cooked but not crispy (it needs to remain flexible)

1 cup (140 g) peeled, diced, and roasted butternut squash

1 teaspoon olive oil

3 ounces (85 g) fresh (soft) goat cheese, crumbled

8 large eggs

¼ teaspoon fine sea salt

¼ teaspoon freshly ground black pepper

1. Preheat the oven to 400°F (205°C). Have on hand a standard-size 12-cup nonstick muffin pan.

2. Line 8 of the muffin cups with the bacon, using 1 slice per cup. Divide the butternut squash among the bacon cups, then drizzle with the oil and sprinkle on the goat cheese.

3. Crack the eggs into a large bowl, season with the salt and pepper, whisk well, and pour into the bacon-lined cups, filling each about three-quarters full.

4. Place the muffin pan in the oven and bake until the eggs are firm, puffed, and golden brown, about 15 minutes.

5. Remove the pan from the oven, let the muffins cool a bit, then remove the muffins from the pan and enjoy warm. Store the remaining cups in the refrigerator for up to 1 week. Enjoy cold or reheat individually as desired.

VARIATIONS

Use a range of different ingredients to fill the egg cups before pouring in the whisked eggs and baking:

► Crumbled or diced cooked Italian sausage, diced roasted red peppers, and crumbled feta cheese

► Diced or shredded cooked chicken, sliced cooked asparagus, and shredded mozzarella cheese

► Diced roasted Mediterranean vegetables and grated Parmesan cheese

► Crumbled cooked sausage of choice, chopped cooked broccoli, and crumbled blue cheese

► Sliced roast beef and diced and caramelized red onions

NUTRITION FACTS (PER SERVING)

CALORIES	FAT	PROTEIN	NET CARBS	CARBS
133	9g	10g	2g	3g
	61%	30%	6%	

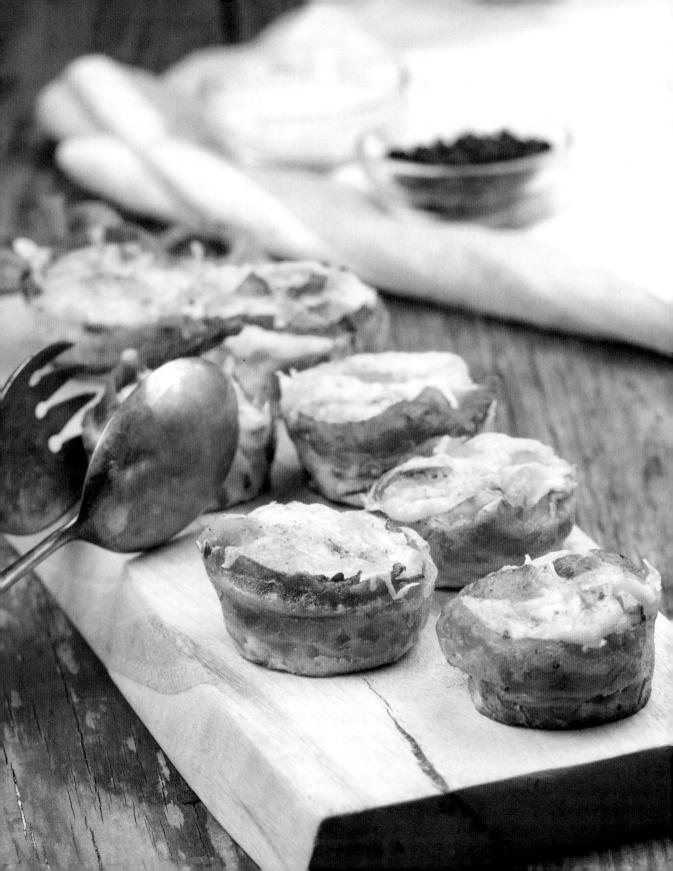

ZUCCHINI, SAUSAGE & MELTED CHEESE CASSEROLE

PREP TIME: 10 minutes
COOKING TIME: 30 minutes
MAKES 8 servings

This versatile casserole, which is similar to a frittata, makes a great brunch, or it can be made ahead and stored in the refrigerator for quick and easy breakfasts during the week.

1 tablespoon olive oil

4 medium zucchinis

Fine sea salt and freshly ground black pepper

1 pound (450 g) spicy bulk Italian sausage (made with no grain fillers)

7 ounces (200 g) fontina cheese, shredded

6 large eggs

½ cup (120 ml) heavy cream

Crispy cooked bacon slices, cut into 1-inch (2.5-cm) pieces, for garnish (optional)

1. Preheat the oven to 400°F (205°C). Heat the oil in a large frying pan over medium-high heat.

2. Slice the zucchini, add it to the pan with the oil, and season with ⅛ teaspoon each of salt and pepper. Cook the zucchini for 5 minutes or until soft and starting to brown, then remove from the pan and set aside.

3. Add the sausage meat to the pan and sauté until fully cooked and golden brown.

4. Line an 8-inch (20-cm) round baking pan (or similar vessel) with parchment paper, leaving some parchment overhanging. Evenly distribute the zucchini and sausage in the pan and sprinkle with the fontina cheese (reserving a small handful for the top of the casserole).

5. Crack the eggs into a mixing bowl, season with ¼ teaspoon each of salt and pepper, add the cream, and whisk well. Pour the egg mixture over the zucchini-sausage mixture and sprinkle the reserved fontina on top. Place the pan in the oven and bake until the egg mixture is firm and the top of the casserole golden brown, about 30 minutes.

6. Top with crispy bacon slices, if desired. Lift the casserole out of the pan, cut into 8 pieces, and serve immediately or store in the refrigerator for up to 4 days and reheat as desired.

NUTRITION FACTS (PER SERVING)

CALORIES	FAT	PROTEIN	NET CARBS	CARBS
356	28g	20g	5g	6g
	71%	22%	6%	

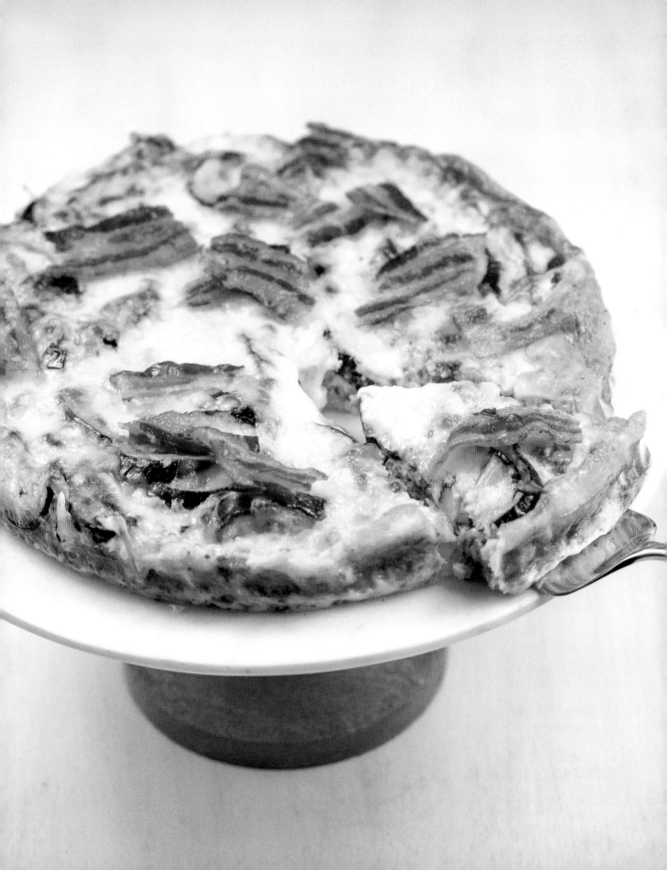

VANILLA-ALMOND GRANOLA

PREP TIME: 10 minutes

COOKING TIME: 35 minutes + 1 hour to cool

MAKES Twenty ¾-cup (145-g) servings

This delicious granola is a low-carb dream—a sweet alternative to the more common savory breakfast options. Granola really does not need oats to be delicious and satisfying; this grain-free version is nutrient-rich and provides long-lasting energy. Top with full-fat yogurt or ice-cold unsweetened almond milk and fresh berries.

1 cup (100 g) raw walnuts

1 cup (100 g) raw pecans

2 cups (220 g) almond flour

1 cup (80 g) unsweetened coconut flakes

¾ cup (145 g) granulated low-carb sweetener of your choice (see Note)

½ cup (65 g) dried apricots, chopped (optional—they contain sugar)

½ cup (40 g) golden flaxseed meal

½ cup (65 g) pumpkin seeds

½ cup (120 ml) water

¼ cup (60 ml) coconut oil, melted, plus more for the parchment

2 teaspoons vanilla extract

½ teaspoon ground cinnamon

Full-fat yogurt or almond milk, for serving (optional)

Fresh berries, for serving (optional)

1. Preheat the oven to 300°F (150°C). Line a sheet pan with parchment paper and grease the paper with coconut oil.

2. Place the walnuts in a food processor and press the pulse button a few times to roughly chop them. Your goal is a rough chop, not ground nuts or nut butter, so watch closely! Remove the walnuts to a large mixing bowl. Repeat with the pecans, then place them in the bowl with the walnuts.

3. Add the remaining ingredients to the bowl with the nuts and mix well, using your hands. Transfer the mixture to the baking sheet and lightly press into an even layer.

4. Bake for 15 minutes, then remove the pan from the oven, stir the granola with a large spoon, and press it back down onto the sheet. Bake for another 15 to 20 minutes, or until fragrant and lightly browned on the surface. Switch off the oven and let the granola cool completely in the oven, about 1 hour. It will crisp up as it cools.

5. When the granola has fully cooled, use your hands to crumble it up into small chunks. Serve with full-fat yogurt or unsweetened almond milk and fresh berries. Store the granola in an airtight container in a cool, dark place, such as the pantry, for up to 1 month.

NOTE

Feel free to reduce the amount of sweetener to taste.

NUTRITION FACTS (PER SERVING)

CALORIES	FAT	PROTEIN	NET CARBS	CARBS
218	18g	5g	3g	14g
	74%	9%	6%	

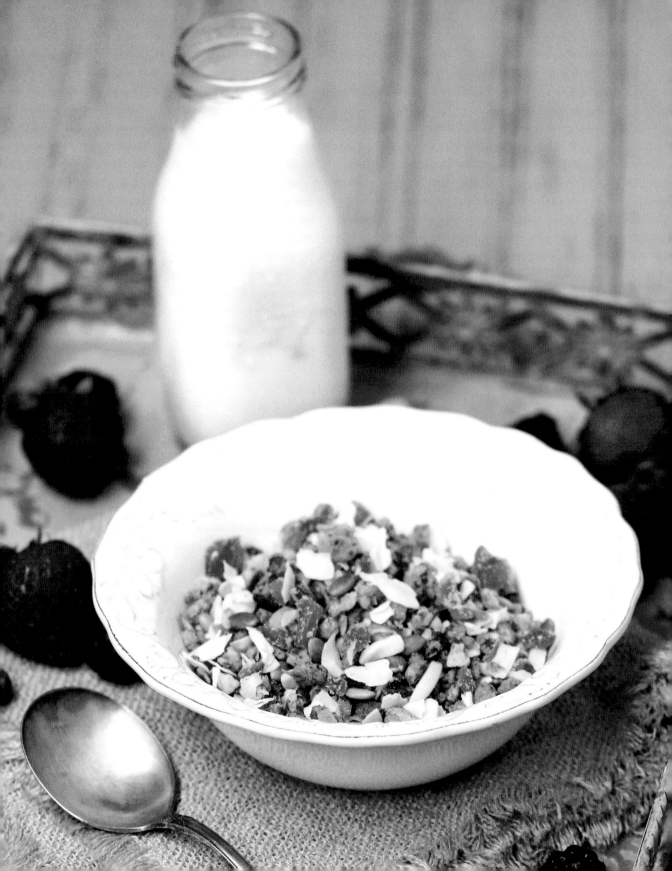

OVERNIGHT BLUEBERRY & CHIA BREAKFAST PUDDING

PREP TIME: 5 minutes + 4 hours to chill

MAKES 6 servings

Chia seeds have been used for centuries by the indigenous populations of Mexico and Guatemala, mainly in beverages. Chia naturally thickens liquids when soaked, creating a thick, creamy texture. This is a fantastic, filling breakfast that takes very little effort to prepare.

2 cups (480 ml) unsweetened almond milk

1 cup (130 g) fresh blueberries

6 tablespoons granulated low-carb sweetener of your choice (see Note)

½ cup (120 ml) heavy cream

½ cup (95 g) white chia seeds

Pinch of fine sea salt

Additional fresh blueberries and/or other fresh berries of choice, for garnish

1. Place the almond milk, blueberries, and sweetener in a blender and blend until the blueberries are broken down and the mixture is smooth. Transfer to a medium-size mixing bowl.

2. Add the cream, chia seeds, and salt and whisk until well combined. Cover the bowl with plastic wrap and refrigerate overnight or for at least 4 hours.

3. When you are ready to serve the pudding, remove from the refrigerator and whisk well; the chia seeds will have swelled and the mixture should have thickened to about the consistency of yogurt.

4. Spoon the pudding into individual serving glasses and top with fresh berries. Store leftovers in the fridge for up to 4 days.

NOTE

Feel free to reduce the amount of sweetener to taste.

VARIATION: VANILLA CHIA BREAKFAST PUDDING

► Simply omit the blueberries and add 1 teaspoon of vanilla extract.

NUTRITION FACTS (PER SERVING)

CALORIES	FAT	PROTEIN	NET CARBS	CARBS
200	14g	5g	4g	17g
	63%	10%	8%	

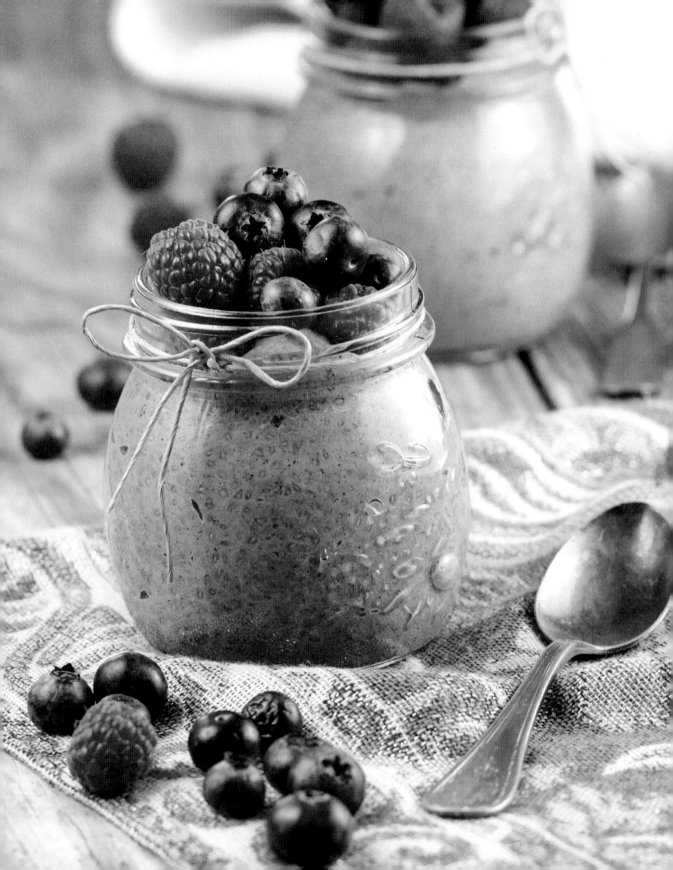

CHEDDAR & ALMOND FLOUR BISCUITS

PREP TIME: 10 minutes
COOKING TIME: 20 minutes
MAKES 8 biscuits (1 per serving)

These moist, savory biscuits make an excellent breakfast or quick snack. Serve them warm with salted butter.

2 cups (220 g) almond flour

2 teaspoons baking powder

½ teaspoon fine sea salt

Pinch of cayenne pepper

6 ounces (170 g) sharp or extra-sharp cheddar cheese, shredded, divided

2 large eggs, beaten

½ stick (¼ cup/55 g) unsalted butter, softened

Salted butter, for serving

1. Preheat the oven to 350°F (177°C). Grease 8 cups of a standard-size 12-cup nonstick muffin pan.

2. In a large bowl, whisk together the almond flour, baking powder, salt, and cayenne pepper. Set aside ¼ cup (30 grams) of the cheese for the tops of the biscuits. Add the remaining cheese, eggs, and butter to the dry ingredients and mix with a rubber spatula until well combined.

3. Divide the mixture evenly among the greased muffin cups, filling each about two-thirds full, and top each with a sprinkle of the reserved cheddar cheese.

4. Place the muffin pan in the oven and bake until the biscuits have doubled in size and are golden, 15 to 20 minutes.

5. Cool the biscuits slightly in the pan, then turn out onto a cooling rack and enjoy warm with salted butter. Store any leftovers in an airtight container in the refrigerator for up to 4 days.

NUTRITION FACTS (PER SERVING)

CALORIES	FAT	PROTEIN	NET CARBS	CARBS
322	28g	12g	4g	7g
	78%	15%	5%	

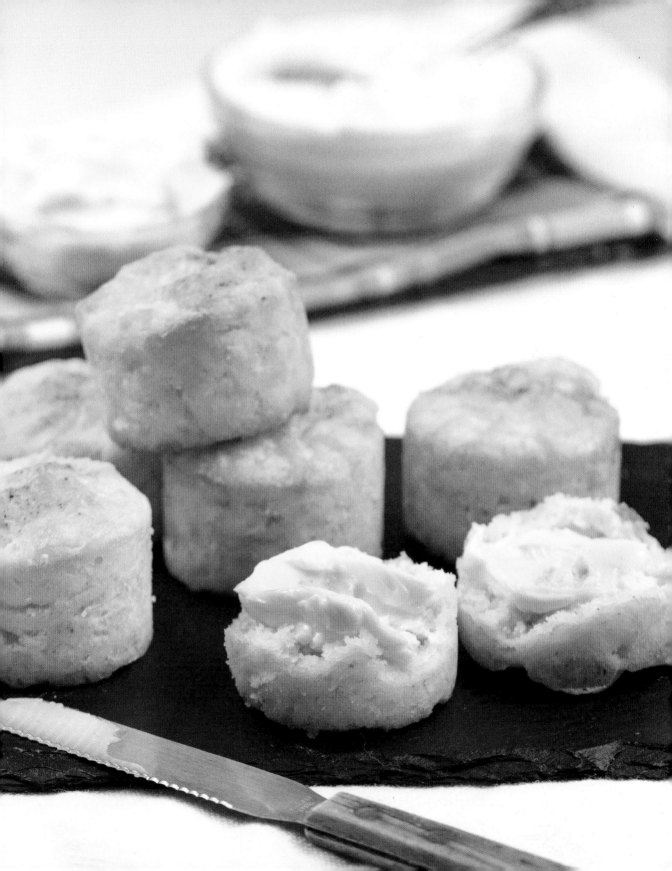

CHEESY CAULIFLOWER "GRITS"
WITH GARLICKY PORTOBELLO MUSHROOMS

PREP TIME: 10 minutes
COOKING TIME: 30 minutes
MAKES 4 servings

Cheesy grits make an excellent savory breakfast. This recipe uses a sprinkle of real corn grits for flavor and texture, but the bulk of the dish is grated cauliflower. A warm bowl of these "grits" with sautéed mushrooms and a bit of crispy bacon is a winning weekend breakfast.

GRITS

½ stick (¼ cup/55 g) unsalted butter

¼ white onion, finely diced

2 cloves garlic, minced

1 tablespoon coarsely ground corn grits or polenta (not quick-cook)

Florets from ½ head cauliflower, riced (see page 136)

½ cup (120 ml) all-natural salted chicken stock

½ cup (120 ml) heavy cream

¼ teaspoon smoked paprika

Pinch of cayenne pepper

A few dashes of Tabasco sauce

½ cup (55 g) shredded cheddar cheese

½ cup (55 g) grated Parmesan cheese

Fine sea salt and freshly ground black pepper

MUSHROOMS

2 large portobello mushrooms

2 tablespoons olive oil

½ stick (¼ cup/55 g) unsalted butter

2 cloves garlic, minced

1 teaspoon fresh thyme leaves, chopped, or ¼ heaping teaspoon dried thyme leaves

Fine sea salt

12 slices crispy cooked bacon, for serving (optional)

Fresh thyme (sprigs or leaves) or chopped fresh parsley, for garnish

1. Prepare the "grits": Place the butter, onion, and garlic in a large saucepan and sauté over medium heat for 2 to 3 minutes, until softened.

2. Add the corn grits and continue to sauté for 2 minutes. Add the cauliflower and cook for a further 2 minutes, stirring well.

3. Add the chicken stock and cream and bring to a boil, then reduce the heat to a steady simmer. Add the spices and hot sauce and continue to simmer for 15 to 20 minutes, until the liquid has reduced to a creamy sauce and the cauliflower and grits are tender.

4. While the grits are cooking, prepare the mushrooms: Slice the portobellos into ½-inch (1.25-cm) strips, place in a large frying pan with the oil and butter, and fry over medium heat for about 5 minutes. Add the minced garlic and thyme and continue to cook for 4 to 5 minutes more, until the mushrooms are golden brown and caramelized. Season to taste with salt.

5. When the grits are done, add the cheddar and Parmesan cheeses and continue to cook for 5 minutes, until the cheese is melted and evenly distributed, stirring often. Season to taste with salt and pepper and immediately divide among four serving plates.

6. Top the creamy grits with the mushrooms and add crispy bacon, if desired. Garnish with thyme or parsley and serve. Store any leftovers for up to 3 days in the refrigerator and reheat as desired.

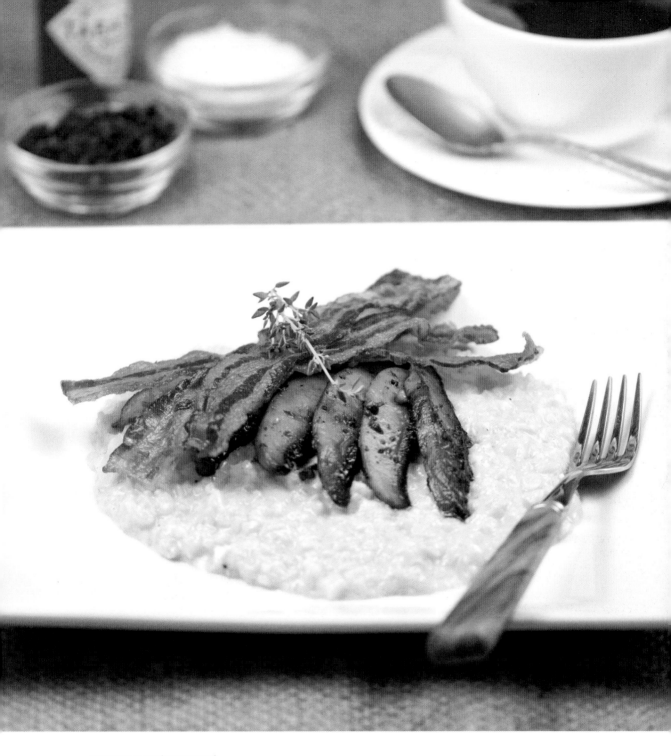

NUTRITION FACTS (PER SERVING)				
CALORIES	FAT	PROTEIN	NET CARBS	CARBS
632	56g	19g	9g	13g
	80%	12%	6%	

CHEF'S TIP

▶ Store corn grits or polenta in an airtight container in the freezer for up to 6 months.

HIGH-PROTEIN BREAKFAST SMOOTHIES

Smoothies are a great way to get all of your nutrients and energy for the morning in a quick format that is easy to take on the go.

BERRY BLITZ
PROTEIN SMOOTHIE

PREP TIME: 5 minutes
MAKES 4 servings

2 cups (480 ml) unsweetened almond milk

2 cups (480 ml) ice

½ cup (75 g) unsweetened whey protein powder

½ cup (65 g) hulled and sliced fresh strawberries

½ cup (60 g) fresh raspberries

½ cup (60 g) fresh blackberries

⅓ cup (38 g) raw almonds

¼ cup (32 g) fresh blueberries

Granulated low-carb sweetener of your choice (see Note)

GREEN POWER
PROTEIN SMOOTHIE

PREP TIME: 5 minutes
MAKES 4 servings

1 handful of fresh spinach

2 large kale leaves

2 large fresh strawberries, hulled and chopped

2 cups (480 ml) unsweetened almond milk

2 cups (480 ml) ice

½ cup (70 g) fresh raspberries

½ cup (75 g) unsweetened whey protein powder

⅓ cup (38 g) raw almonds

¼ cup (60 ml) heavy cream

Granulated low-carb sweetener of your choice (see Note)

NOTE

Feel free to reduce the amount of sweetener to taste.

1. Place all of the ingredients, except the sweetener, in a high-powered blender and blend for 2 minutes, until smooth and creamy. Taste and add sweetener to your liking. (*Note:* If your blender isn't a high-powdered one, finely chop the kale leaves and pulverize the almonds before adding them to the blender jar. You may need to blend longer to get a smooth texture.)

2. Pour into four 12-ounce (350-ml) glasses and serve immediately.

BERRY BLITZ PROTEIN SMOOTHIE
NUTRITION FACTS (PER SERVING)

CALORIES	FAT	PROTEIN	NET CARBS	CARBS
162	7g	10g	6g	18g
	39%	25%	15%	

GREEN POWER PROTEIN SMOOTHIE
NUTRITION FACTS (PER SERVING)

CALORIES	FAT	PROTEIN	NET CARBS	CARBS
203	13g	11g	5g	16g
	58%	22%	10%	

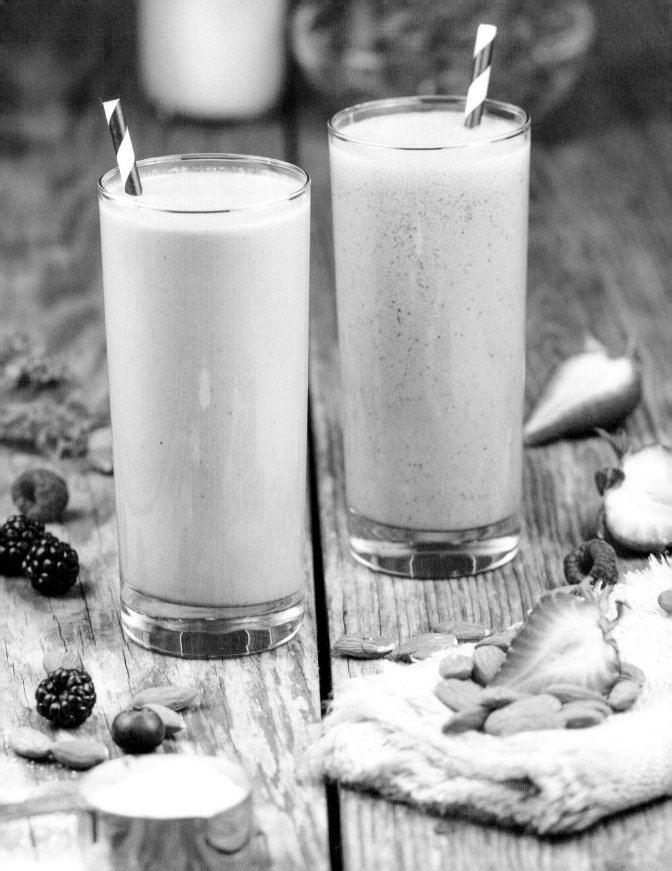

PESTO & TOMATO "FLATBREADS"
WITH CHICKEN PARMESAN CRUST

PREP TIME: 10 minutes
COOKING TIME: 25 minutes
MAKES 4 servings

Making a flatbread crust from chicken may sound a bit strange, but give it a try—this is a delicious, simple solution for a crisp, high-protein base for your favorite toppings. Simply blend Parmesan cheese and chicken, spread into "dough" circles, and bake for ten minutes. The finished product is delicious, satisfying, and healthy. Serve with a side salad for a complete meal.

CHICKEN FLATBREAD CRUST

2 whole boneless, skinless chicken breasts (about 1¾ lbs/675 g)

1 large egg

½ teaspoon fine sea salt

¼ teaspoon freshly ground black pepper

1½ teaspoons fresh oregano leaves, or ½ teaspoon dried oregano leaves

½ teaspoon ground mustard

½ teaspoon onion powder

1½ cups (165 g) grated Parmesan cheese

2 tablespoons extra-virgin olive oil, for drizzling

TOPPINGS

8 teaspoons high-quality store-bought pesto

1 cup (110 g) shredded mozzarella cheese

8 ounces (225 g) fresh (soft) goat cheese, sliced

24 cherry tomatoes, halved

Freshly ground black pepper

1. Preheat the oven to 400°F (205°C). Line 2 sheet pans with parchment paper.

2. Make the crust: Cut the chicken breasts into cubes and place in a food processor. Add the egg, salt, pepper, oregano, ground mustard, and onion powder and process until you have a smooth paste. Add the shredded Parmesan cheese and pulse a few more times, until well incorporated.

3. Divide the chicken mixture into 4 parts and place 2 parts onto each sheet pan, evenly spaced in mounds. Use a pallet knife or the back of a spoon to spread each mound out into tortilla-size circles, about ¼ inch (6 mm) thick. Drizzle the circles with olive oil and place in the oven to bake for 10 minutes, until golden.

4. Remove the sheet pans from the oven and spread 2 teaspoons of the pesto over each flatbread crust. Top each circle with one-quarter of the shredded mozzarella and goat cheese slices, then finish with cherry tomato halves (12 per circle) and a grind of black pepper.

5. Place the flatbreads back in the oven and bake for 15 minutes, until golden brown and bubbly.

6. Remove the sheet pans from the oven and let the flatbreads cool slightly, then cut into quarters and serve. Store any leftovers in the refrigerator for up to 3 days and reheat as desired.

NUTRITION FACTS (PER SERVING)

CALORIES	FAT	PROTEIN	NET CARBS	CARBS
577	41g	47g	4g	5g
	64%	33%	3%	

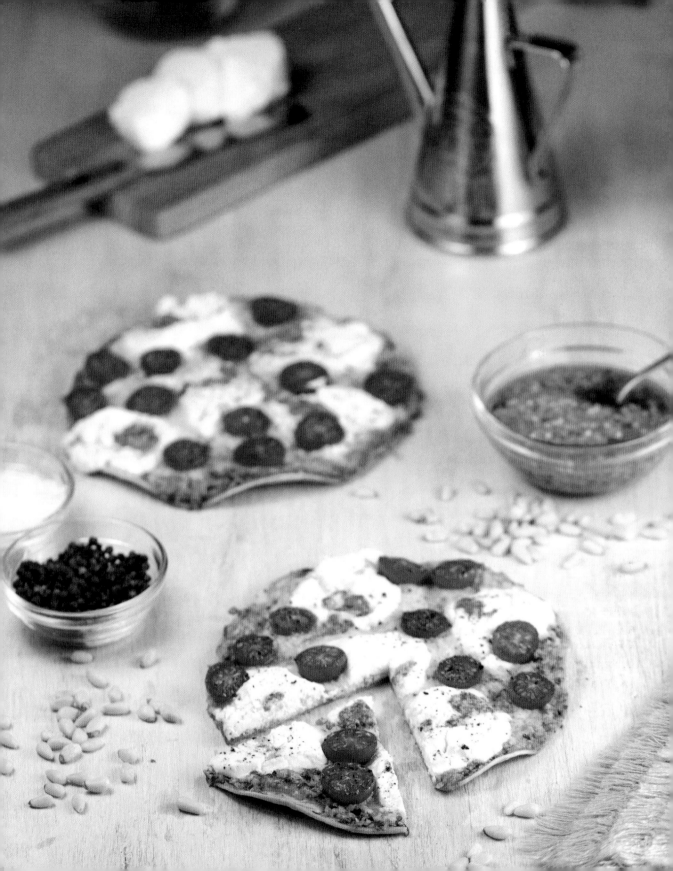

CREAMY CHICKEN-MUSHROOM SOUP

PREP TIME: 10 minutes
COOKING TIME: 55 minutes
MAKES 6 servings

This is a spectacularly delicious soup, but you need to be a mushroom lover to enjoy it as the soup has an intensely rich and earthy mushroom flavor. Make a large batch in advance and simply reheat for a quick, wholesome lunch during the week.

POACHED CHICKEN

6 cups (1.4 liters) all-natural salted chicken stock

1 whole boneless, skinless chicken breast (about 14 ounces)

SOUP

1 tablespoon olive oil

2 tablespoons unsalted butter

4 portobello mushrooms, diced

2 stalks celery, diced

3 cloves garlic, minced

2 cups (480 ml) heavy cream

1 teaspoon fresh thyme leaves, finely chopped

Fresh parsley, for garnish (optional)

Sautéed sliced portobello mushroom, for garnish (optional)

CHEF'S TIP

▶ For a fancy presentation, swirl a tablespoon of crème fraîche into each bowl of soup.

1. Place the chicken stock in a large saucepan and bring to a boil. Reduce the heat to a steady simmer, then add the chicken breast. Cover with a lid and poach gently for 20 minutes, or until the chicken is fully cooked. Remove the chicken from the pan (reserve the stock) and set aside.

2. Make the soup: Heat the oil and butter in a large saucepan over medium-high heat. Once hot, add the vegetables and cook, stirring constantly, for 5 minutes, until tender. Add the cream, thyme, and 3 cups (720 ml) of the reserved chicken stock. Bring to a boil, then reduce the heat to a rolling simmer.

3. Dice the cooked chicken, add to the soup, and continue to cook for 20 to 25 minutes, until thick and creamy. Garnish with parsley and sautéed mushroom, if desired, and serve. Store any leftovers in the refrigerator for up to 3 days.

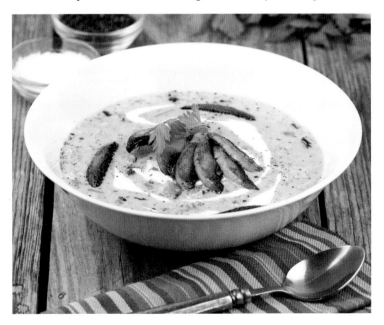

NUTRITION FACTS (PER SERVING)

CALORIES	FAT	PROTEIN	NET CARBS	CARBS
454	39g	21g	5g	6g
	77%	19%	4%	

CREAMY TOMATO-BASIL SOUP

PREP TIME: 10 minutes
COOKING TIME: 25 minutes
MAKES 6 servings

This aromatic soup features a classic tomato-and-basil flavor combination. Using canned diced tomatoes makes this recipe really easy, but feel free to use fresh ripe tomatoes if you prefer. Serve with toasted Low-Carb Almond Bread (page 134) for a delicious, hearty lunch.

1 tablespoon olive oil

2 tablespoons unsalted butter

2 stalks celery, diced

½ white onion, chopped

3 cloves garlic, chopped

1 (28-oz/785-g) can diced tomatoes, or 1 pound (450 g) fresh tomatoes, diced

2 cups (480 ml) heavy cream

2 cups (480 ml) all-natural salted chicken stock

1 large handful of fresh basil leaves, chopped

Heavy cream, for garnish

Torn fresh basil, for garnish

Freshly ground black pepper, for garnish

1. Place a large saucepan over medium-high heat and add the oil and butter. Add the celery, onion, and garlic to the hot oil and cook for 5 minutes, until tender, stirring constantly.

2. Add the diced tomatoes, cream, and chicken stock and bring to a boil. Reduce the heat to a rolling simmer and continue to cook for 20 minutes.

3. Add the chopped basil and continue to cook for 3 more minutes. Remove the pan from the heat and use an immersion blender to purée the soup until smooth and creamy. Pour into serving bowls and garnish with a few drops of cream, some fresh basil leaves, and a sprinkle of freshly ground black pepper. Store any leftovers in the refrigerator for up to 4 days.

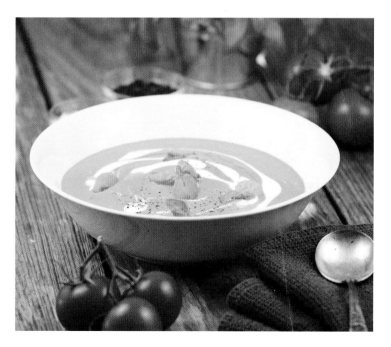

NUTRITION FACTS (PER SERVING)

CALORIES	FAT	PROTEIN	NET CARBS	CARBS
371	35g	4g	9g	10g
	85%	4%	10%	

PHILLY CHEESESTEAK LETTUCE WRAPS

PREP TIME: 10 minutes
COOKING TIME: 15 minutes
MAKES 4 servings

For those not in the know, a Philly cheesesteak is a simple delicacy that originates from Philadelphia—a sandwich comprising finely sliced steak, sautéed onions and bell peppers, and processed cheese sauce, served in a soft white hoagie roll. In this version, the processed cheese sauce is replaced with real melted cheese and the bread is exchanged for large crunchy romaine lettuce leaves, which cuts the carbs dramatically and still delivers an extremely satisfying meal.

2 (8-oz/225-g) boneless rib-eye steaks

2 tablespoons olive oil

2 red bell peppers, sliced

½ white onion, sliced

3 cloves garlic, minced

2 cups (220 g) shredded full-fat cheese (any combination you like—half provolone and half Gruyère works well)

8 large romaine lettuce leaves

SPECIAL EQUIPMENT

Cocktail skewers

1. Place the steaks in the freezer for 30 to 40 minutes (very cold meat is easier to slice).

2. Using a sharp knife, slice the steak into thin strips and set aside.

3. Place a large frying pan over medium-high heat. Add the oil to the pan and heat. Add the sliced red peppers and white onion to the hot oil and sauté for 5 minutes, or until softened. Add the garlic and continue to cook for an additional 3 to 5 minutes, until the vegetables are golden brown and caramelized. Transfer the vegetables to a plate and set aside.

4. Add the sliced steak to the hot frying pan and stir-fry for 2 to 3 minutes, until fully cooked and browned. Add the peppers and onions back to the pan and stir well. Sprinkle the shredded cheese over the steak, cover the pan with a lid, and continue to cook for an additional 2 to 3 minutes, until the cheese is melted and bubbling. Transfer the meat and vegetable mixture to a plate and allow to cool for 3 to 5 minutes.

5. Assemble the wraps: Stack 2 lettuce leaves per wrap and top with a quarter of the steak mixture. Carefully roll the lettuce around the filling, cut each lettuce wrap in half, and secure with cocktail skewers. Serve immediately.

NUTRITION FACTS (PER SERVING)

CALORIES	FAT	PROTEIN	NET CARBS	CARBS
589	41g	42g	8g	13g
	63%	29%	5%	

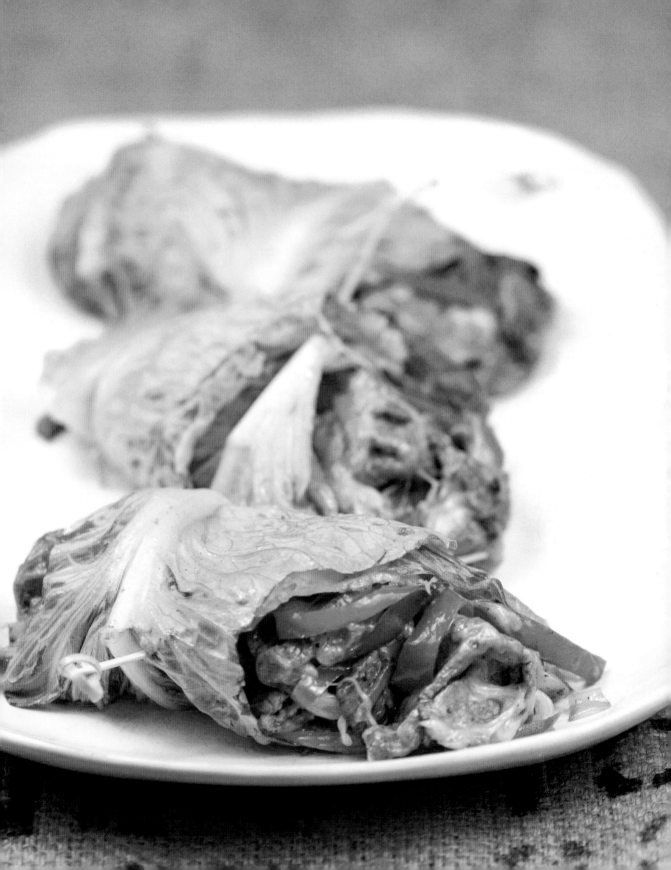

INCREDIBLE KETO PIZZA

PREP TIME: 10 minutes
COOKING TIME: 30 minutes
MAKES 4 servings

Who doesn't like pizza? Pizza may be the food that low-carb, gluten-free, and Paleo dieters miss the most. This pizza crust, made from an ingenious blend of mozzarella cheese and almond flour, tastes very similar to the real thing. It is identical to the recipe for Mozzarella Pastry Dough on page 130, but here is reduced to a manageable size for hand-forming into the perfect thin-crust pizza. Experiment with your favorite toppings!

DOUGH

1 cup (110 g) almond flour

¼ teaspoon fine sea salt

1 teaspoon baking powder

2 tablespoons unsalted butter

½ cup (55 g) grated Parmesan cheese

1 cup (110 g) shredded low-moisture mozzarella cheese

1 large egg

TOPPING

¼ cup (60 ml) store-bought all-natural marinara or pizza sauce (no added sugar)

4 ounces (110 g) fresh mozzarella cheese, sliced

2 ounces (55 g) fresh (soft) goat cheese, crumbled

2 ounces (55 g) blue cheese, crumbled

10 slices pepperoni

4 slices prosciutto, torn, for garnish

Fresh arugula, for garnish

1. Preheat the oven to 400°F (205°C).

2. Make the pizza dough: Place the almond flour, salt, and baking powder in a mixing bowl and whisk thoroughly.

3. Place a large saucepan over low heat and add the butter, Parmesan cheese, and mozzarella cheese. Stirring constantly, melt the butter and cheese (they may look separated at this point, but they will incorporate when mixed with the other ingredients).

4. Pour the cheese-butter mixture into the bowl of a stand mixer fitted with the paddle attachment. With the mixer on low speed, add the almond flour mixture and the egg, then turn the speed to high. Continue to mix for 1 to 2 minutes, until you have smooth, soft dough. Alternatively, you can use an electric hand mixer or good old-fashioned elbow grease, but a stand mixer works best.

5. Allow the dough to cool slightly. Place a large piece of parchment paper on the counter and form the dough into a 12 by 8-inch (30.5 by 20-cm) rectangle directly on the paper. Try to keep the crust as thin as you can.

6. Place the parchment directly onto the middle rack of the oven and par-bake for 10 minutes.

7. Remove the dough from the oven, spread on the marinara sauce, and then add the remaining toppings except the prosciutto and arugula. Place the pizza back in the oven and bake for 15 to 20 minutes, until golden and bubbling.

8. Garnish the hot pizza with the prosciutto slices and fresh arugula and serve immediately. Store leftovers in the refrigerator for up to 3 days.

NUTRITION FACTS (PER SERVING)

CALORIES	FAT	PROTEIN	NET CARBS	CARBS
636	48g	39g	9g	12g
	68%	25%	6%	

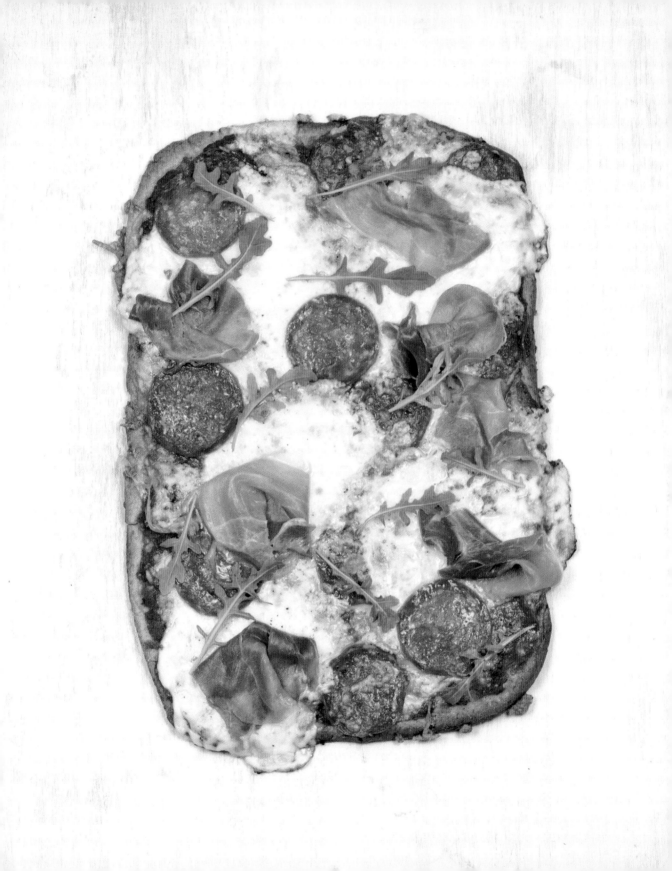

ASIAN-STYLE SHRIMP & VEGETABLE WRAPS
WITH PEANUT-CILANTRO SLAW

PREP TIME: 30 minutes
COOKING TIME: 5 minutes
MAKES 4 wraps (1 per serving)

Rice is typically off-limits on a low-carb diet, but ultra-thin Asian rice paper wraps (also known as *bánh tráng*) are so thin that they really don't contain many carbs at all. They are stretchy when soaked in water and are great for making healthy vegetable and protein-packed rolls. Stuff the wraps with any of your favorite fillings; they are great for boxed lunches and quick snacks as well as meals when paired with this tangy slaw.

COCONUT CURRY POACHED SHRIMP

1 (1-oz/28-g) piece fresh ginger, roughly chopped

1 (14-oz/400-ml) can full-fat unsweetened coconut milk

2 teaspoons curry powder

1 teaspoon fine sea salt

20 raw large shrimp or king prawns, peeled and deveined

4 (8½-in/21½-cm) bánh tráng rice paper wraps

VEGETABLE FILLINGS

1 small handful of mung bean sprouts

1 small handful of fresh cilantro, chopped

½ red bell pepper, sliced into strips

¼ medium cucumber, sliced into strips

3 scallions, sliced into strips

Sesame seeds, for garnish

Soy sauce, for dipping

SLAW

¼ head red cabbage

1 small handful of fresh cilantro leaves, chopped, plus extra for garnish

2 tablespoons 2-Minute Homemade Mayonnaise (page 132)

1 tablespoon creamy all-natural peanut butter (no sugar added)

1 teaspoon soy sauce

1 teaspoon unseasoned rice wine vinegar

½ teaspoon all-natural chili paste

1. Make the poached shrimp: Place all the ingredients, aside from the shrimp, in a saucepan and bring to a boil. Reduce the heat to a simmer, then add the shrimp and gently poach for 5 minutes. Drain the shrimp, then place in a bowl and refrigerate until needed; discard the cooking liquid.

2. Make the rice paper wraps: Soak the wraps in cold water for 30 seconds, then place on a cutting board (they will be pliable and sticky after soaking; work quickly, before they become too tacky). Top each wrap with 5 poached shrimp and one-quarter of each of the filling ingredients. Carefully roll the stuffed wraps into cylinder shapes and store in the refrigerator until needed.

3. Make the slaw: Finely shred the red cabbage and place in a large mixing bowl. Add all the other ingredients, except for the garnishes, and mix well.

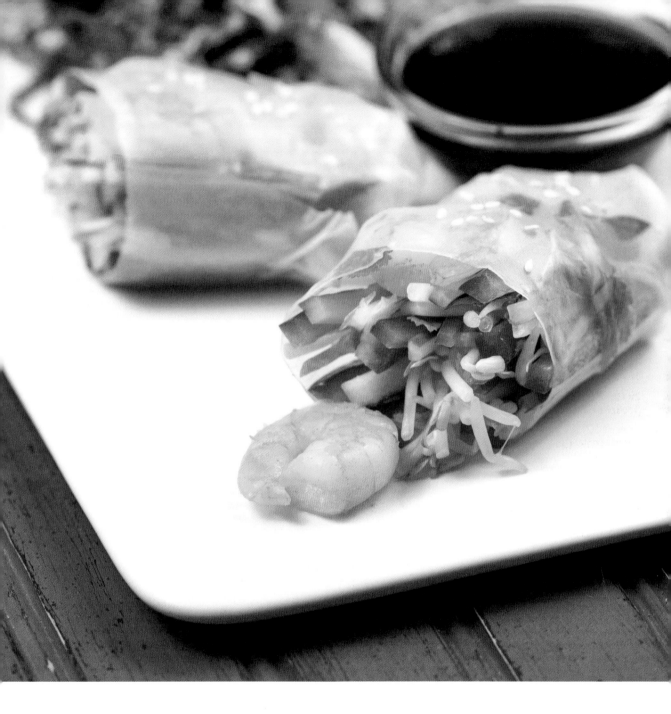

NUTRITION FACTS (PER SERVING)				
CALORIES	FAT	PROTEIN	NET CARBS	CARBS
180	8g	12g	12g	15g
	40%	27%	27%	

4. To serve, slice each rice wrap in half and divide the pieces among 4 serving plates. Place a large scoop of the slaw on each plate and top with some extra cilantro. Sprinkle the wraps with sesame seeds and serve with soy sauce for dipping.

PAN-ROASTED CHICKEN, AVOCADO, APRICOT & PROSCIUTTO SALAD

PREP TIME: 10 minutes
COOKING TIME: 20 minutes
MAKES 4 servings

This colorful salad is full of contrasting flavors; the apricots add a hint of sweetness and tanginess and cut through the rich avocado and prosciutto. Warm, crispy pan-roasted chicken and light Dijon mustard dressing elevate the salad to a refreshing yet wholesome lunch.

CHICKEN

4 boneless, skinless chicken breast halves (about 1¾ lbs/675 g) or boneless, skinless thighs (see Note)

¼ teaspoon fine sea salt

¼ teaspoon freshly ground black pepper

2 tablespoons olive oil

DRESSING

¼ cup (60 ml) white wine vinegar

½ cup (120 ml) extra-virgin olive oil

1 teaspoon Dijon mustard

Fine sea salt and freshly ground black pepper to taste

SALAD

4 large handfuls of arugula

1 large handful of pea shoots (optional)

4 medium ripe apricots, pitted and cut into wedges

2 ripe avocados, peeled and sliced

8 slices prosciutto, roughly torn

Freshly ground black pepper, for garnish

1. Preheat the oven to 400°F (205°C). Season the chicken breasts with the salt and pepper.

2. Place a large ovenproof frying pan over high heat. Add the oil and, once hot, add the chicken breasts. Cook the chicken for 3 minutes on each side, then transfer the frying pan to the oven and continue to cook for 15 minutes, until the chicken is golden brown, crispy, and fully cooked in the center.

3. Make the dressing: Place all ingredients in a mixing bowl and whisk until fully combined and emulsified.

4. Assemble the salad: Place a handful of arugula onto each serving plate. Scatter the pea shoots, apricot wedges, sliced avocado, and torn prosciutto over each pile of arugula.

5. Remove the chicken breasts from the oven, allow to rest for 3 to 5 minutes, and then slice and place on top of each salad. Drizzle the salads with the dressing, garnish with freshly ground black pepper, and serve.

NOTE

Chicken thighs contain more fat, flavor, and calories than breasts.

NUTRITION FACTS (PER SERVING)

CALORIES	FAT	PROTEIN	NET CARBS	CARBS
734	50g	59g	4g	12g
	61%	32%	2%	

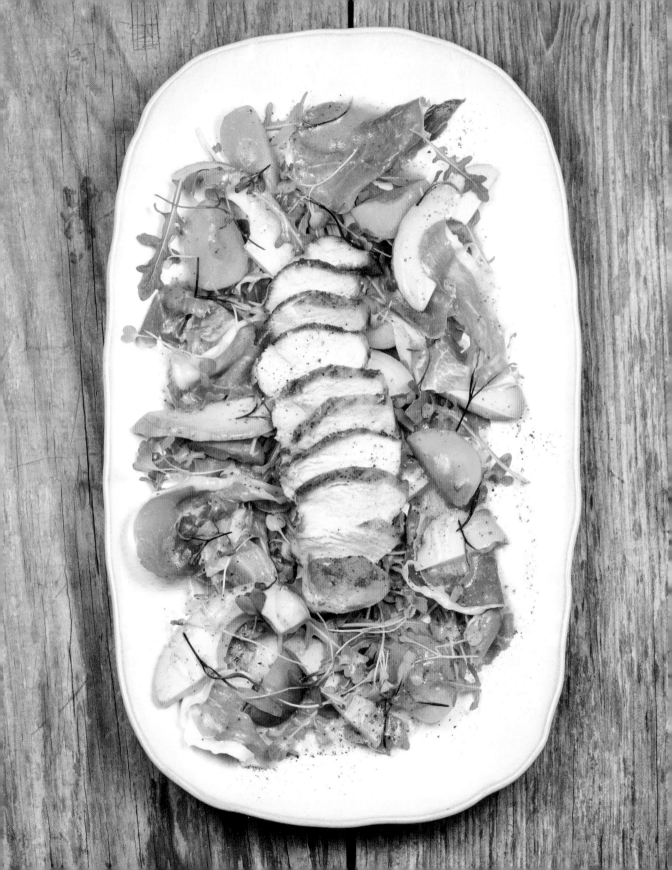

CAESAR SALAD
WITH SEARED SALMON & PARMESAN CRISPS

PREP TIME: 15 minutes
COOKING TIME: 20 minutes
MAKES 4 servings

Caesar salad is always a crowd-pleaser. Anchovies, traditional in Caesars, add a real kick of umami flavor. Little-known Caesar salad factoid: it was actually invented in Mexico! Parmesan crisps are added in this version as a superior replacement for croutons.

CAESAR DRESSING

2 cloves garlic, minced

1 tablespoon grated Parmesan cheese

1½ teaspoons Dijon mustard

2 large egg yolks

Juice of ½ lemon

2 anchovy fillets (packed in oil), roughly chopped

1¼ cups (300 ml) extra-virgin olive oil

Fine sea salt and freshly ground black pepper

PARMESAN CRISPS

1 cup (110 g) freshly grated Parmesan cheese (from a block, not powdered)

SALMON

2 tablespoons olive oil

4 (6-oz/170-g) skinless salmon fillets, ideally wild-caught

¼ teaspoon fine sea salt

¼ teaspoon freshly ground black pepper

SALAD

2 romaine lettuce hearts

12 marinated white anchovy fillets (boquerones), for garnish

Lemon wedges, for serving

1. Make the dressing: Place the garlic, Parmesan cheese, mustard, egg yolks, lemon juice, and anchovies in a food processor and blend until very smooth.

2. With the motor running, trickle in the olive oil very slowly, until fully emulsified and creamy (this should take about 1½ minutes). Transfer the dressing to a jar and season with salt and pepper to taste. If the dressing is thicker than you would like, add 1 to 2 tablespoons of boiling water to thin it out.

3. Make the crisps: Preheat the oven to 350°F (177°C) and line a sheet pan with parchment paper. Spread the Parmesan cheese onto the sheet in a thin layer, ensuring there are no gaps.

4. Place the sheet pan in the oven and bake for 4 to 5 minutes, until golden brown and bubbly. Remove the sheet pan from the oven and, using a metal spatula, immediately remove the molten cheese from the parchment paper to a cooling rack. The cheese layer will become crispy as it cools; when cooled completely, snap the layer into small crisps.

5. Cook the salmon: Place a large frying pan over medium-high heat and add the olive oil. Season the salmon fillets evenly with the salt and pepper and, once the oil is hot, add the salmon to the pan. Cook for 5 minutes on the first side, until golden and crispy, then flip and continue cooking for 2 to 3 minutes more, until the salmon is cooked through (or less if you like your salmon medium-rare).

6. Prepare the salad: Trim the base of the lettuce hearts, separate the leaves, and wash well. Place the leaves in a large bowl, pour the dressing over them, and toss. Divide the salad among 4 large plates and top with the warm salmon. Garnish with the anchovies and Parmesan crisps and serve with lemon wedges. Store any leftover salmon in the refrigerator for up to 2 days.

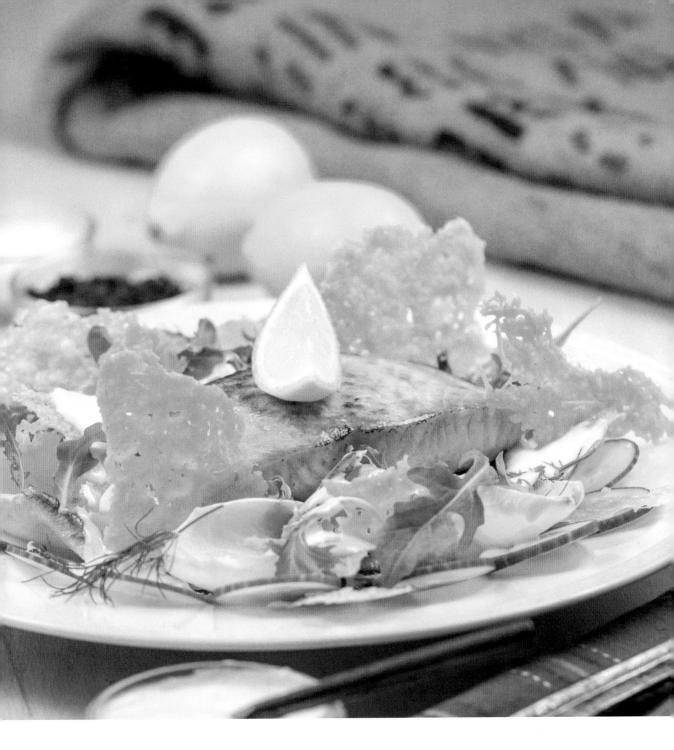

NUTRITION FACTS (PER SERVING)				
CALORIES	FAT	PROTEIN	NET CARBS	CARBS
886	70g	52g	5g	12g
	71%	23%	2%	

CHEF'S TIP

► For this particular recipe, it's important to use freshly grated Parmesan—it melts better and creates better crisps.

BUNLESS BURGERS
WITH HALLOUMI FRIES

PREP TIME: 15 minutes

COOKING TIME: 25 minutes

MAKES 4 servings

You can't beat the fresh taste of a high-quality homemade beef burger. These burgers take ten minutes or less to put together and are packed with juicy flavor. The crispy halloumi fries are made by simply deep-frying halloumi cheese—a low-carb french fry alternative packed with flavor and protein.

BURGER PATTIES

2 pounds (900 g) grass-fed ground beef (80% lean)

2 teaspoons Dijon mustard

1 teaspoon fine sea salt

1 teaspoon freshly ground black pepper

BURGER TOPPINGS

2 tablespoons olive oil

½ red onion, sliced

Fine sea salt and freshly ground black pepper

2 ounces (60 g) fresh (soft) goat cheese, crumbled

FRIES

High-heat oil for deep-frying, such as coconut oil or avocado oil (about 3 cups/720 ml)

1 (8.8-oz/250-g) package halloumi cheese, sliced into fry-size pieces

SIDE SALAD (OPTIONAL)

4 large handfuls of mixed salad greens

2-Minute Homemade Mayonnaise (page 132), for dressing the salad

1. Combine all the ingredients for the burger patties in a large bowl and use your hands to mix until thoroughly combined.

2. Divide the burger meat evenly into 4 balls, then use your hands to press into patties about 5 inches (12.75 cm) in diameter and ½ inch (1.25 cm) thick. Preheat a grill or cast-iron griddle pan to high heat.

3. While the grill is heating up, make the red onion topping: Place the olive oil in a frying pan over medium heat and add the red onion slices. Sauté the onions for about 5 to 10 minutes. Season to taste with salt and pepper.

4. Cook the burgers on the preheated grill or cast-iron griddle pan for about 5 minutes on the first side, then flip it and cook 5 minutes on the other side for medium done burgers.

5. Make the halloumi fries: In a large heavy saucepan, heat a generous amount of oil (about 3 cups) to 350°F (177°C) over medium-high heat. (You want about 2 inches (5 cm) of oil in the pan and 3 inches (7.5 cm) or more of headspace above the oil.) Add all of the halloumi pieces to the hot oil and cook for about 5 minutes, until golden brown and crispy. Drain the fries on paper towels.

6. Top the cooked burgers with the onions and crumbled goat cheese. Serve with a side salad, if desired. Store any leftovers in the refrigerator for up to 3 days.

NUTRITION FACTS (PER SERVING)

CALORIES	FAT	PROTEIN	NET CARBS	CARBS
716	52g	60g	2g	2g
	65%	34%	1%	

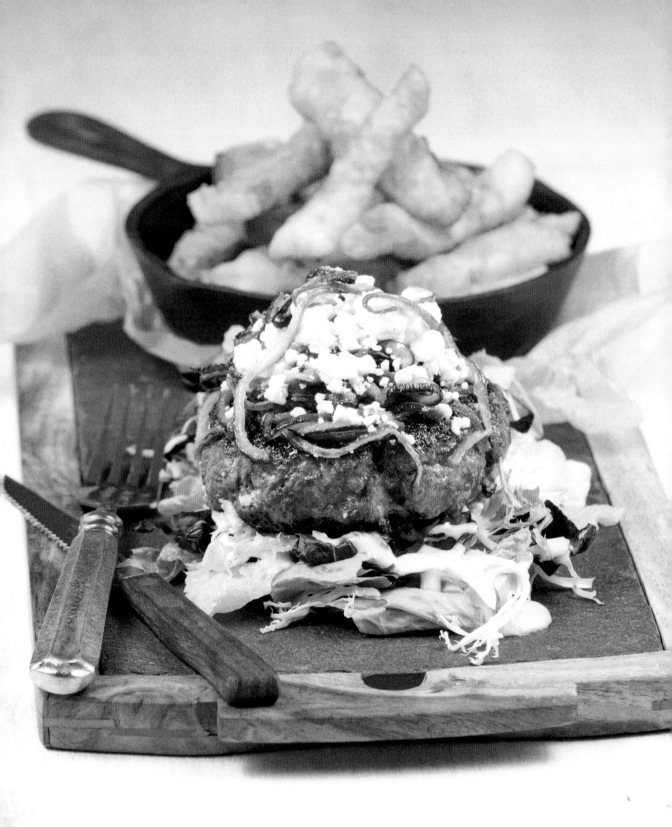

BACON-CHEDDAR PINWHEELS

PREP TIME: 10 minutes + 15 minutes for the pastry dough

COOKING TIME: 30 minutes

MAKES 22 pinwheels (1 per serving)

Crisp bites of warm golden-brown pastry stuffed with cheddar and bacon—yum! This mouthwatering party appetizer (or meal when paired with a salad) is versatile and surprisingly very low carb. Once baked, the pinwheels can be garnished with extra toppings of your choice, such as cream cheese and smoked salmon. Use the directions below to make an endless array of flavor varieties by filling the pinwheels with your own ingredient combinations.

1 recipe Mozzarella Pastry Dough (page 130)

12 slices crispy cooked bacon, chopped

8 ounces (225 g) sharp or extra-sharp cheddar cheese, shredded

4 ounces (110 g) Parmesan cheese, grated

1. Preheat the oven to 350°F (177°C) and line a sheet pan with parchment paper.

2. Make the pastry dough according to recipe instructions. Place the dough on a clean work surface and roll it out into a large rectangle about ¼ inch (6 mm) thick. Use a little bit of almond flour for dusting if the pastry becomes sticky.

3. Sprinkle the bacon and cheddar over the pastry and, working with one of the long sides, carefully roll it into a long cylinder shape.

4. Slice the cylinder into 22 round discs and place them onto the baking sheet. Sprinkle the Parmesan cheese over the pinwheels and bake for 30 minutes, until golden brown and crispy. Serve immediately.

5. Store leftover pinwheels in an airtight container at room temperature for 2 to 3 days. To reheat, place in a preheated moderate oven for 5 to 8 minutes, or until piping hot and crispy.

NUTRITION FACTS (PER SERVING)

CALORIES	FAT	PROTEIN	NET CARBS	CARBS
231	19g	12g	3g	3g
	74%	21%	5%	

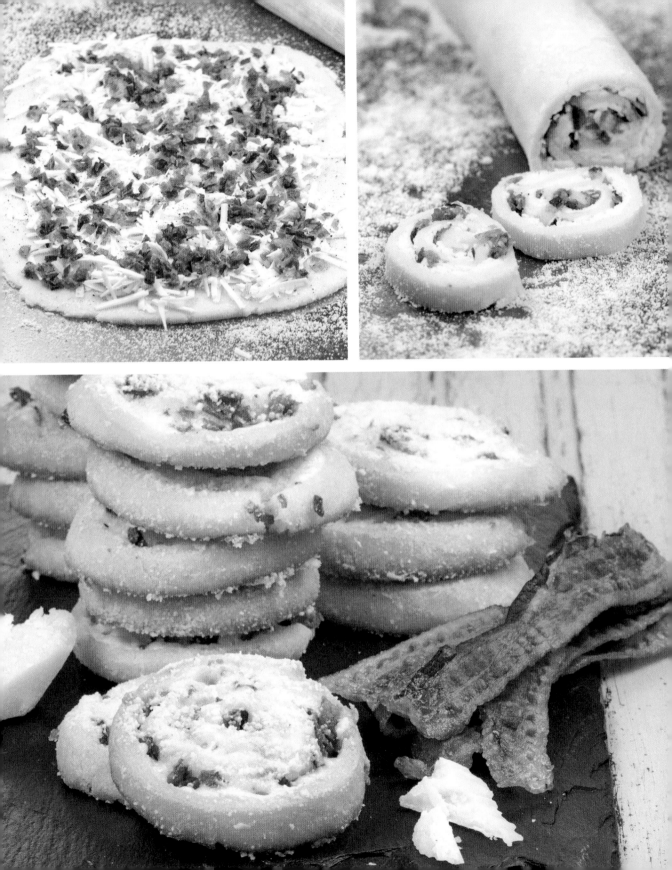

PARMESAN ROASTED MIXED NUTS

PREP TIME: 5 minutes
COOKING TIME: 45 minutes
MAKES 12 servings

Nuts are a classic low-carb snack, but store-bought flavored mixes often feature additives and sugars. This homemade nut mix is delicious, crunchy, and cheesy, and it can be made with any of your favorite nuts.

4 tablespoons olive oil, divided

PARMESAN COATING

1½ cups (165 g) grated Parmesan cheese

1 teaspoon fine sea salt

1 teaspoon onion powder

1 teaspoon smoked paprika

½ teaspoon dried ground oregano

¼ teaspoon cayenne pepper

2 large egg whites

NUT MIX

1 cup (135 g) raw almonds

1 cup (145 g) raw peanuts

½ cup (65 g) raw Brazil nuts

½ cup (65 g) raw macadamia nuts

½ cup (50 g) raw pecan halves

½ cup (65 g) raw hazelnuts

1. Preheat the oven to 325°F (163°C). Line a sheet pan with parchment paper and drizzle with 2 tablespoons of the oil.

2. Make the Parmesan coating: Place the Parmesan, salt, and spices in a bowl and mix well until combined.

3. Whisk the egg whites in a separate medium-sized bowl until they form soft peaks.

4. Add the mixed nuts and the Parmesan coating mixture to the egg whites and stir well until the nuts are thoroughly coated with the mixture.

5. Sprinkle the nuts onto the prepared sheet pan and drizzle the remaining 2 tablespoons of oil over the top.

6. Place the sheet pan in the oven and bake for 15 minutes. Stir the nut mixture well and continue to bake for 5 to 10 minutes more, until golden and aromatic. Switch off the oven and leave the nuts inside with the door ajar for 20 minutes.

7. Remove the nuts from the oven and cool completely in the pan, then store in an airtight container at room temperature for up to 1 week.

NUTRITION FACTS (PER SERVING)

CALORIES	FAT	PROTEIN	NET CARBS	CARBS
330	29g	12g	4g	9g
	79%	15%	5%	

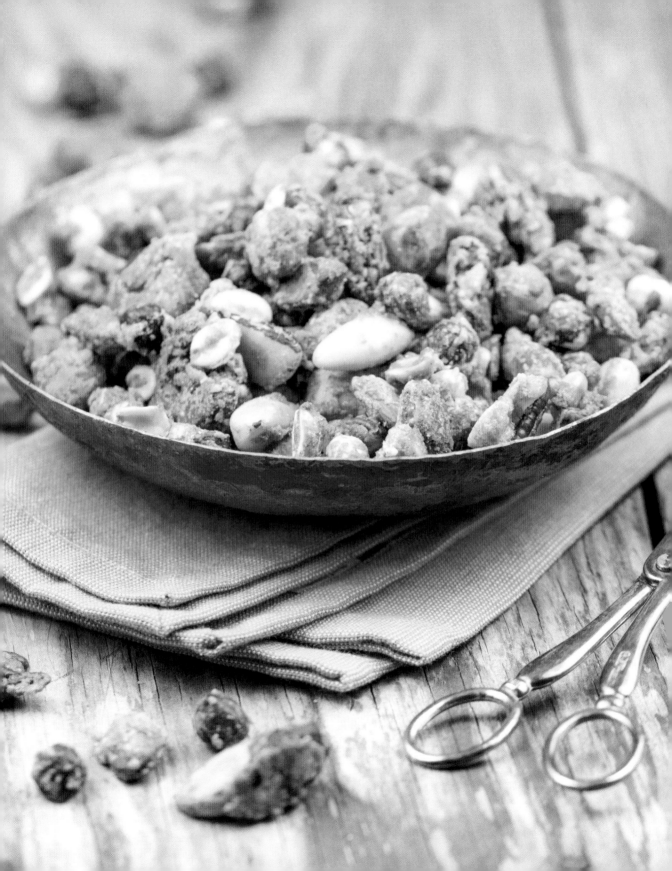

CHICKEN TIKKA SKEWERS
WITH CILANTRO-LIME DIPPING SAUCE

PREP TIME: 15 minutes + 1 hour to marinate

COOKING TIME: 30 minutes

MAKES 6 servings

These flavor-packed skewers make a fantastic party appetizer. This recipe uses store-bought tikka masala curry paste, so they are super easy to make. If you are ambitious, you can make your own curry paste. The cooling cilantro dipping sauce adds a sharp and tangy contrast to the robust flavors of the spiced chicken.

CHICKEN TIKKA

1 whole boneless, skinless chicken breast (about 14 oz/400 g)

½ cup (120 ml) full-fat yogurt

3 tablespoons all-natural Indian tikka masala curry paste

Juice of ½ lemon

½ teaspoon fine sea salt

CILANTRO-LIME DIPPING SAUCE

¾ cup (180 ml) full-fat yogurt

½ cup (120 ml) 2-Minute Homemade Mayonnaise (page 132)

Zest and juice of 2 limes

3 tablespoons chopped fresh cilantro

¼ teaspoon freshly ground black pepper

¼ teaspoon fine sea salt

Stevia to taste (optional)

Chopped fresh cilantro, for garnish

SPECIAL EQUIPMENT

Bamboo skewers, soaked in water for 15 minutes

1. Marinate the chicken: Cut the chicken breasts into 1-inch (2.5-cm) cubes and place in a large mixing bowl. Add the rest of the ingredients for the chicken, stir well, and refrigerate for 1 hour.

2. Make the dipping sauce: Simply mix all of the ingredients in a bowl and store in the refrigerator until needed.

3. Preheat the oven to 400°F (205°C) and line a sheet pan with parchment paper. Thread 2 or 3 pieces of chicken onto each bamboo skewer and place the skewers on the sheet pan. Place the pan in the oven and bake the chicken for 30 minutes, until golden brown and no longer pink in the center. Serve the skewers with a bowl of the dipping sauce, garnished with chopped fresh cilantro. Store any leftovers in the refrigerator for up to 3 days.

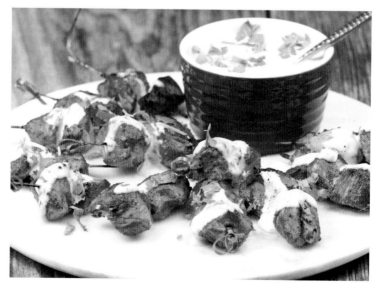

NUTRITION FACTS (PER SERVING)

CALORIES	FAT	PROTEIN	NET CARBS	CARBS
269	17g	23g	3g	6g
	57%	34%	4%	

NO-BAKE
COCOA PEANUT BUTTER PROTEIN BALLS

PREP TIME: 15 minutes + 1 hour to chill

COOKING TIME: 5 minutes

MAKES 12 protein balls (1 per serving)

These protein-packed bites are a quick and easy snack to keep in the refrigerator for a sweet energy boost. Take them in the car or on a hike!

DRY MIX

¾ cup (82 g) almond flour

¼ cup (32 g) whey protein powder

¼ cup (20 g) unsweetened shredded coconut

3 tablespoons unsweetened cocoa powder

2 tablespoons chia seeds

⅛ teaspoon fine sea salt

SYRUP

¼ cup (60 ml) water

¼ cup (48 g) granulated low-carb sweetener of your choice (see Note)

2 tablespoons unsalted butter

1 teaspoon vanilla extract

¼ cup (60 g) creamy all-natural peanut butter (no sugar added)

Crushed toasted peanuts, for garnish (optional)

1. Place all of the ingredients for the dry mix in a mixing bowl and combine.

2. Place all the ingredients for the syrup in a saucepan over medium heat. Bring to a boil, then reduce the heat to a simmer and cook until syrupy, about 5 minutes.

3. Pour the syrup over the dry ingredients, then add the peanut butter and stir until fully combined. Cover and refrigerate for 1 hour.

4. Use a tablespoon to scoop the chilled mixture into 12 portions and roll between your hands to form balls. Coat the balls with crushed peanuts, if desired, and store in an airtight container in the refrigerator for up to a week or in the freezer for up to a month.

NOTE

Feel free to reduce the amount of sweetener to taste.

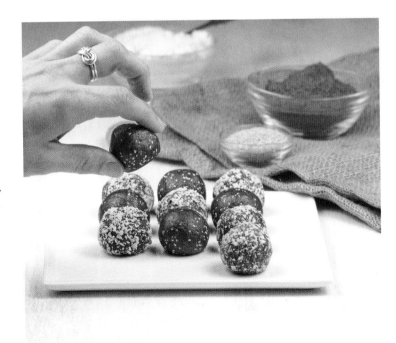

NUTRITION FACTS (PER SERVING)

CALORIES	FAT	PROTEIN	NET CARBS	CARBS
142	10g	6g	2g	7g
	63%	17%	6%	

CRISPY SESAME SHRIMP "TOAST"

PREP TIME: 15 minutes + 1 hour to freeze
COOKING TIME: 10 minutes
MAKES 6 servings

Sesame shrimp toast is a popular Chinese takeout item and usually consists of a flavorful shrimp paste spread on bread, coated in sesame seeds and deep-fried. This low-carb version skips the bread and uses shrimp paste alone; it's a fantastic accompaniment to a stir-fried main course or as a punchy umami appetizer on its own.

SHRIMP PASTE

10 ounces (285 g) raw shrimp, peeled and deveined

1 large egg white

1 scallion, chopped

2 cloves garlic, chopped

High-heat oil for deep-frying, such as coconut oil or avocado oil (about 3 cups/720 ml)

"BREADING"

1 cup (110 g) almond flour

¼ cup plus 2 tablespoons (55 g) sesame seeds

EGG WASH

1 large egg

Black sesame seeds, for garnish (optional)

Scallions, thinly sliced on the diagonal, for garnish (optional)

Soy sauce, for serving

1. Line a sheet pan with parchment paper, leaving some overhanging. Place all of the shrimp paste ingredients in a high-powered blender or food processor and blend until smooth. Spread the paste in an even layer in the bottom of the lined sheet pan. Place the pan in the freezer for 1 hour.

2. In a large heavy saucepan, heat a generous amount of oil (about 3 cups/700 ml) to 350°F (177°C) over medium-high heat. (You want about 2 inches/5 cm of oil in the pan and 3 inches/7.5 cm or more of headspace above the oil.)

3. While the oil is heating, prepare the breading and egg wash: Mix the almond flour and sesame seeds together in a large bowl and beat the egg in a separate small bowl.

4. Remove the shrimp paste from the freezer and, using the parchment, transfer it to a cutting board. Slice it into triangles. Working quickly, dip each triangle into the beaten egg, then into the almond flour mixture, and then gently drop in the oil. Deep-fry the "toasts" in batches for 3 to 5 minutes, until golden brown and crispy, then drain on paper towels and sprinkle with sea salt.

5. Serve immediately, garnished with black sesame seeds and sliced scallions, if desired, and with soy sauce for dipping.

NUTRITION FACTS (PER SERVING)

CALORIES	FAT	PROTEIN	NET CARBS	CARBS
270	22g	12g	3g	6g
	73%	18%	4%	

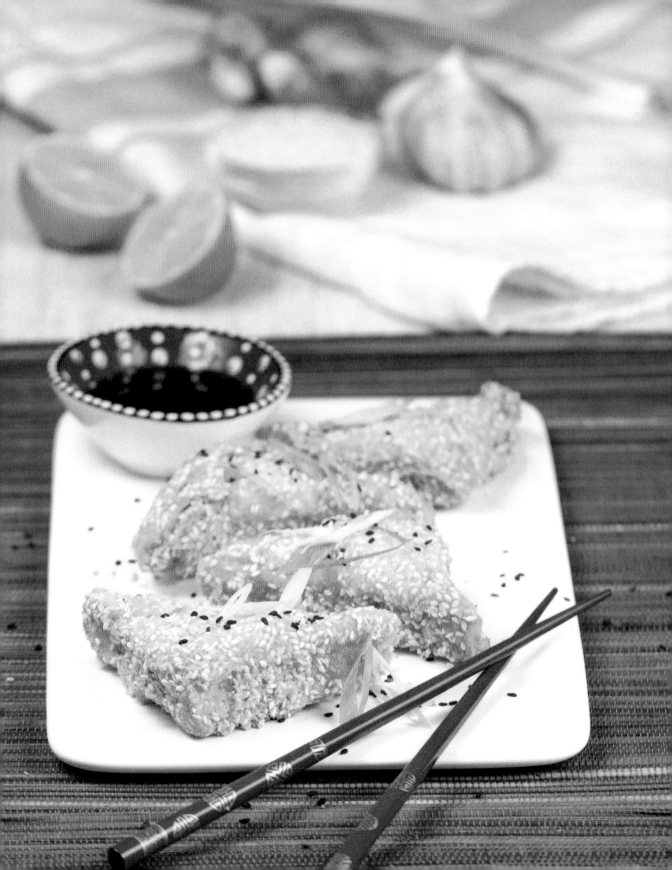

CRISPY BONELESS CHICKEN WINGS
WITH BUFFALO RANCH DIP

PREP TIME: 15 minutes + 30 minutes to marinate
COOKING TIME: 30 minutes
MAKES 4 servings

There is something very satisfying about the crispy skin, tender meat, and tangy Buffalo sauce of Buffalo chicken wings. You may be aware of the increasingly popular boneless "wings," which are essentially chicken nuggets with breading, jam-packed full of carbs. Here's a recipe for an equally satisfying low-carb alternative with a great crunch—they are yummy!

1 whole boneless, skinless chicken breast (about 14 ounces), cut into 1-inch (2.5-cm) cubes

MARINADE

½ cup (120 ml) full-fat buttermilk

¼ cup (60 ml) Buffalo wing hot sauce (see Note)

¼ teaspoon fine sea salt

¼ teaspoon freshly ground black pepper

"BREADING"

1 cup (110 g) almond flour

1 cup (110 g) grated Parmesan cheese

EGG WASH

2 large eggs, beaten

BUFFALO DRIZZLE

3 tablespoons Buffalo wing hot sauce (see Note)

⅓ cup (80 ml) olive oil

CREAMY BUFFALO DIP

¼ cup plus 2 tablespoons (90 ml) 2-Minute Homemade Mayonnaise (page 132)

¼ cup (60 ml) full-fat sour cream

1 tablespoon Buffalo wing hot sauce (see Note)

¼ teaspoon smoked paprika

¼ teaspoon freshly ground black pepper

1. Place the chicken breast cubes in a large mixing bowl with all the marinade ingredients, stir well, and marinate for 30 minutes in the refrigerator.

2. After the chicken has marinated for 15 minutes, preheat the oven to 450°F (232°C) and line a sheet pan with parchment paper.

3. Prepare the breading and egg wash: Mix the almond flour and Parmesan cheese in a large mixing bowl and beat the eggs in a small bowl.

4. Take a chicken cube and shake off the excess marinade, dip it in the egg, and then roll it in the almond flour mixture, until well coated. Place the breaded chicken cube on the lined sheet pan. Repeat with the rest of the chicken, egg wash, and breading.

5. Mix the drizzle ingredients together and drizzle the mixture over the chicken using a spoon. Place the sheet pan in the oven and bake the chicken for 30 minutes, until golden brown.

6. Mix all the dip ingredients together and serve alongside the crispy chicken pieces. Store any leftovers in the refrigerator for up to 3 days.

NOTE

Make sure to purchase an all-natural, no-sugar-added Buffalo sauce, available online and at natural food markets such as Whole Foods. Or make your own low-carb version. (We recommend a recipe on the site Allrecipes.com. Search for "Buffalo Chicken Wing Sauce" and select the recipe submitted by Chef John.)

NUTRITION FACTS (PER SERVING)				
CALORIES	FAT	PROTEIN	NET CARBS	CARBS
624	52g	28g	7g	11g
	75%	18%	4%	

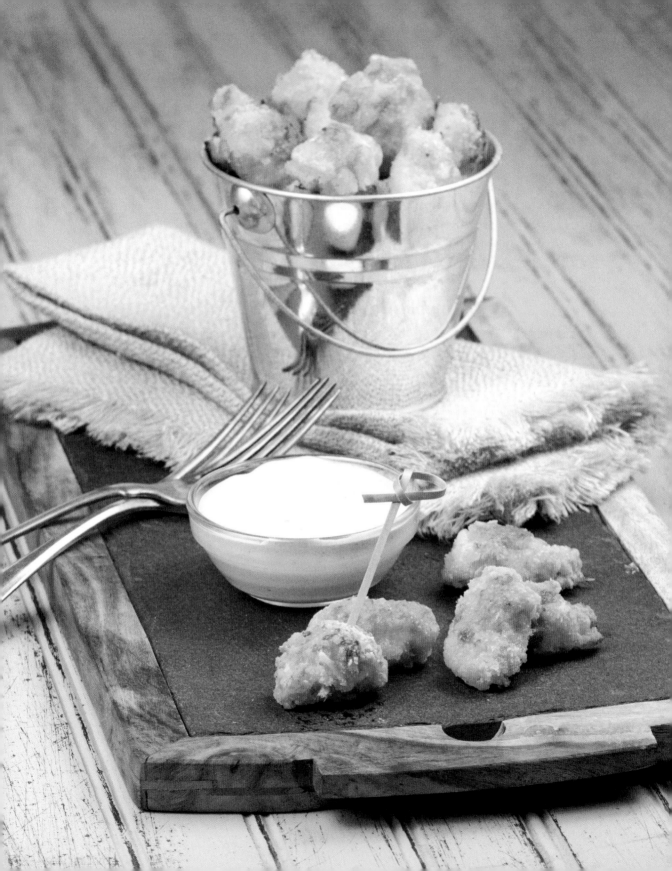

INDIAN-STYLE
COCONUT BUTTER CHICKEN

PREP TIME: 10 minutes + 1 hour to marinate

COOKING TIME: 25 minutes

MAKES 4 servings

A rich and creamy curry offers a slight kick of spice without being overpowering. This also happens to be one of the easiest curries to make: just throw marinated chicken in a frying pan, add cream and tomato sauce, and simmer until the chicken is tender and the sauce is thick. This makes a great weeknight dinner when paired with cauliflower "rice" (page 136). You can even drop the chicken in the marinade in the morning so that it's ready to cook when you get home from work.

MARINADE

½ cup (120 ml) full-fat yogurt

Juice of ½ lemon

5 cloves garlic, minced

2 tablespoons grated fresh ginger

2 teaspoons chopped fresh curry leaves (optional, but it adds fantastic flavor)

2 teaspoons garam masala

2 teaspoons ground mustard

1 teaspoon turmeric powder

1 teaspoon ground cumin

½ teaspoon cayenne pepper

¼ teaspoon ground cardamom

CURRY

1½ pounds (675 g) skinless, boneless chicken breasts or thighs, cut into bite-size pieces (see Note)

1 tablespoon coconut oil

½ teaspoon fine sea salt

1 cup (240 ml) unsweetened all-natural tomato sauce

1 cup (240 ml) heavy cream

½ stick (¼ cup/55 g) unsalted butter

1 batch Simple Cauliflower "Rice" (page 136), for serving

Fresh cilantro, for garnish

1. Combine the marinade ingredients in a large mixing bowl. Add the chicken, stir well, and let marinate in the refrigerator for a minimum of 1 hour or up to 8 hours.

2. Heat the oil in a large frying pan over high heat and add the marinated chicken. Sauté for 5 minutes, until the chicken is browned.

3. Add the salt, tomato sauce, cream, and butter and stir well. Simmer the mixture on low heat for 20 minutes, until the chicken is fully cooked and tender. Taste for seasoning and add salt if needed.

4. Serve the curry with cauliflower "rice" and garnish with cilantro. Store any leftovers in the refrigerator for up to 3 days.

NOTE

Chicken thighs contain more fat, flavor, and calories than breasts.

NUTRITION FACTS (PER SERVING)

CALORIES	FAT	PROTEIN	NET CARBS	CARBS
549	37g	45g	8g	9g
	61%	33%	6%	

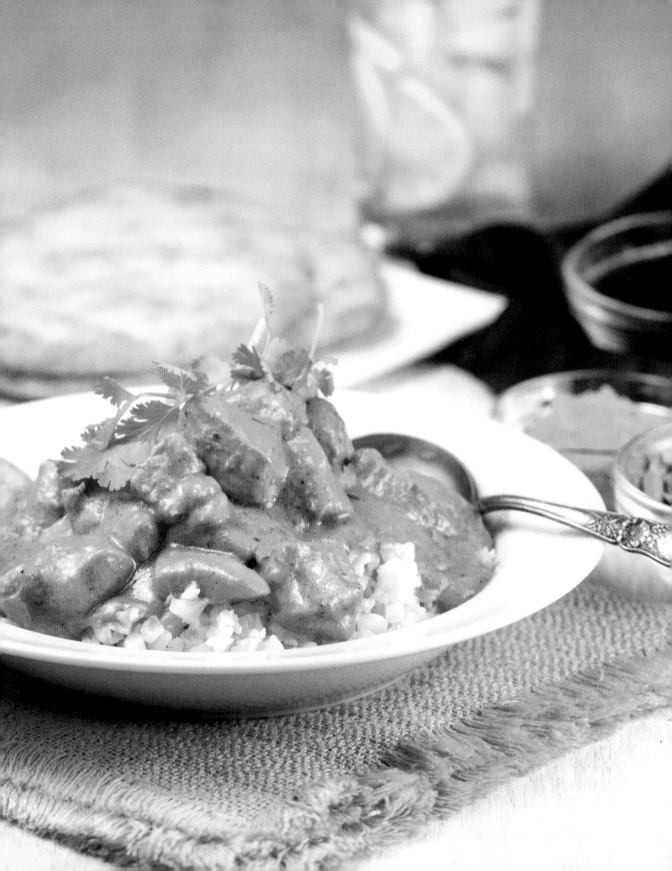

MACADAMIA-CRUSTED HALIBUT
WITH ORANGE-SESAME SALAD

PREP TIME: 15 minutes
COOKING TIME: 25 minutes
MAKES 4 servings

This Asian-style salad is fresh and light tasting, yet substantial. Halibut is encrusted with crushed macadamia nuts and baked, which results in a texture similar to that of a traditional panko-breaded fish.

HALIBUT

¾ cup (100 g) raw macadamia nuts

½ cup (55 g) grated Parmesan cheese

4 (8-oz/225-g) skinless halibut fillets

¼ teaspoon fine sea salt

¼ teaspoon freshly ground black pepper

1 large egg, beaten

3 tablespoons olive oil

SALAD

1 large orange

4 large handfuls of mixed salad leaves

1 (2-inch/5-cm) piece cucumber, sliced

DRESSING

3 tablespoons light olive oil

2 tablespoons fresh orange juice

1 tablespoon toasted (dark) sesame oil

1 tablespoon unseasoned rice wine vinegar

1 tablespoon soy sauce

1 tablespoon minced fresh ginger

1 tablespoon sesame seeds

Fresh cilantro, for garnish

1. Preheat the oven to 400°F (205°C). Line a sheet pan with parchment paper.

2. Place the macadamia nuts in a food processor and process until they resemble finely textured bread crumbs. Add the Parmesan and pulse to mix in, then transfer to a plate or shallow bowl.

3. Season the halibut fillets evenly with the salt and pepper. Dip each fillet in the beaten egg, then dredge the fillets in the macadamia-Parmesan mixture on all sides until fully coated. Place the fillets on the baking sheet and drizzle with the olive oil. Place the baking sheet in the oven and cook for 20 to 25 minutes, until golden brown and crispy and opaque in the center.

4. Meanwhile, peel and segment the orange for the salad and set aside.

5. Make the dressing: Place all ingredients in a mixing bowl and whisk well until fully combined.

6. Divide the salad leaves among 4 serving plates. Top with the orange segments and cucumber slices and drizzle some of the dressing on each serving. Place the cooked halibut fillets on the plates, directly on top of the salad or to the side, and garnish with cilantro.

NUTRITION FACTS (PER SERVING)

CALORIES	FAT	PROTEIN	NET CARBS	CARBS
624	40g	51g	7g	15g
	58%	33%	4%	

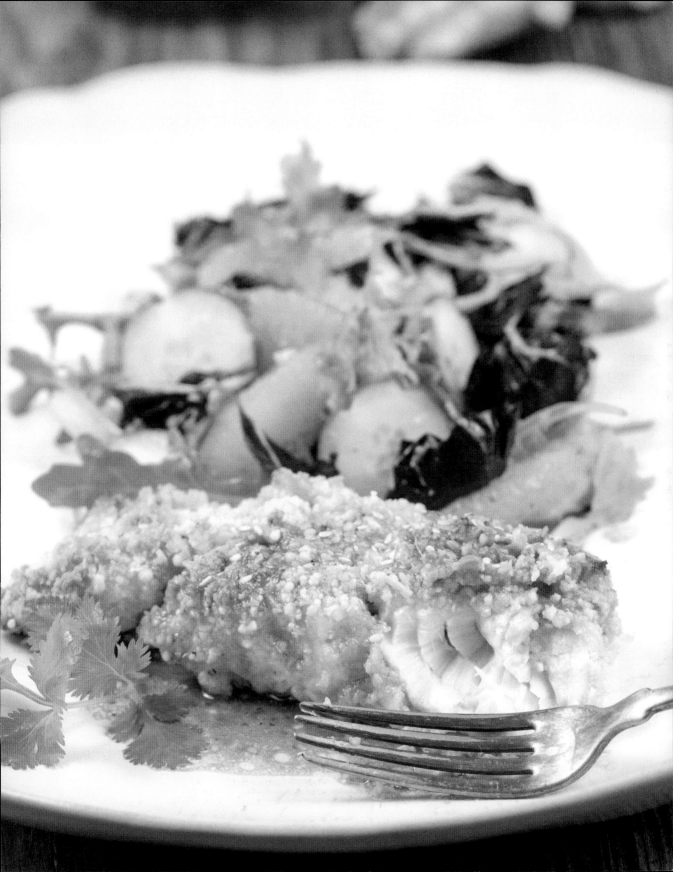

JUICY TURKEY SWEDISH MEATBALLS

PREP TIME: 20 minutes
COOKING TIME: 30 minutes
MAKES 4 servings

These easy-to-make baked turkey meatballs are served in a creamy sauce flavored with bacon, mustard, and Parmesan cheese. They taste like the most delicious Swedish meatballs you've ever had. Serve the meatballs over zucchini "noodles" for an indulgent dinner.

2 large zucchinis

MEATBALLS

¼ white onion, finely diced

2 cloves garlic, minced

2 tablespoons olive oil, divided

1 teaspoon chopped fresh thyme leaves

1 tablespoon chopped fresh oregano leaves

2 pounds (900 g) ground turkey meat (not lean)

3 tablespoons grated Parmesan cheese

½ teaspoon fine sea salt

Pinch of freshly ground black pepper

1 large egg

BACON SAUCE

6 slices bacon, chopped

¼ white onion, diced

2 cloves garlic, minced

½ cup (120 ml) all-natural salted chicken stock

1 tablespoon chopped fresh parsley

½ teaspoon whole-grain mustard (no sugar added)

Fine sea salt and freshly ground black pepper

2 cups (480 ml) heavy cream

2 tablespoons grated Parmesan cheese

Grated Parmesan cheese, for garnish

Fresh chopped parsley, for garnish

1. Preheat the oven to 400°F (205°C). Line a sheet pan with aluminum foil.

2. Use a spiralizer, julienne peeler, or vegetable peeler to cut the zucchinis into "noodles." Set aside.

3. Make the meatballs: Fry the onion and garlic in a tablespoon of the olive oil over medium heat for 5 minutes, until softened. Add the herbs and continue to cook for another 2 minutes. Remove from the heat, place the mixture in a large mixing bowl, and allow to cool.

4. Add the ground turkey, Parmesan cheese, seasoning, and egg to the mixing bowl. Use your hands to combine the ingredients thoroughly.

5. Form the mixture into 24 meatballs, rolling them into compact balls with your hands. Place the meatballs on the sheet pan, drizzle with the remaining tablespoon of olive oil, and place the pan in the oven to bake for 20 minutes, until golden brown and cooked through.

6. Make the sauce: In a large saucepan, cook the bacon over high heat for 5 minutes, until crispy, then add the onion and garlic and cook for 5 more minutes, until softened. Add the chicken stock, parsley, mustard, and seasoning and bring the mixture to a boil. Cook for 5 minutes, until the chicken stock has mostly evaporated, then add the cream and Parmesan cheese and reduce the heat to a simmer. Cook for 10 minutes, until the sauce has thickened.

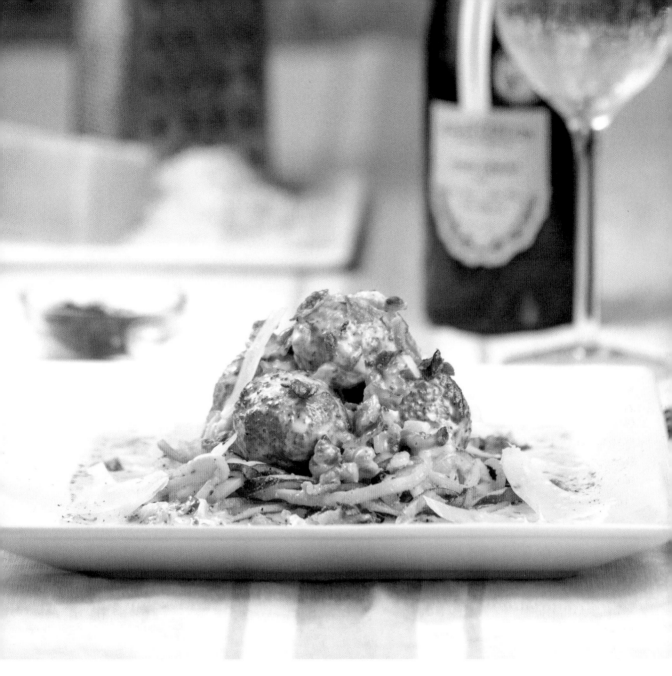

NUTRITION FACTS (PER SERVING)				
CALORIES	FAT	PROTEIN	NET CARBS	CARBS
1030	90g	49g	6g	6g
	79%	19%	2%	

7. Remove the meatballs from the oven and add them to the sauce. Simmer the meatballs in the sauce for a few minutes to ensure they are piping hot. Divide the zucchini "noodles" evenly among 4 plates and top with the meatballs and sauce. Sprinkle with extra Parmesan and chopped parsley. Store any leftovers in the refrigerator for up to 3 days.

ZUCCHINI, RICOTTA & PARMESAN LASAGNA

PREP TIME: 10 minutes

COOKING TIME: 1 hour 30 minutes

MAKES 8 servings

This family-size low-carb lasagna is a great make-ahead dish to reheat as needed. Layers of baked zucchini replace traditional pasta noodles, and add a lovely texture to the finished dish; you'll barely even notice you aren't eating pasta. For a dinner party, serve the lasagna with a simple Caesar salad with Parmesan crisps (see page 166 for the recipe, but omit the salmon).

ZUCCHINI "PASTA" LAYER

6 large zucchinis, sliced lengthwise into ¼-inch (6-mm)-thick planks (a mandoline works perfectly for this)

Fine sea salt and freshly ground black pepper

¼ cup (60 ml) olive oil

BOLOGNESE MEAT SAUCE

2 pounds (900 g) grass-fed ground beef (80% lean)

½ white onion, chopped

6 cloves garlic, minced

1 teaspoon dried oregano leaves

1 teaspoon chopped fresh thyme leaves, or ¼ heaping teaspoon dried thyme leaves

½ teaspoon freshly ground black pepper

1 (28-oz/785-g) can diced tomatoes

1 cup (240 ml) all-natural salted chicken stock

RICOTTA & PARMESAN LAYER

20 ounces (565 g) full-fat ricotta cheese

8 ounces (225 g) Parmesan cheese, grated, plus extra for the top

Fine sea salt and freshly ground black pepper

1. Prepare the "pasta" layer: Preheat the oven to 350°F (177°C). Line 3 sheet pans with parchment paper. Place the zucchini slices on the baking sheets in a single layer. Season well with salt and pepper and drizzle with the oil. Place in the oven and bake for 45 minutes, flipping the slices after 20 minutes. The idea is to dry out the zucchini as much as possible so that the finished lasagna is not soggy. When the zucchini is done, remove it from the oven and turn the temperature up to 400°F (205°C).

2. Meanwhile, make the Bolognese: Place a large saucepan over high heat. Put the ground beef in the pan and cook for about 5 minutes, until browned, crumbling the meat as it cooks. Drain the excess oil, then add the onion, garlic, herbs, and pepper; continue to cook the mixture for 5 more minutes, until the onion has softened.

3. Add the diced tomatoes and chicken stock to the beef mixture. Bring to a boil, then reduce the heat to a steady simmer and continue to cook for an additional 30 minutes, until the sauce has thickened, stirring often.

4. Make the ricotta-Parmesan layer: Mix the two ingredients together and season to taste.

5. Assemble the lasagna: Line a 12 by 8-inch (30.5 by 20-cm) baking pan with parchment paper. Start with a layer of meat sauce, then alternate layers of zucchini slices, cheese mixture, and meat sauce, finishing with the cheese mixture on top. Sprinkle some extra grated Parmesan on the top of the lasagna and bake for 40 minutes, until golden brown and bubbling.

6. Serve hot. Store leftovers in the refrigerator for up to 4 days.

NUTRITION FACTS (PER SERVING)				
CALORIES	FAT	PROTEIN	NET CARBS	CARBS
395	23g	35g	10g	12g
	52%	35%	10%	

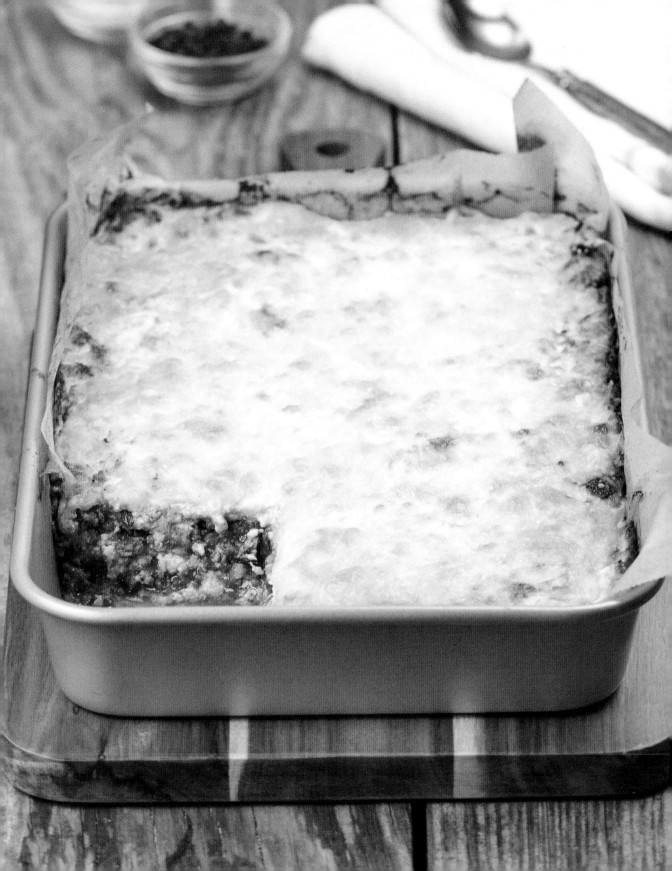

PESTO-MOZZARELLA CHICKEN
WITH CAPRESE SALAD

PREP TIME: 15 minutes

COOKING TIME: 25 minutes

MAKES 4 servings

Rich, flavorful pesto and creamy mozzarella make a classic flavor combination and a winning weeknight dinner. Chicken breasts are the base for a layer of pesto that is topped with mozzarella then baked until golden brown and bubbling. An heirloom tomato and mozzarella caprese salad is a simple pairing.

CHICKEN

1 whole boneless, skinless chicken breast (about 14 ounces)

¼ teaspoon fine sea salt

¼ teaspoon freshly ground black pepper

4 tablespoons (60 ml) store-bought pesto (see Note)

8 ounces (225 g) fresh mozzarella cheese, sliced

CAPRESE SALAD

3 large heirloom tomatoes

8 ounces (225 g) fresh mozzarella cheese

2 tablespoons extra-virgin olive oil

2 tablespoons store-bought pesto

Fine sea salt and freshly ground black pepper

FOR GARNISH

1 handful of fresh arugula

3 tablespoons pine nuts, toasted

1. Preheat the oven to 400°F (205°C). Line a sheet pan with parchment paper.

2. Slice the chicken breasts in half horizontally to make a total of 4 large, flat pieces. Place the chicken on the sheet pan and season evenly with the salt and pepper. Spread each chicken piece with 1 tablespoon of the pesto and top with the mozzarella cheese slices, dividing them evenly among the chicken. Bake for 25 minutes, or until the chicken is cooked through (it will be opaque throughout) and the mozzarella is golden and bubbling.

3. Meanwhile, make the caprese salad: Wash and slice the tomatoes, then slice the mozzarella cheese. Alternate the tomato slices with mozzarella slices in a fan-shaped arrangement on four serving dishes. Drizzle with the olive oil and pesto and season with salt and pepper to taste.

4. Serve the cooked chicken with the caprese salad and top with fresh arugula and a sprinkling of pine nuts. Store any leftovers in the refrigerator for up to 3 days.

NOTE

When buying store-bought pesto, be sure to check the ingredient label to make sure it is free of sugar. Make your own pesto if you are ambitious!

NUTRITION FACTS (PER SERVING)

CALORIES	FAT	PROTEIN	NET CARBS	CARBS
658	42g	58g	10g	12g
	57%	35%	6%	

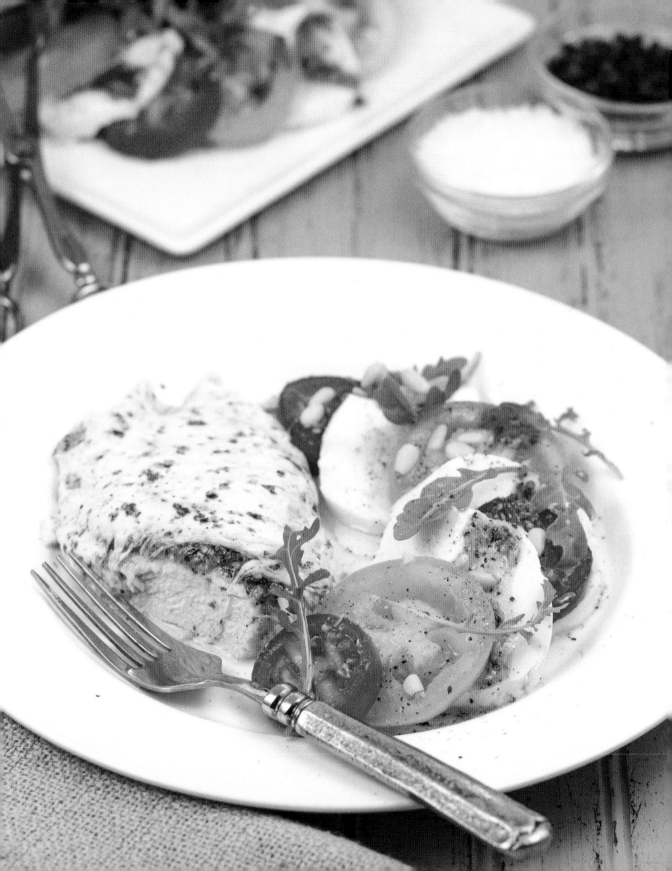

PORK LOIN SCHNITZEL
WITH TOMATO PESTO & MOZZARELLA

PREP TIME: 20 minutes + 1 hour to marinate
COOKING TIME: 35 minutes
MAKES 4 servings

Layers of creamy mozzarella and tangy tomato pesto broiled on top of breaded pork loin cutlets...Need we say more? For a balanced meal, serve this with a side of your favorite low-carb vegetables or a salad.

PORK SCHNITZEL

1 pound (450 g) boneless pork loin

1 cup (240 ml) full-fat buttermilk

Fine sea salt and freshly ground black pepper

1½ cups (165 g) almond flour

1½ cups (165 g) grated Parmesan cheese

2 large eggs

¼ cup (60 ml) olive oil

TOPPINGS

8 tablespoons store-bought tomato pesto

8 ounces (225 g) fresh mozzarella, sliced

Chopped fresh parsley, for garnish

1. Preheat the oven to 450°F (232°C). Line a sheet pan with parchment paper.

2. Slice the pork loin into 4 pieces (you can ask your butcher to do this for you when you buy it) and place each piece between 2 layers of plastic wrap. Use a rolling pin to pound the pork into ¼-inch (6-mm)-thick cutlets. Place the meat in a mixing bowl, add the buttermilk, and stir well to coat. Marinate for 1 hour (this helps tenderize the meat, but you can skip this step if you are short on time).

3. Remove the pork from the buttermilk and pat dry with paper towels. Season well with salt and pepper.

4. In a large mixing bowl, combine the almond flour and Parmesan cheese and mix well. In a small bowl, beat the eggs. Dip the pork cutlets in the beaten eggs and then in the almond flour mixture, making sure the cutlets are thoroughly coated on both sides. Transfer the cutlets to the prepared sheet pan and drizzle with the oil.

5. Bake the cutlets for 30 minutes, or until golden brown and no longer pink in the center, then remove from the oven.

6. Top each pork cutlet with 2 tablespoons of tomato pesto and one-quarter of the mozzarella slices. Turn on the broiler and, once it is fully hot, broil the pork cutlets for 5 minutes, until the cheese is melted, golden, and bubbling.

7. Remove the pan from the broiler and place the cutlets on individual serving plates. Garnish with fresh parsley and serve. Store any leftovers in the refrigerator for up to 3 days.

NUTRITION FACTS (PER SERVING)

CALORIES	FAT	PROTEIN	NET CARBS	CARBS
835	59g	62g	9g	14g
	64%	30%	4%	

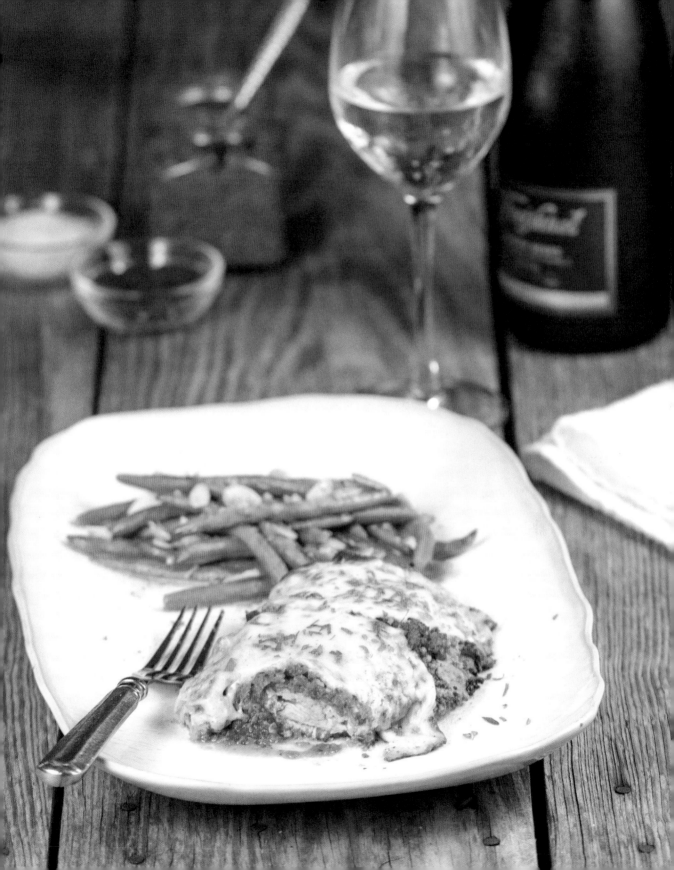

ALMOND & PARMESAN-CRUSTED BAKED SALMON
WITH BRAISED BROCCOLINI

PREP TIME: 10 minutes
COOKING TIME: 20 minutes
MAKES 4 servings

Before we found out about the benefits of a LCHF diet, panko breadcrumb–crusted salmon was one of our favorite midweek dinners. This new and improved recipe uses the same concept of fresh salmon fillets with a crunchy, flavorful topping, but it replaces the panko crumbs with a mixture of almonds and Parmesan cheese. This is a fantastic quick dinner.

SALMON

4 (6-oz/170-g) skin-on salmon fillets, ideally wild-caught

¼ teaspoon fine sea salt

¼ teaspoon freshly ground black pepper

¼ cup (60 ml) olive oil

PARMESAN CRUST

1 cup (110 g) grated Parmesan cheese

½ cup (55 g) almond flour

½ cup (42 g) sliced or chopped raw almonds

1 teaspoon chopped fresh dill

1 egg white

Pinch of fine sea salt

Pinch of freshly ground black pepper

BRAISED BROCCOLINI

2 tablespoons unsalted butter

2 (8-oz/225-g) bunches broccolini, stalks trimmed

½ cup (120 ml) all-natural salted chicken stock

4 ounces (110 g) cherry tomatoes

Fine sea salt and freshly ground black pepper

Zest of ½ lemon, cut into thin strips, for garnish (optional)

1. Preheat the oven to 400°F (205°C). Season the salmon fillets evenly with the salt and pepper, then place the fillets on a sheet pan.

2. Mix all the ingredients for the Parmesan crust in a large mixing bowl until fully combined.

3. Top each salmon fillet with the Parmesan crust mixture and press down lightly. Drizzle generously with the oil and place in the oven to bake for 20 minutes, or until opaque in the center.

4. Meanwhile, prepare the broccolini: Place a large frying pan over medium-high heat. Melt the butter in the hot pan until frothy, then add the broccolini and stir-fry for 2 to 4 minutes.

5. Add the chicken stock, cherry tomatoes, and a pinch each of salt and pepper, then cover the pan with a lid and cook for an additional 3 minutes.

6. Remove the lid and continue to cook over high heat for about 5 minutes, until the liquid has evaporated and the broccolini is tender and glazed.

7. Serve the cooked salmon over the broccolini. Garnish with lemon zest, if desired. Store any leftovers in the refrigerator for up to 3 days.

NUTRITION FACTS (PER SERVING)

CALORIES	FAT	PROTEIN	NET CARBS	CARBS
739	51g	54g	9g	16g
	62%	29%	5%	

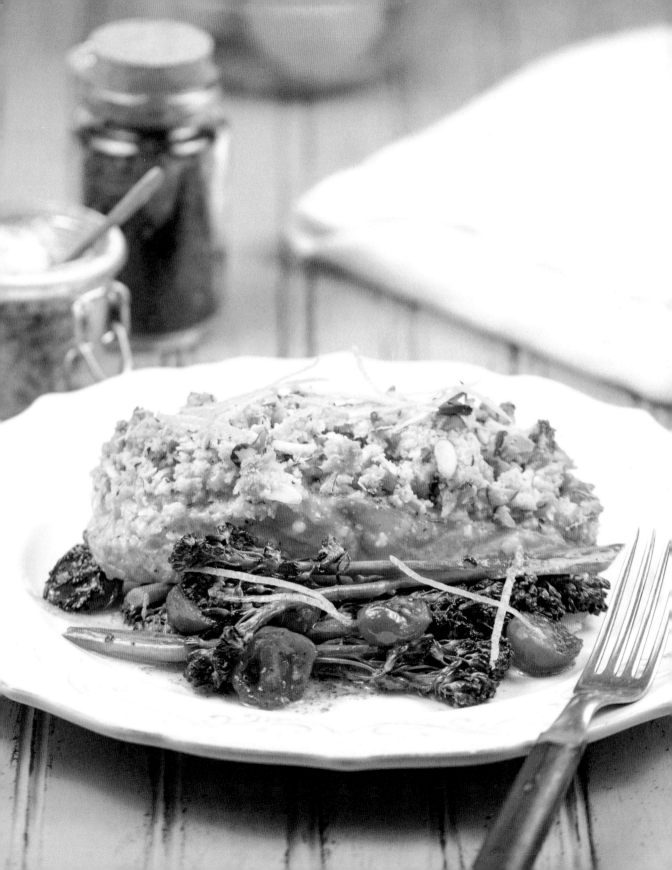

SHRIMP FRIED CAULIFLOWER "RICE"

PREP TIME: 15 minutes
COOKING TIME: 20 minutes
MAKES 4 servings

Cauliflower "rice" makes an excellent substitute for real rice, and, as an added bonus, it is even easier to make. This flavorful Asian-style fried "rice" is ready in 35 minutes—a great weeknight dinner. If you are feeling adventurous and have extra time, serve the "rice" with our delicious sesame shrimp "toast" (page 176) for a Chinese takeaway-like experience, minus the carbs and guilt.

3 tablespoons coconut oil

2 tablespoons minced ginger

3 cloves garlic, minced

½ red bell pepper, diced

1 pound (450 g) raw shrimp (preferably tail-on), peeled and deveined

1 pound (450 g) riced cauliflower (see Note)

1 teaspoon curry powder

1 teaspoon all-natural chili paste

½ cup (120 ml) all-natural salted chicken stock

2 tablespoons unsalted butter

¼ teaspoon fine sea salt

1 large handful of fresh cilantro, chopped

½ cup (50 g) mung bean sprouts

3 scallions, sliced on the diagonal

Lime wedges, for serving

NOTE

To rice cauliflower, see Step 1 of the recipe for Simple Cauliflower "Rice" on page 136; to get 1 pound (450 g) of riced cauliflower you will need 1 medium head of cauliflower (about 1½ lbs/675 g). Use store-bought riced cauliflower to save time if you can find it.

1. Place a large frying pan or wok over high heat, add the oil, ginger, garlic, and red bell pepper, and stir-fry for 5 minutes. Add the shrimp and continue to cook for 2 to 3 minutes more, until no longer translucent.

2. Add the riced cauliflower, curry powder, chili paste, chicken stock, butter, and salt and cover with a lid. Cook the mixture for 5 minutes, then remove the lid and continue to stir-fry for another 3 to 5 minutes, until the cauliflower is tender and the dish is aromatic.

3. Divide the fried "rice" among 4 serving plates and sprinkle with the cilantro, mung bean sprouts, and scallions. Serve with lime wedges.

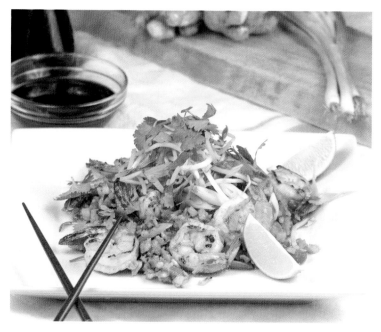

NUTRITION FACTS (PER SERVING)

CALORIES	FAT	PROTEIN	NET CARBS	CARBS
223	11g	19g	8g	12g
	44%	34%	14%	

SLOW COOKER BEEF STEW

PREP TIME: 15 minutes
COOKING TIME: 8 hours
MAKES 6 servings

Spend fifteen minutes of your morning preparing this stew and you'll have a wonderful, hearty dinner waiting for you when you get home! Low-carb cooking does not have to be labor-intensive. The addition of radishes may sound strange, but after slow-cooking, they lose their peppery bite and taste very similar to steamed new potatoes.

1¾ pounds (800 g) boneless chuck steak

2 tablespoons olive oil

10 ounces (280 g) radishes, peeled

6 cloves garlic, minced

½ white onion, diced

1 (14½-oz/400-g) can diced tomatoes

1 cup (240 ml) heavy cream

½ cup (120 ml) all-natural salted chicken stock

2 teaspoons ground mustard

Chopped fresh parsley, for garnish

1. Preheat a slow cooker to high.

2. Cut the chuck steak into 2-inch (5-cm) cubes. Heat a large frying pan over high heat, then pour the oil into the hot pan; when the oil is hot, add the steak cubes and brown on all sides for 5 minutes.

3. Place the browned meat and all the other ingredients in the slow cooker. Cover with the lid and cook on high for 8 hours.

4. After 8 hours of cooking, stir well, garnish with chopped parsley, and serve. Store leftovers in the refrigerator for up to 3 days.

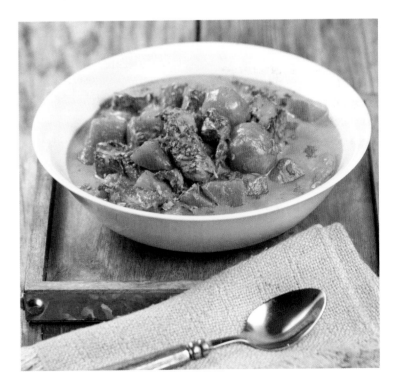

NUTRITION FACTS (PER SERVING)

CALORIES	FAT	PROTEIN	NET CARBS	CARBS
374	26g	28g	6g	7g
	63%	30%	6%	

PROVOLONE & HAM-STUFFED PORK TENDERLOIN

PREP TIME: 20 minutes
COOKING TIME: 40 minutes
MAKES 6 servings

Smoky melted cheese and cured ham make a simple and delightful filling for this crowd-pleasing meal. Serve the pork with a big green salad and, voilà, you have a perfect dinner for Sunday or any other day of the week!

1 boneless pork tenderloin (about 1½ lbs/675 g)

¼ teaspoon fine sea salt

¼ teaspoon freshly ground black pepper

1 pound (450 g) smoked full-fat provolone cheese, shredded

6 thin slices ham, preferably cured (see Note)

3 tablespoons olive oil

NOTE

For health and flavor, always buy high-quality ham, cut off the bone; avoid processed, reformed ham.

1. Preheat the oven to 400°F (205°C). Line a sheet pan with parchment paper.

2. Butterfly the pork tenderloin lengthwise and place between 2 sheets of plastic wrap (or ask your butcher to do this). Use a rolling pin to smash the meat into 1 flat piece, about ¼ inch (6 mm) in thickness.

3. Season the tenderloin with the salt and pepper and sprinkle the provolone cheese on top. Layer the ham over the cheese, then roll the tenderloin into a long roll and secure with cocktail skewers.

4. Place a large frying pan over high heat. Pour the oil into the pan and, once hot, add the tenderloin roll. Sear for 2 to 3 minutes on each side, until golden.

5. Transfer the roll to the prepared sheet pan and place in the oven. Cook for 35 minutes, or until golden brown and no longer pink in the middle.

6. When the tenderloin is cooked, remove it from the oven and allow to rest for 5 minutes. Cut into 1-inch (2.5-cm) slices and serve. Store any leftovers in the refrigerator for up to 3 days.

NUTRITION FACTS (PER SERVING)

CALORIES	FAT	PROTEIN	NET CARBS	CARBS
474	30g	48g	3g	3g
	57%	41%	3%	

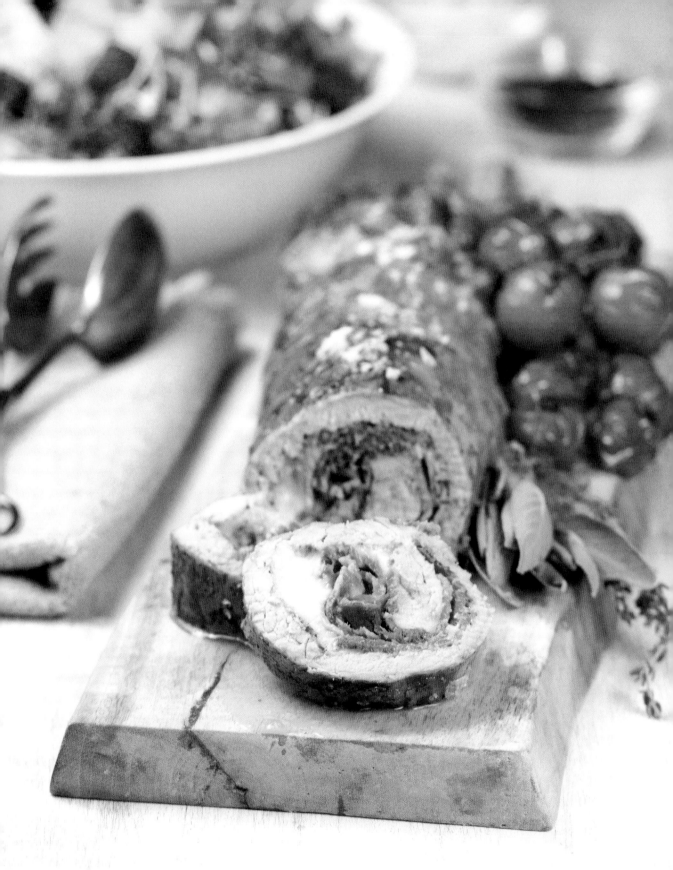

ONE-PAN THAI COCONUT CHICKEN & VEGETABLE BAKE

PREP TIME: 15 minutes + 1 hour to marinate
COOKING TIME: 45 minutes
MAKES 6 servings

This meal of spicy and sweet chicken pieces and roasted squash makes a great family-style centerpiece when served with a big bowl of cauliflower "rice" (page 136)—a simple yet satisfying dinner that involves minimal prep time. You will love how the coconut-coated chicken pieces come out: crispy on the outside and tender on the inside.

CHICKEN

1 whole boneless, skinless chicken breast (about 14 oz/400 g), or 2 boneless, skinless thighs, cut into 1-inch (2.5-cm) cubes (see Note)

6 ounces (170 g) coconut cream

2 tablespoons all-natural Thai red curry paste

½ cup (40 g) unsweetened shredded coconut

3 tablespoons coconut oil, melted

VEGETABLES

1 large yellow zucchini or summer squash, cut into ½-inch (1.25-cm) dice

1 large zucchini, cut into ½-inch (1.25-cm) dice

2 cloves garlic, minced

1 cup (140 g) peeled and cubed butternut squash

2 tablespoons olive oil

2 tablespoons all-natural Thai red curry paste

¼ teaspoon fine sea salt

¼ teaspoon freshly ground black pepper

GARNISH

1 handful of fresh cilantro, roughly chopped

1 handful of fresh basil, roughly chopped

2 tablespoons unsweetened shredded coconut

2 limes, halved or quartered

1 batch Simple Cauliflower "Rice" (page 136), for serving

1. Marinate the chicken: Place the chicken breast cubes, coconut cream, and curry paste in a large mixing bowl, stir well, and refrigerate for 1 hour to marinate.

2. Preheat the oven to 400°F (205°C). Have on hand a nonstick sheet pan or grease a metal sheet pan with coconut oil.

3. Remove the chicken cubes from the bowl, roll them in the shredded coconut, and set aside.

4. Prepare the vegetables: Place the zucchini, garlic, and butternut squash on the sheet pan. Add the olive oil and curry paste and mix well using your hands. Ensure that all the vegetables are covered in the oil and curry paste mixture, then season them with the salt and pepper. Bake the vegetables for 15 minutes.

5. Remove the sheet pan from the oven and add the coconut-crusted chicken pieces. Drizzle the chicken with the melted coconut oil and place the sheet pan back in the oven to cook for 30 minutes more, until the chicken is golden brown and no longer pink in the center.

6. Remove the pan from the oven, then garnish with the fresh cilantro and basil, shredded coconut, and lime halves or wedges. Bring the sheet pan right to the table and serve alongside a bowl of hot, steamed cauliflower "rice."

NOTE

Chicken thighs contain more fat, flavor, and calories than breasts.

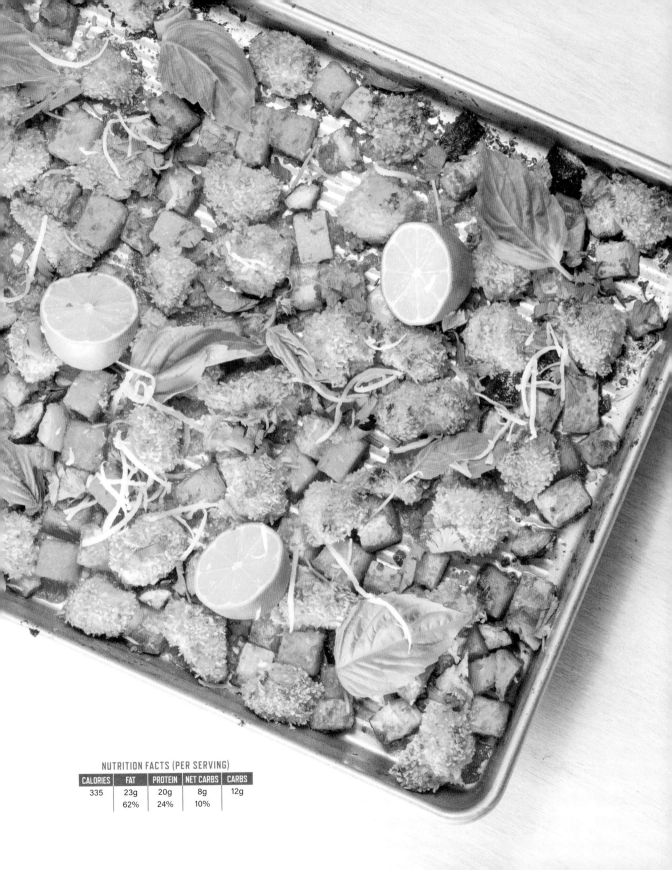

NUTRITION FACTS (PER SERVING)

CALORIES	FAT	PROTEIN	NET CARBS	CARBS
335	23g	20g	8g	12g
	62%	24%	10%	

SEARED LIVER
WITH BACON & WILD MUSHROOMS

PREP TIME: 15 minutes + 1 hour to marinate
COOKING TIME: 25 minutes
MAKES 4 servings

If you are a liver lover, you are going to really like this dish, and if you're not, give it a try anyway; this recipe may convert you! Liver is a fantastic source of nutrients and pairs beautifully with earthy morel mushrooms—or you can substitute any other mushroom of your choice for similar results. For a complete meal, serve with your favorite low-carb vegetables or a salad.

4 (4-oz/110-g) calves' liver steaks

1 cup (240 ml) full-fat buttermilk

4 tablespoons (60 ml) olive oil, divided

6 slices bacon, finely chopped

5 cloves garlic, minced

4 ounces (110 g) morel mushrooms or other mushrooms of your choice

1 cup (240 ml) all-natural salted chicken stock

1 stick (½ cup/110 g) cold unsalted butter, cubed

Fine sea salt and freshly ground black pepper

2 tablespoons chopped fresh parsley, or a handful of pea shoots, for garnish

1. Place the liver in a mixing bowl and add the buttermilk. Stir well and let marinate for 1 hour (this improves the flavor of the liver).

2. Heat a large frying pan over medium heat, then pour 2 tablespoons of the oil into the pan. When the oil is hot, add the bacon and sauté for 5 to 8 minutes, until golden brown. Add the garlic and morels and cook for 3 to 5 minutes more, until the mushrooms are tender.

3. Add the chicken stock and bring to a boil, then reduce the heat to a steady simmer and cook for about 5 minutes, until the liquid has reduced by two-thirds.

4. Reduce the heat to low and whisk in the cold butter until emulsified. You should have a smooth, buttery sauce. Slide the pan off the heat and move to the back of the stove to keep warm.

5. Remove the liver from the buttermilk and pat dry with a paper towel. Heat the remaining 2 tablespoons of oil in a frying pan over high heat. Season the liver steaks well with salt and pepper, then pan fry for about 2 minutes on each side; the liver should still be slightly pink in the middle (be careful not to overcook it since it can become dry, chewy, and grainy).

6. To serve family style, cut the steaks crosswise into ½-inch (1.25-cm) strips and place on a platter, then spoon the morel-butter sauce over the top and garnish with chopped parsley. Or divide the liver steaks among four serving plates, spoon the morel-butter sauce over the steaks, and garnish with chopped parsley. Store any leftovers in the refrigerator for up to 3 days.

NUTRITION FACTS (PER SERVING)

CALORIES	FAT	PROTEIN	NET CARBS	CARBS
619	51g	31g	8g	9g
	74%	20%	5%	

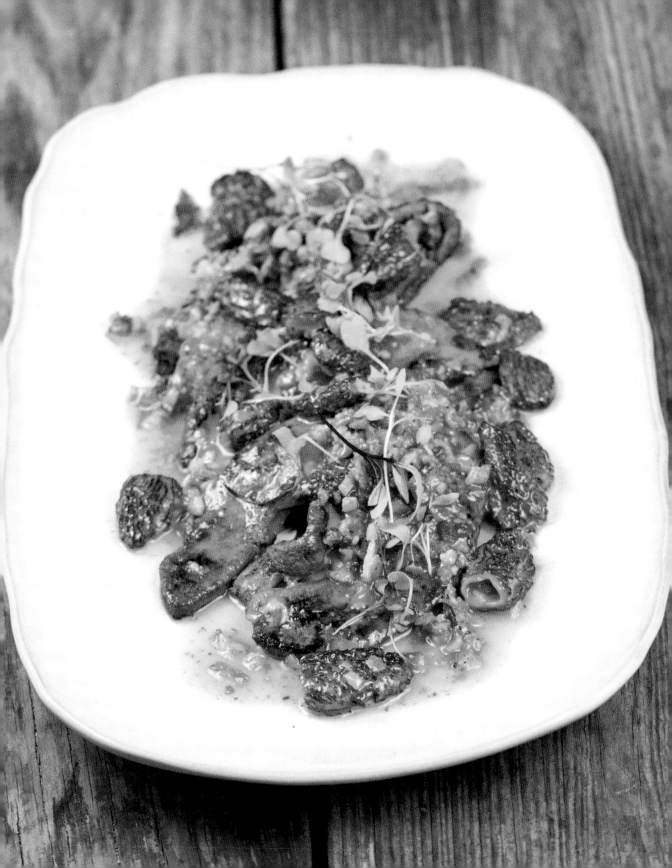

SLOW COOKER
CHICKEN IN CREAMY BACON SAUCE

PREP TIME: 10 minutes
COOKING TIME: 8 hours
MAKES 4 servings

This is an all-time favorite recipe, converted to a slow cooker method. The low and slow cooking ensures tender, flavorful chicken. Simply brown the chicken and bacon, put all ingredients in a slow cooker before work, and come home to a wonderful-smelling house and an irresistible dinner. For a complete, wholesome meal, pair this with any low-carb vegetable. Our favorite choice is grilled asparagus.

2 tablespoons olive oil

4 boneless, skinless chicken breast halves (about 1¾ lbs/780 g) or boneless, skinless chicken thighs (see Note)

¼ teaspoon fine sea salt

¼ teaspoon freshly ground black pepper

8 slices bacon, diced

1 cup (240 ml) heavy cream

½ cup (120 ml) all-natural salted chicken stock

1 teaspoon chopped fresh thyme leaves, or ¼ heaping teaspoon dried thyme leaves

½ teaspoon ground mustard

Chopped fresh parsley or a handful of pea shoots, for garnish

1. Preheat a slow cooker to high.

2. Heat a large frying pan until hot and add the oil. Season the chicken breasts evenly with the salt and pepper and add to the pan. Cook the chicken for 2 to 3 minutes on each side, until golden brown. Add the chopped bacon and cook for 2 minutes more, until crispy.

3. Place the browned chicken breasts, bacon, and all other ingredients in the slow cooker. Secure the lid and leave to cook on high for 8 hours.

4. After 8 hours, stir the ingredients well and season to taste. Garnish with fresh parsley and serve. Store any leftovers in the refrigerator for up to 3 days.

NOTE

Chicken thighs contain more fat, flavor, and calories than breasts.

NUTRITION FACTS (PER SERVING)

CALORIES	FAT	PROTEIN	NET CARBS	CARBS
573	37g	58g	2g	2g
	58%	40%	1%	

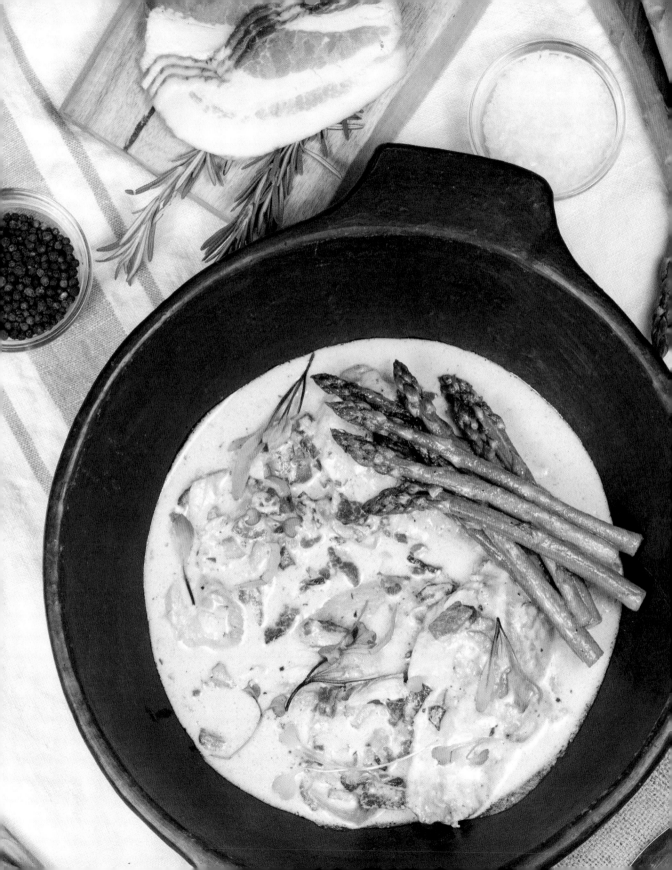

SQUID "PASTA"
WITH PAN-SEARED COD, CHORIZO & SPINACH

PREP TIME: 10 minutes + 2 hours to tenderize
COOKING TIME: 15 minutes
MAKES 4 servings

Make sure you use the freshest squid you can find for this delicious, summery dinner. Fresh fish should not taste fishy at all. Frozen squid will work, too, though fresh is preferred. Follow the directions carefully to end up with tender, not chewy, squid!

1 pound (450 g) cleaned squid tubes (fresh or frozen)

1 cup (240 ml) whole milk

3 tablespoons olive oil, divided

4 ounces (110 g) Spanish-style dry-cured chorizo sausage, sliced

5 ounces (140 g) fresh spinach

2 tablespoons unsalted butter

Fine sea salt and freshly ground black pepper

4 (6-oz/170-g) skinless cod fillets

Chopped fresh parsley, for garnish

Lemon wedges, for serving

1. Prepare the squid: Place a tube on a cutting board with a short end facing you. Slice lengthwise through one side to open it up into a large rectangle of flesh (do not cut all the way though, which would leave you with 2 pieces). Discard any remaining membrane inside the squid.

2. Cover the rectangle with a piece of plastic wrap. Use a metallic or wooden meat tenderizer or rolling pin to gently smash the squid into a uniformly thick layer—this will also soften its texture. Make sure that the squid pieces remain whole and aren't broken up.

3. Repeat this process for all the squid tubes, placing them in a large mixing bowl as you go. Cover the squid with the milk and place in the fridge for at least 2 hours to tenderize.

4. When you are ready to cook, remove the squid from the milk and pat dry using paper towels. Cut the pieces lengthwise into thin noodle-size strips.

5. Place a large frying pan over medium heat and pour 1 tablespoon of the oil into the pan. Add the chorizo and cook until crispy, 3 to 5 minutes. Add the spinach and butter and cook until the spinach is wilted. Add the squid and cook for about 1 more minute, stirring constantly, until the squid is opaque. Season well with salt and pepper, then slide off the heat and move to the back of the stove to keep warm.

6. Prepare the cod: Season each fillet with a generous pinch of salt and pepper. Place a large frying pan over high heat and pour the remaining 2 tablespoons of oil into the pan. Once hot, add the cod and pan-fry the fish for 5 minutes, until crispy and golden, then flip and cook for 2 to 3 minutes more, until no longer translucent in the center.

7. Divide the squid "pasta" evenly among 4 serving plates and top with the hot cod.

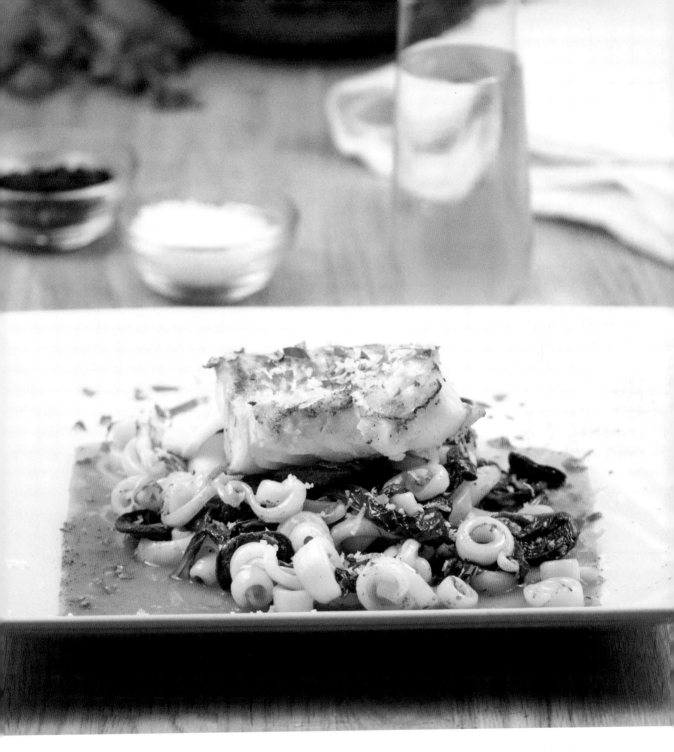

NUTRITION FACTS (PER SERVING)				
CALORIES	FAT	PROTEIN	NET CARBS	CARBS
362	14g	53g	5g	6g
	35%	59%	6%	

8. Garnish with chopped parsley and serve with a lemon wedge. Store any leftovers in the refrigerator for up to 2 days.

DOUBLE CHOCOLATE PUDDING

PREP TIME: 10 minutes + 3 hours to chill

COOKING TIME: 15 minutes

MAKES 4 servings

This rich chocolate pudding combines a chocolate egg custard and a silky chocolate sauce for a double chocolatey match made in heaven. Pudding can be dressed up as an excellent no-fuss dinner-party dessert or dressed down as a simple sweet snack to keep in the refrigerator. For a particularly pretty presentation, you can swirl the sauce into the pudding, and then top with the cream and berries.

PUDDING

2 teaspoons powdered unflavored gelatin

2 cups (480 ml) heavy cream, divided

½ cup (95 g) granulated low-carb sweetener of your choice

½ stick (¼ cup/55 g) unsalted butter

6 tablespoons (30 g) unsweetened cocoa powder

Pinch of fine sea salt

4 large egg yolks

1 teaspoon vanilla extract

CHOCOLATE SAUCE

½ cup (120 ml) heavy cream

3 tablespoons granulated low-carb sweetener of your choice

1 tablespoon unsweetened cocoa powder

Pinch of fine sea salt

FOR GARNISH

Fresh berries

Additional heavy cream

1. Make the pudding: Sprinkle the gelatin over ½ cup (120 ml) of the cream, whisk with a fork, and let rest for 5 minutes to bloom.

2. In a saucepan over medium heat, heat the remaining 1½ cups (360 ml) of the cream, sweetener, butter, cocoa powder, and salt almost to the point of boiling, whisking often.

3. While the cream mixture is heating, place the egg yolks in a large mixing bowl and lightly beat until well combined.

4. While whisking rapidly, slowly pour the hot cream mixture into the bowl with the egg yolks. Add the bloomed gelatin mixture and continue to whisk.

5. Return the cream-egg mixture to the saucepan and continue to cook over low heat, stirring constantly, until the mixture thickens and lightly coats the back of a spoon. Whisk in the vanilla extract.

6. Pour the mixture into a heatproof bowl. Place plastic wrap directly on the surface of the pudding to stop a skin from forming, let cool slightly, then place the pudding in the refrigerator until fully cooled and firm, about 3 hours.

7. Make the sauce: Place all the ingredients in a small saucepan and simmer over medium heat for 5 minutes, until thickened, stirring continuously. Pour the sauce into a small heatproof jar and place in the refrigerator to cool before using.

8. When ready to serve, remove the chilled pudding from the refrigerator and whisk well until it is smooth and glossy (you can do this by hand for a great biceps workout, or with an electric beater).

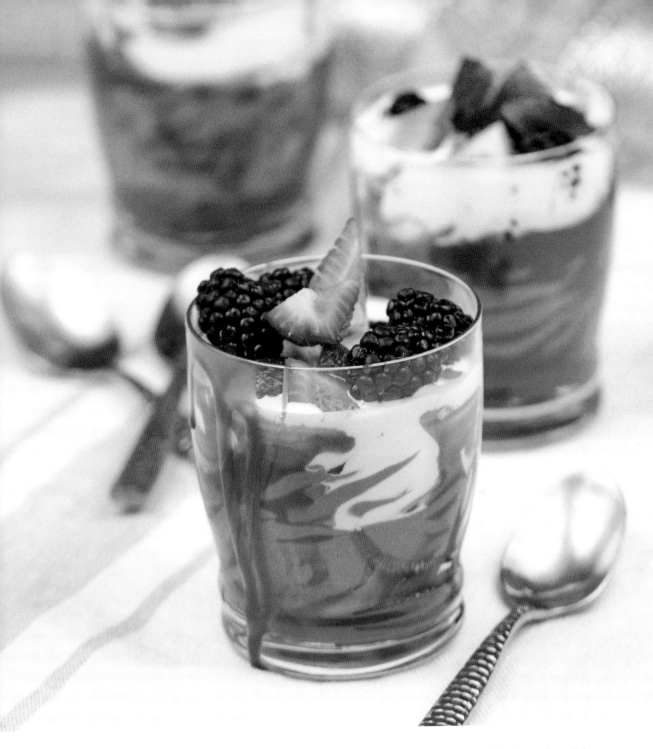

NUTRITION FACTS (PER SERVING)				
CALORIES	FAT	PROTEIN	NET CARBS	CARBS
745	71g	17g	8g	22g
	86%	9%	4%	

9. Divide the pudding among 4 individual serving dishes. Drizzle the cooled chocolate sauce on each serving and top with cream and fresh berries.

BLUEBERRY CUSTARD TART

PREP TIME: 20 minutes +
3 hours to chill

COOKING TIME: 55 minutes

MAKES one 9-inch (23-cm) tart
(12 servings)

This tart is a crowd-pleasing recipe that's perfect for picnics and summery lunches. It features the ingenious mozzarella pastry dough, which results in a buttery crust that tastes very similar to traditional pastry, and a velvety egg custard filling that is similar in texture to crème brûlée. Fresh berries and whipped cream top it off.

CRUST

1 recipe Mozzarella Pastry Dough (page 130)

BLUEBERRY CUSTARD FILLING

5 large egg yolks

2 large eggs

1½ cups (360 ml) heavy cream

1 cup (150 g) fresh blueberries

½ cup (120 ml) whole milk

½ cup (95 g) granulated low-carb sweetener of your choice

TOPPING

1 cup (240 ml) heavy cream

1 cup (150 g) fresh blueberries

1. Preheat the oven to 300°F (150°C).

2. Make the pastry dough according to the recipe instructions on page 130. Line a 9-inch (23-cm) round pie dish with the dough and cover it with parchment paper. Place the crust in the oven to par-bake for 15 minutes.

3. Make the filling: Place all the ingredients in a blender and blend on high until smooth, 2 to 3 minutes, then pour into the crust and return to the oven.

4. Bake the tart for 30 to 40 minutes, until the custard is just set but still has a slight wobble in the center. Chill for at least 3 hours or preferably overnight.

5. When the tart is fully chilled, whip the cream, spread over the top, and finish with a layer of fresh blueberries. Enjoy the tart cold and store in the refrigerator for up to 3 days.

NUTRITION FACTS (PER SERVING)

CALORIES	FAT	PROTEIN	NET CARBS	CARBS
509	45g	15g	8g	14g
	80%	12%	6%	

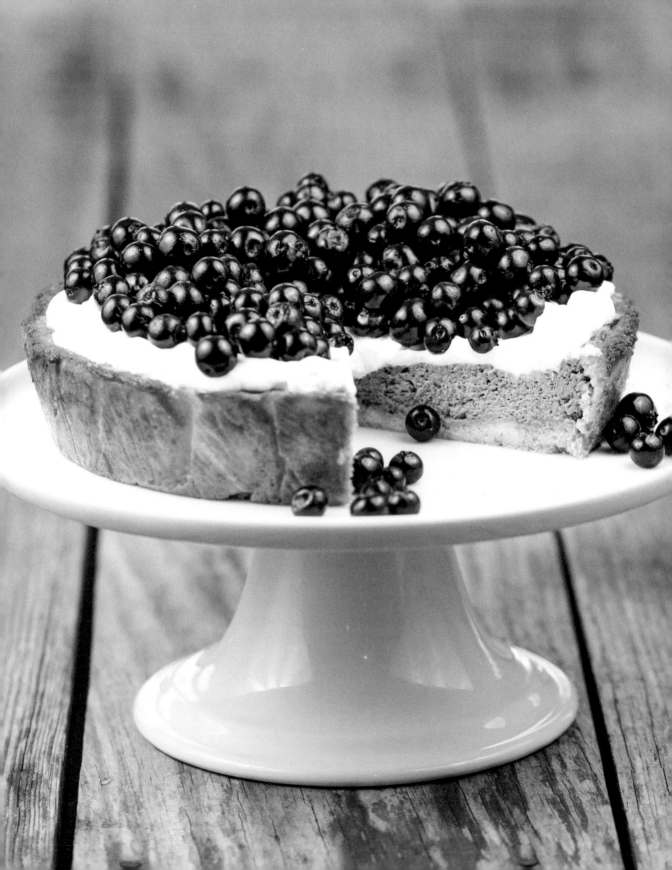

NO-BAKE STRAWBERRY CHEESECAKE
WITH ALMOND-MACADAMIA CRUST

PREP TIME: 35 minutes + 3 hours to chill
COOKING TIME: 5 minutes
MAKES one 8- or 10-inch (20- or 25-cm) cheesecake (12 servings)

This is one of our favorite cheesecake recipes. It is much lighter and silkier than a baked cheesecake, and because it is no-bake, it is simple and quick to make. Make this delicious and attractive cheesecake for a celebration or a family gathering and be the star of the party!

FILLING

3 cups (700 ml) heavy cream, divided

1 tablespoon powdered unflavored gelatin

4 ounces (110 g) full-fat cream cheese, softened

8 ounces (225 g) mascarpone cheese, softened

Seeds of 1 vanilla bean

¾ cup (145 g) granulated low-carb sweetener of your choice

CRUST

1 cup (135 g) raw macadamia nuts

2 cups (220 g) almond flour

¾ stick (6 tablespoons/85 g) unsalted butter, melted

¼ cup (48 g) granulated low-carb sweetener of your choice

1 teaspoon ground cinnamon

Pinch of fine sea salt

FOR GARNISH

1 pound (450 g) fresh strawberries, hulled and sliced

3 tablespoons chopped raw pistachios

1. Grease an 8- or 10-inch (20- or 25-cm) cheesecake pan (with a removable bottom), then line the bottom with parchment paper and grease the paper.

2. Bloom the gelatin for the filling: Pour ½ cup (120 ml) of the cream into a small saucepan, then sprinkle the gelatin over the top; whisk with a fork and let rest for 5 minutes.

3. Meanwhile, make the crust: Place the macadamia nuts in a food processor and process until the consistency resembles fine breadcrumbs. Transfer the macadamia nuts to a large mixing bowl, then add the almond flour, melted butter, granulated sweetener, cinnamon, and salt; mix the ingredients together with a wooden spoon until evenly combined.

4. Place the crust mixture in the prepared pan and press it into the bottom and up the sides to form a crust. Place the pan in the refrigerator to chill while you make the filling.

5. Place the saucepan with the bloomed gelatin-cream mixture over low heat and warm through until the gelatin is dissolved. Transfer the mixture to a small bowl and let cool to room temperature, about 10 minutes.

6. Place the cream cheese, mascarpone, vanilla bean seeds, and granulated sweetener in the bowl of a stand mixer fitted with the whisk attachment (or use an electric hand whisk and a large bowl). Whisk the cream cheese mixture for a few minutes, until it becomes light and creamy.

7. While whisking on low speed, slowly add the remaining 2½ cups (600 ml) of cream to the cream cheese mixture (this helps the consistency of the batter to stay smooth). When all of the cream has been added, turn the mixer to full power and whisk until the mixture takes on the consistency of stiff whipped cream.

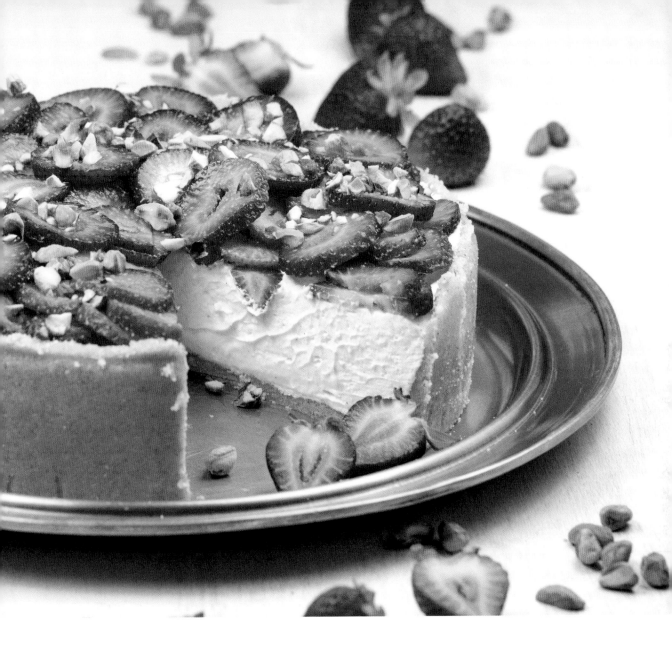

NUTRITION FACTS (PER SERVING)				
CALORIES	FAT	PROTEIN	NET CARBS	CARBS
591	56g	10g	8g	18g
	85%	7%	5%	

8. When the gelatin-cream mixture is cool, add it to the cheesecake mixture and, using a wooden spoon, stir very well to ensure that it is fully incorporated. Transfer the filling to the cheesecake pan and smooth the top with a spoon. Place the cheesecake in the refrigerator to chill for at least 3 hours.

9. When ready to serve, remove the cake from the pan and top with the sliced strawberries and a sprinkling of chopped pistachios. Store the cheesecake in an airtight container in the refrigerator for up to 4 days.

NO-CHURN
AVOCADO & SALTED PISTACHIO ICE CREAM

PREP TIME: 10 minutes + 3 hours to freeze

MAKES 8 servings

Avocados are often thought of as a savory food, but the creamy texture and mild flavor are wonderful complements to smooth, silky desserts like ice cream and cheesecake. This easy no-churn ice cream combines healthy fats with a hint of lemon juice to offset the richness; it's a great energy-boosting treat.

3 large ripe avocados, pitted and peeled

Juice of ½ lemon

¾ cup (145 g) granulated low-carb sweetener of your choice

2½ cups (600 ml) heavy cream, divided

⅓ cup (41g) shelled, salted pistachios, roughly chopped

Fresh sliced strawberries, for garnish

Whole shelled pistachios, for garnish

1. Line a 10-inch (25-cm) square baking pan with parchment paper. Place the prepared avocado, lemon juice, sweetener, and half of the cream in a blender and blend on high until completely smooth, about 1 minute. Remove the mixture from the blender and place in a large mixing bowl.

2. Whisk the remaining cream into soft peaks and fold into the avocado mixture. Add the chopped pistachios and transfer to the prepared pan.

3. Freeze for at least 3 hours before serving.

4. Use an ice cream scoop to serve the ice cream and garnish with sliced strawberries and pistachios.

5. Store the remaining ice cream in the freezer for up to 1 month.

NUTRITION FACTS (PER SERVING)

CALORIES	FAT	PROTEIN	NET CARBS	CARBS
393	38g	4g	4g	17g
	87%	4%	4%	

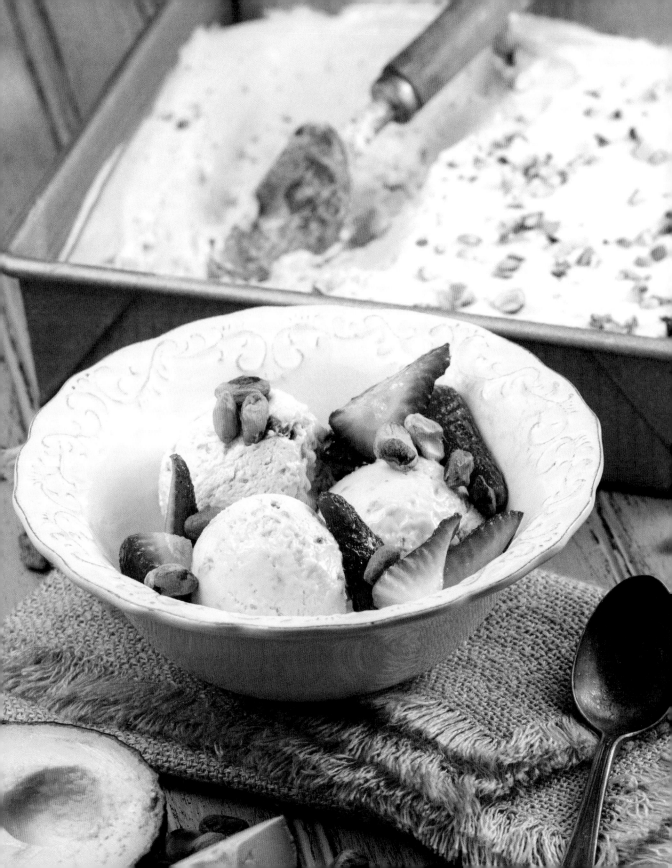

MINI RHUBARB CUSTARDS

PREP TIME: 20 minutes + 3 hours to chill
COOKING TIME: 20 minutes
MAKES 6 servings

The combination of rhubarb and custard is a very British, very delicious, tried-and-true pairing. Rhubarb is in season in the spring and increasingly available in the United States, so look for it at your local grocery store. Rhubarb is tart, but when cooked into a sweetened compote it becomes mellow and tangy; it's the perfect complement to a creamy custard.

CUSTARD

2 teaspoons powdered unflavored gelatin

2 cups (480 ml) heavy cream, divided

½ cup (95 g) granulated low-carb sweetener of your choice

Seeds of 1 vanilla bean

½ stick (¼ cup/55 g) unsalted butter

Generous pinch of fine sea salt

4 large egg yolks

RHUBARB LAYER

1 pound (450 g) rhubarb stalks, washed and chopped

½ cup (95 g) granulated low-carb sweetener of your choice

½ cup (120 ml) water

½ stick (¼ cup/55 g) unsalted butter

Chopped raw pistachios, for garnish

1. Make the custard: Sprinkle the gelatin over ½ cup (120 ml) of the cream, whisk with a fork, and let bloom for 5 minutes.

2. Place the remaining 1½ cups (360 ml) of cream, sweetener, vanilla bean seeds, butter, and salt in a saucepan over medium heat. Bring the cream mixture to almost boiling, whisking often to combine the ingredients thoroughly.

3. While the cream is heating, place the egg yolks in a large mixing bowl and lightly beat until well combined. While whisking rapidly, slowly pour the hot cream mixture into the bowl with the egg yolks. Add the bloomed gelatin mixture and continue to whisk.

4. Return the cream-egg-gelatin mixture to the saucepan and continue to cook over low heat, stirring constantly, until the mixture thickens and lightly coats the back of a spoon.

5. Pour the mixture into a heatproof bowl. Place plastic wrap directly on the surface to prevent a skin from forming, let cool slightly, then place the custard in the refrigerator for about 3 hours, until fully cooled.

6. Make the rhubarb layer: Place all the ingredients in a saucepan and bring to a boil over medium heat, then reduce to a light simmer and cook for 5 to 10 minutes, until the rhubarb is tender. Pour the mixture into a bowl, cover, and place in the refrigerator to cool for at least 3 hours.

7. Assemble the custards: Remove the custard mixture from the refrigerator and whisk well until smooth and glossy (you can do this by hand for a great biceps workout, or with a stand mixer or an electric beater).

8. Divide the rhubarb mixture among 6 ramekins or glasses and top with the custard. Sprinkle a few chopped pistachios on the tops for garnish. Store leftover custards, covered, in the refrigerator for up to 4 days.

NUTRITION FACTS (PER SERVING)

CALORIES	FAT	PROTEIN	NET CARBS	CARBS
381	36g	6g	4g	18g
	85%	6%	4%	

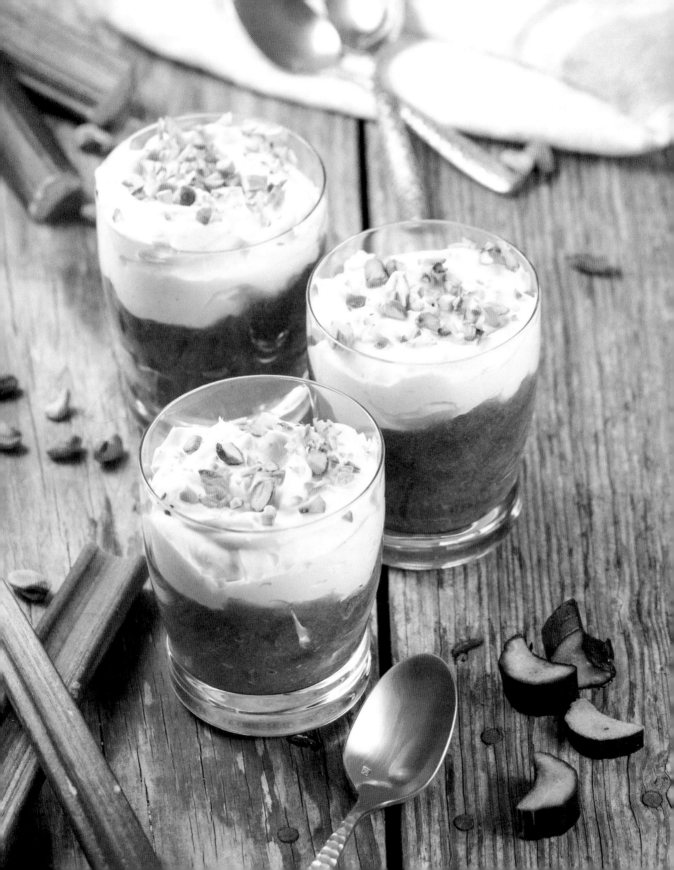

STRAWBERRY CHEESECAKE KETO "FAT BOMBS"

PREP TIME: 20 minutes + 1 hour to freeze
COOKING TIME: 25 minutes
MAKES 36 fat bombs (1 per serving)

Fat bombs are delicious little morsels loaded with healthy fats and calories—sweet treats that supply a boost of energy without the carb crash. These cheesecake fat bombs combine a smooth strawberry-laced base with crunchy almond-coconut cookie crumbs.

STRAWBERRY SAUCE

10 ounces (285 g) fresh strawberries, hulled and roughly chopped

5 tablespoons (60 g) granulated low-carb sweetener of your choice

1 tablespoon water

CRUNCHY COOKIE CRUMBS

1 large egg white

1 cup (110 g) almond flour

½ cup (40 g) unsweetened shredded coconut

3 tablespoons granulated low-carb sweetener of your choice

½ stick (¼ cup/55 g) unsalted butter

½ teaspoon ground cinnamon

½ teaspoon baking powder

Generous pinch of fine sea salt

FAT BOMB BASE

12 ounces (340 g) cream cheese, softened

¾ cup (110 g) whey protein powder

1 stick (½ cup/110 g) unsalted butter

1. Preheat the oven to 325°F (163°C). Line both a sheet pan and a 9-inch (23-cm) square baking pan with parchment paper, leaving some paper overhanging the square baking pan.

2. Make the strawberry sauce: Place the strawberries, sweetener, and water in a saucepan over medium heat. Bring the mixture to a boil, then reduce to a low simmer and cook for 10 minutes, until thickened. Remove the pan from the heat and let cool.

3. Make the cookie crumbs: Place all the ingredients in a large bowl and stir by hand until well combined. Spread the mixture out on the lined sheet pan, press down to form a smooth layer, and bake for 15 minutes, until golden brown. Remove the pan from the oven and cool, then crumble into small chunks. Remove 3 tablespoons of the crumbs and reserve for a garnish.

4. Place the fat bomb base ingredients in the bowl of a stand mixer, add the strawberry sauce, and whisk on high speed for 5 minutes, until smooth and creamy. Alternatively, use an electric hand mixer.

5. Add the cookie crumbs and lightly stir by hand with a spoon until well combined (do not use a mixer as you want the cookie crumbs to remain chunky).

6. Transfer the mixture to the prepared baking pan and sprinkle with the reserved cookie crumbs. Place in the freezer until firm, at least 1 hour. Lift the fat bomb batter out of the pan and slice into 36 small squares. Store the fat bombs in the freezer for up to 1 month and enjoy guilt-free ice cream–like treats whenever you like, straight from the freezer!

NUTRITION FACTS (PER SERVING)

CALORIES	FAT	PROTEIN	NET CARBS	CARBS
115	10g	4g	2g	4g
	78%	14%	7%	

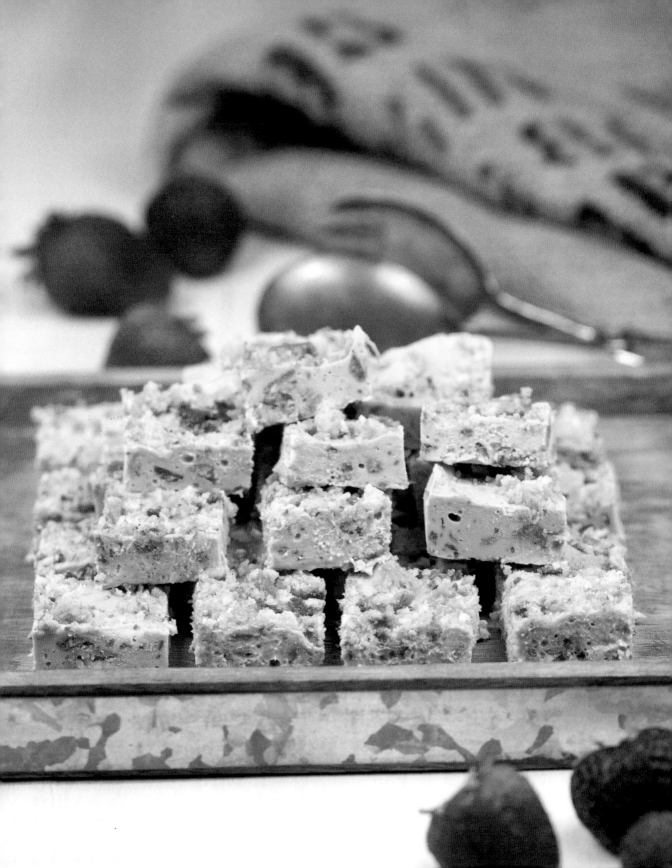

BUTTER "CAPPUCCINO"

PREP TIME: Less than 5 minutes
MAKES 2 servings

Butter coffee is an excellent jump start to your day. Blending high-quality, nutrient-rich fats into strong coffee offers sustained energy and keeps you sated for long periods.

2 cups (480 ml) strong-brewed hot coffee (dark roast works well)

¼ cup (60 ml) heavy cream, warmed

2 tablespoons unsalted butter, softened

Stevia or other low-carb sweetener (optional; we prefer ours unsweetened)

Ground cinnamon, for garnish

1. Place all the ingredients in a high-powered blender. (You can use a regular blender to make this, but the coffee won't be as frothy.)

2. Blend on high until smooth and frothy, about 1 minute.

3. Divide the mixture between two 8-ounce (240-ml) mugs, sprinkle each with a pinch of ground cinnamon, and serve immediately.

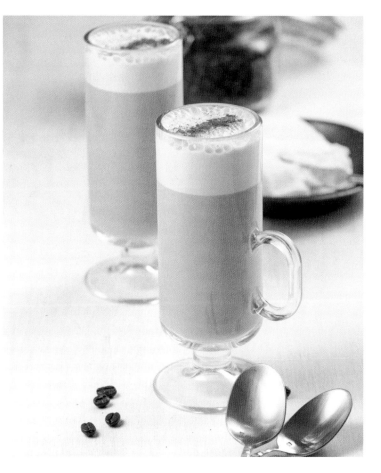

NUTRITION FACTS (PER SERVING)

CALORIES	FAT	PROTEIN	NET CARBS	CARBS
213	23g	1g	1g	4g
	97%	2%	2%	

VANILLA BEAN FRAPPÉ
WITH WHIPPED CREAM

PREP TIME: 5 minutes

MAKES 2 servings

This delightful concoction is very similar to the famous Starbucks Vanilla Bean Frappuccino, which is notorious for containing an astonishing amount of sugar.

1¼ cups (300 ml) heavy cream

1½ cups (360 ml) ice

1 cup (240 ml) unsweetened almond milk

¼ cup (48 g) granulated low-carb sweetener of your choice

Seeds of ½ vanilla bean

Whipped cream, for garnish

1. Place all the ingredients in a blender and blend on high until smooth and creamy, about 1 minute.

2. Pour the mixture into two 12-ounce (360-ml) serving glasses and top with whipped cream.

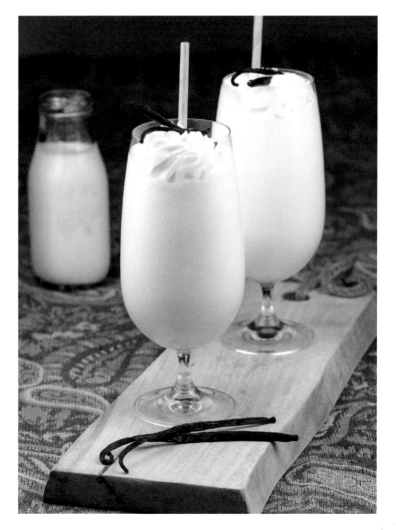

NUTRITION FACTS (PER SERVING)

CALORIES	FAT	PROTEIN	NET CARBS	CARBS
542	56g	5g	5g	18g
	93%	4%	4%	

CUCUMBER & RASPBERRY MOJITO MOCKTAIL

PREP TIME: 5 minutes
MAKES 2 servings

This refreshing "mocktail" can also be made into a real mojito with the addition of a bit of white rum or vodka. The flavors of mint and cucumber with a hint of raspberry make this an ideal summer beverage—virgin or not!

6 lime wedges

10 mint leaves

6 slices cucumber

2 tablespoons granulated low-carb sweetener of your choice

½ cup (60 g) fresh raspberries

Crushed ice, to top

Seltzer water, to top

2 fresh mint sprigs, for garnish

1. Divide the lime wedges, mint, cucumber, and sweetener between two tall 12-ounce (360-ml) glasses with sturdy bottoms. Muddle (crush and mix) the ingredients with a cocktail muddler or the handle of a wooden spoon.

2. Put ¼ cup (30 g) of the raspberries in each glass and fill three-quarters full with crushed ice. Top each glass with seltzer water, stir well, and finish with additional crushed ice and a sprig of fresh mint. Serve immediately with a straw.

NOTE

If you prefer a boozy alternative, add 1½ ounces (45 ml) of white rum or vodka to each glass with the raspberries.

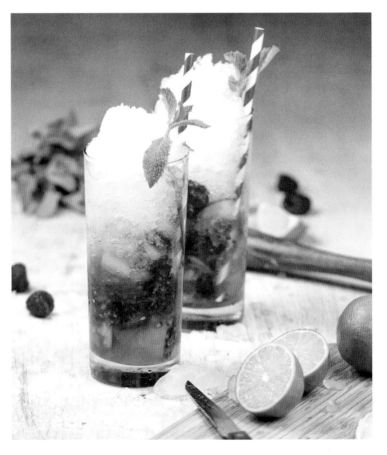

NUTRITION FACTS (PER SERVING)

CALORIES	FAT	PROTEIN	NET CARBS	CARBS
39	0g	1g	3g	12g
	0%	10%	31%	

INDULGENT
CHOCOLATE MILKSHAKE

This rich, creamy milkshake is a perfect pick-me-up when you don't have time to make a dessert. Simply throw all the ingredients in a blender for one minute. If you have the time and the desire, top with whipped cream, nuts, and a sprinkle of cocoa powder.

1½ cups (360 ml) ice

1 cup (240 ml) unsweetened almond milk

1 cup (240 ml) heavy cream

¼ cup (20 g) unsweetened cocoa powder

¼ cup (48 g) granulated low-carb sweetener of your choice

FOR GARNISH (OPTIONAL)

Whipped cream

Chopped toasted nuts of your choice

Sprinkle of unsweetened cocoa powder

1. Place all the ingredients in a blender and blend on high until smooth and creamy, about 1 minute.

2. Pour into two 12-ounce (360-ml) serving glasses and top with whipped cream, chopped nuts of your choice, and sprinkle of cocoa powder, if you wish.

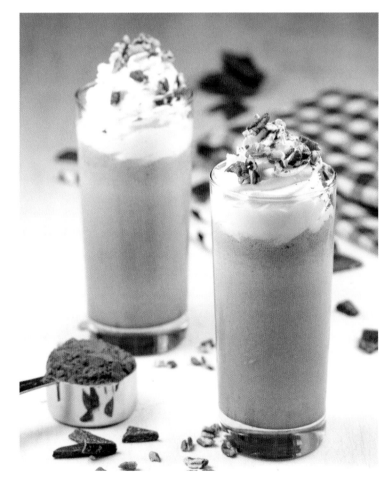

NUTRITION FACTS (PER SERVING)

CALORIES	FAT	PROTEIN	NET CARBS	CARBS
490	46g	6g	7g	22g
	84%	5%	6%	

3

EAT RICH, LIVE LONG: THE DEEPER DIVE

"Hyperinsulinemia [high insulin] adversely affects almost all degenerative diseases. That includes coronary artery disease, hypertension, cancer, stroke, diabetes, of course, obesity, autoimmune disorders, and mental disease and decline."

—Dr. Ron Rosedale

CHAPTER 10

MOST OF US HAVE DIABETES:
INSULIN AS A MASTER GAUGE OF CHRONIC DISEASE

There are two rules of Longevity Club. The first rule of Longevity Club is, respect your insulin. The second rule of Longevity Club is … respect your insulin.

Okay, so that's obviously paraphrased from *Fight Club*. It is entirely appropriate.

This chapter is perhaps the most important one in the book. There is no more important factor in weight loss and longevity than your insulin status—period. The single unifying factor among people who live to over one hundred years of age is a low insulin status.[1]

Insulin status is central to the modern epidemic of obesity and ill health. The profound importance of this truth is finally being recognized in the scientific literature.[2] We have a terrifying obesity epidemic, intimately linked to high insulin. We have an exploding type 2 diabetes epidemic—also related to high insulin. We have a growing Alzheimer's epidemic, with some leading researchers now calling the disease "type 3 diabetes" because it's related to insulin resistance in the brain. And rates of cardiovascular disease are steadily growing out of control—yet another high-insulin issue.

We have failed to focus on the primary root causes of all these problems while distracting ourselves with surrogate sideshows.

THE ROOT CAUSES OF MANY DISEASES

Heart disease is the world's biggest cause of premature death. It beats all cancers combined, although cancer rates are catching up. Similar root causes drive both diseases, and many others. We must look at the young victims of heart disease to find out what the most important causes are. As mentioned in Chapter 4, teenagers who have the insulin dysregulation of MIRS can exhibit fifteen times the risk for heart disease by the time they reach their forties. Compare this to the statistical noise of cholesterol's predictive power.

In 2015, the cardiology field was beginning to recognize the central importance of diabetic physiology in driving cardiovascular disease. Scientists had known for some time that diabetes drove heart disease like nothing else. But they also believed that diabetes was not overly common, even though rates had been climbing for years—there appeared to be many other important causes to focus on. But the 2015 EuroAspire study revealed the reality.[3]

In the EuroAspire study, researchers took a random sample of coronary artery disease (CAD) patients ages eighteen to eighty across twenty-four countries of Europe. (This paper uses the term "coronary artery disease" while we tend to use "coronary heart disease"; they're essentially the same.)

First, they needed to take out the CAD patients who already had full-blown diabetes. Nearly a third of them turned out to be known type 2 diabetics. They didn't need to look any closer at these guys. The study team already knew that type 2 diabetes massively drives coronary disease.[4]

But what was going on with the remaining folks, the apparently nondiabetic coronary-diseased people? What did their blood glucose metrics look like when scrutinized?

These "nondiabetics" were riddled with diabetes.

Figure 10.1. More than a third of CAD victims were already diagnosed diabetics, but more than three-quarters were essentially diabetic. Source: V. Gyberg et al., "Screening for Dysglycaemia in Patients with Coronary Artery Disease as Reflected by Fasting Glucose, Oral Glucose Tolerance Test, and HbA1c: A Report from EUROASPIRE IV—a Survey from the European Society of Cardiology," *European Heart Journal* 36, no. 19 (2015): 1171–77.

Coronary Disease Victims, Ages 18–80, Across All of Europe

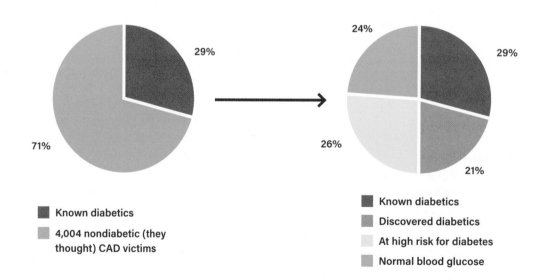

A shocking picture emerged.

► Nearly a third of the "nondiabetics" were found to have full-blown diabetes. They are shown in the orange segment in Figure 10.1.

► Over a third more were found to be at "high risk for diabetes" (yellow). Which, by the way, *is* having diabetes—"high risk for diabetes" is a misleading way of putting it. Even though standard lab tests for diabetes focus on blood glucose, you can be diabetic while your glucose metrics remain normal if you have elevated levels of insulin, which would keep your glucose under some control. By the time your glucose metrics show that you're at "high risk for diabetes," your blood glucose has actually been spiraling for some time—it's just that now your insulin can no longer control it. (This is why testing insulin levels is a much better way of evaluating diabetes risk.)

► The remaining third appeared to have reasonable blood glucose metrics (green). But, as mentioned above, blood glucose is a very weak measure for identifying diabetes. You need to use insulin measures to properly test for this disease. We predict that if insulin had been properly tested, many of these people would have insulin-signaling issues. In other words, they would be shown to be essentially diabetic.

Diabetes is a vascular disease. It manifests itself specifically through vascular damage. Here's how renowned pathologist Dr. Joseph R. Kraft, whose pivotal work on insulin response we'll discuss shortly, put it: "Based upon my several thousand autopsy examinations, the pathology of diabetes is vascular. The initial manifestation of the pathology of diabetes is atherosclerosis. The pathology begins when the blood sugars are normal."[5] Blood sugar may be normal in these cases, but insulin isn't.

The reality is that coronary artery disease is overwhelmingly the vascular disease of diabetes. To avoid it, you mainly have to ensure that you are the exact opposite of diabetic—that you're insulin sensitive. There are other elements, but being insulin sensitive will mostly put you in the clear. The focus on cholesterol has been a weapon of mass distraction from the real cause of CAD for more than fifty years. We can't get that time back—the millions who were lost shall remain lost.

Another landmark study released in 2015 provides another bombshell. It reveals that *the majority of adult Americans are now essentially diabetic.*[6] The distinction between prediabetes and diabetes is arbitrary and misleading— it's based only on how much the diabetic problem has progressed. Currently prediabetes is only called diabetes when you have *late-stage* insulin dysfunction and your blood glucose has finally gone out of control. We don't make a distinction between prediabetes and diabetes, because doing so makes no sense whatsoever. The diabetic disease state is an insulin disease state—one of hyperinsulinemia (high insulin) and accompanying insulin resistance. And the reality is that most Americans now have some form of it, no matter what it's called. The more hyperinsulinemia and insulin resistance you have, the higher your risk of death, not just from cardiovascular disease but also from a dizzying range of common diseases that drive early mortality, including Alzheimer's, cancer, and other diseases of the liver, kidneys, and other organs.

FORGET GLUCOSE—THINK INSULIN

How did we reach a point where the majority of adult Americans are now essentially diabetic—a situation in which the rising rates of cardiovascular and other diseases are being driven by this modern epidemic?

We must always remind ourselves that type 2 diabetes is a disease of hyperinsulinemia and insulin resistance, not a disease of blood sugar. (And throughout this chapter, when we refer to "diabetes," we mean type 2 diabetes—it's the form of diabetes that can be prevented through diet and the form that's ravaging America today.) It is fundamentally a disease of damaged insulin signaling. Therefore, the correct way to diagnose the problem is to scrutinize blood insulin metrics, which is rarely done.

How did the research on how diabetes works not lead to routine insulin testing as part of a regular checkup? The problem is that a major symptom of late-stage diabetes is elevated blood glucose. Tragically, it was possible to measure glucose long before measuring insulin became simple to do. As a result, diabetes became mistakenly defined as a disease of blood glucose levels. The implications of the mistake have been devastating.

True, an elevated fasting blood glucose is very damaging to the body's blood vessels and organs. But high blood glucose only develops after decades of high insulin have already wreaked havoc—by then it's too late for most people. Countless people who don't even know they have diabetes die of cardiovascular disease and other diseases long before they get any warning. To find out in time that you are heading for the rocks, you need to focus on your insulin signaling. It will tell you when the problem starts.

People with full-blown diabetes exhibit increased rates of most chronic diseases. This is to be expected. This occurs because a diabetic state is ultimately a state of accelerated aging. The usual effects of aging are, among others, oxidative stress, cellular damage, and failing repair mechanisms.

Diabetes hypercharges these processes, which is why it has such grim implications for mortality. The legions of undiagnosed diabetics around us are all suffering from the results of this accelerated aging: elevated risk for cancer, arthritis, Alzheimer's, and more. They also suffer greatly from vascular damage and chronic infection, which lead to limb amputations, loss of eyesight, and other dreadful afflictions—the list goes on and on. Because most American adults now share this insulin-regulation disease, the majority of them are experiencing chronic afflictions long before they should. This situation is the primary cause of early mortality.

INSULIN: A BILLION YEARS IN THE DRIVER'S SEAT

Insulin is one of the oldest molecules in the biology of life on our planet. Many estimates put its origins in the primordial past—more than eight hundred million years ago.

Life on Earth began in the oceans. Success was determined by what could reproduce most effectively. Glucose was the primary fuel source a bil-

---

LOW INSULIN AND HIGH CARB?

Historically, the many tribal populations that consumed low-carb or keto diets (Maasai, Inuit/Yupik, !Kung, and others) achieved very low insulin with ease. In fact, one study suggests that "nearly 9 out of 10 of the diets of hunter-gatherer groups had less than a third of calories coming from carbohydrates."[7] But interestingly, even tribal populations eating a higher-carb whole-foods diet often have good health and low insulin. For example, the indigenous Kitavan people in Papua New Guinea are the clichéd paragon of slimness, health, and long life—in spite of eating significant quantities of whole-food, non-refined carbohydrates. Despite the carbohydrate in their diet, they achieved very low insulin levels. But their unparalleled application of the other rules enabled them to manage the glucose load.

Sadly, trying to achieve low insulin with a high-carb diet by following the other rules is a risky strategy in the modern environment, outside the hunter-gatherer lifestyle—adherence is difficult and failure widespread. There is no question that the low-carb approach is vastly more appropriate and workable for our modern population. It is a no-brainer due to the massive advantage it brings. So there may be different routes to optimal health, but the smart people go with the superior route. And the target always remains the same:

Achieve low insulin.

---

lion years ago. Early life-forms developed nutrient-sensing molecules that would enable rapid reproduction when glucose was plentiful. They would also trigger a lockdown survival mode when it was not. Although much has since changed, these fundamentals remain. The most crucial of these nutrient-sensing molecules was insulin.

Organisms became more complex with time and the changing environment. While early life-forms didn't require oxygen to use glucose—there was no oxygen in the atmosphere back then—as oxygen increased in the atmosphere, organisms evolved to use it to produce energy. The earliest oxygen-using cells were mitochondria, and with time they were incorporated into other organisms. They gave these mother organisms the ability to burn fat as a fuel, using oxygen to do so. We humans now have trillions of these mitochondria in our bodies. Without them and their fat-burning ability, we would cease to exist. They are our power plants, built into our bodies during a billion years of development.

Insulin was the first nutrient sensor and triggered rapid growth when glucose was plentiful. Other sensors developed later as the organisms became more complex. We now have insulin (for glucose), mTOR (for protein), and leptin (for fat). The interplay of these sensors is critically important. Insulin and leptin are hormones released by our pancreas and our fat cells, respectively. mTOR is like a complex microprocessor that responds to dietary protein directly, but also to all other dietary elements through insulin and other diet-driven signals—it integrates the signals from many other feedback loops. All three sensors work together to keep our bodies running optimally. They manage the harsh nutritional environments we encounter. When their signaling is damaged, disease results.

When dietary glucose is kept moderate or low, our bodies perceive that a challenging environment exists because we evolved from single-cell organisms that were forced to rely totally on glucose. Like those early life-forms, the body focuses on extending life through many mechanisms in order to survive until conditions improve. We can tap into this ancient machinery for our longevity advantage.

Insulin also promotes growth—beneficial growth when insulin is at appropriate levels, bad kinds of growth when it is too high. An example is the dangerous "growth" of our blood vessel walls in diabetes and cardiovascular disease, as they swell from inflammatory insults and debris buildup. Here's another example: when insulin and glucose are high, exposing us to factors that disrupt our cellular-signaling systems, our cells tend toward triggering their ancient genetic desire to reproduce as fast as possible. We now have a name for this kind of phenomenon. We call it "cancer."

INSULIN THE MASTER HORMONE

The power of hormones becomes clear if you consider the example of adrenaline. Anyone who has experienced panic knows what it feels like: rocketing fear, racing heart, explosive perspiration. Hormones carry massively powerful effects.

Insulin is also a hormone, one released by the pancreas. Here's how it works: When carbohydrate foods reach your upper intestine, they trigger another key hormone, glucose-dependent insulinotropic polypeptide (GIP). This carb-driven spurt of GIP streaks to your pancreas and to your fat cells. In the pancreas, it triggers a surge of insulin release. In fat cells, it gets things ready for fat-storage mode.

The surge of insulin flashes around your body, triggering your cells to get ready to absorb glucose. It stops the release of other hormones, such as glucagon, in order to prevent inappropriate glucose production in your liver. It tells the hypothalamus in your brain that glucose is on the way in order to control your appetite. It tells your body to stop burning fat and preferentially burn the glucose coming down the hatch—glucose is dangerous if it remains at a high level in the bloodstream, so it must be prioritized for burning immediately or be turned into body fat for storage. Insulin does all this and much more. It is truly the master regulator of your body.

If you keep your insulin levels low, all these signals are highly effective. Your body will stay exquisitely sensitive to insulin's messages. This is pivotal for longevity and slimness. There are many strategies for keeping your insulin low. Here are a couple of the most important approaches, all of which were discussed at length in Parts 1 and 2:

► Don't consume too much carb, which is mainly made up of glucose.

► Don't consume processed carb or processed vegetable oils.

► Absolutely don't ingest carbs along with fatty foods—a very bad combo indeed.

► Don't consume too much fructose.

► Do not eat frequently—rather, eat well-spaced meals. Snacking screws up your insulin signaling.

Excessive carb drives excessive insulin. Processed carb in particular leads to explosive GIP release in the gut—driving truly excessive insulin. Carb and fat together really jack up GIP and consequently insulin. Fructose drives insulin problems in the liver, promoting bad cholesterol along the way. These are the main mechanisms that a low-carb, high-fat diet tackles.

There are also emerging studies that show that gut microbiome problems—issues with the balance of good and bad bacteria in your gut—can also drive insulin dysregulation.[8] In fact they may be very significant drivers in the modern population. Luckily, the steps to improve your microbiome are largely the same steps you would take to tackle insulin problems directly.

Finally, insulin acts as a master gauge to flag many other things that are damaging your body. Insulin and insulin resistance both rise in response to chronic stress, poor sleep, smoking, air pollution, infections, and many other insults.

The bottom line? Respect your insulin—and do everything you can to keep it low and healthy.

DR. REAVEN KNEW THE SCORE

What is the consequence of not respecting your insulin—of triggering it too much and too often? In short, you will embark on a long steady descent into chronic disease. You'll also greatly reduce your ability to maintain a healthy body weight. There's no beating the science on this one.

Gerald M. Reaven is an American endocrinologist and professor emeritus in medicine at the Stanford University School of Medicine. Reaven's work on insulin resistance and diabetes goes back to the 1970s. He created the term *metabolic syndrome* to describe humankind's epidemic insulin dysfunction (we've referred to it as metabolic insulin resistance syndrome, MIRS—see page 47). After decades of work, he understood the enormous implications of this problem. In 2012, he finally conducted a study to verify how massively important it really was. The results surprised even him.[9]

Reaven and his team randomly selected 208 apparently healthy middle-aged people. None were obese. Not one of them had a body mass index over 30, the standard cutoff for obesity. The research team measured their insulin status using an extremely accurate method (SSPG). The method was very important to get right. One of the reasons that the importance of insulin is grossly underestimated is that poor methods have been and are being used to measure it. Reaven did not make this mistake.

The team split the participants into three groups based on their insulin status: low, medium, and high. Then they monitored them for more than six years to see how they fared. Here's what the researchers found: *all that really mattered was insulin status.*

	LOW Insulin Resistance	MEDIUM Insulin Resistance	HIGH Insulin Resistance
Disease	0	10	24
Death	0	2	4
Total tragedy	0	12	28

Figure 10.2. Our future health depends on our place on the insulin spectrum. Source: F. S. Faccini, N. Hua, F. Abbasi, and G. M. Reaven, "Insulin Resistance as a Predictor of Age-Related Diseases," *Journal of Clinical Endocrinology & Metabolism* 86, no. 8 (2001): 3574–78.

As you can see in Figure 10.2, the one-third who were lowest in insulin had no incidence of disease or death. The middle third had twelve disease diagnoses; of those, two had died by the end of the study. The upper third had twenty-eight disease diagnoses; of those, four died. The diseases seen in the participants were the usual ones that have been connected to insulin issues for decades: type 2 diabetes (5), heart disease (7), cancer (9), hypertension (12), and stroke (4). As mentioned, most diseases of aging are intricately connected to insulin and its connected biochemical pathways. When it is not causing problems, insulin acts as a master gauge of these diseases.

It is important to note that when a study uses a moderate sample size like this and participants are chosen in a fair and random manner, the conclusions cannot be questioned. More than two hundred people, correctly sampled, is a sample size plenty large enough to statistically prove the relevance of variables.

The team carried out a thorough analysis of the data. No factor among the many other measurements taken was significant, other than insulin—the insulin-resistance measure was the key. When corrected for this factor, cholesterol levels and other supposedly important variables collapsed. The team's conclusion: "The fact that an age-related clinical event developed in approximately 1 out of 3 healthy individuals in the upper tertile of insulin resistance at baseline, followed for an average of 6 years, whereas no clinical events were observed in the most insulin-sensitive tertile, should serve as a strong stimulus to further efforts to define the role of insulin resistance in the genesis of age-related diseases."

Cholesterol has never predicted disease the way insulin does. Cholesterol doesn't even properly predict heart disease alone, never mind the other diseases. For associational studies to carry weight, a variable's "risk multiplier" should exceed 2x—the variable should at least double the risk. If the risk multiplier exceeds 5x, there is likely something pretty serious going on. What was the risk multiplier for insulin resistance here? *40x!* The risk multiplier for high LDL was 1.001x—there was no statistical significance. Reaven's study can be put alongside massive volumes of mechanistic and other data gathered previously on the connection between insulin dysregulation and disease. He has elegantly demonstrated that insulin, a nearly billion-year-old molecule, dominates our disease landscape.

THE INSULIN-CENTRIC STRATEGY FOR LOSING WEIGHT AND LIVING LONGER

We are not simply "healthy" or "unhealthy" when it comes to insulin. We are all on a spectrum of health. There are, for sure, many causes of chronic disease, but most can be managed by focusing on insulin metrics. This is why insulin dysregulation is the biggest thing you need to address. When you address this you will improve your health enormously.

The diagram on the facing page may help you visualize how the population is spread across the insulin spectrum.

We can be anything from truly nondiabetic (left) through to full-blown diabetic (right), or anywhere in between. We estimate that those safely at the left are in the minority nowadays.

You will also notice that there are relatively healthy fat people in the safe zone. There are also very unhealthy slim people in the dangerous zone. This illustrates a hugely important fact: it is not your body weight that dictates your fate. Your health depends on the health of your fat tissue, not the quantity of it.

Insulin sensitivity starts with cells: just like the body as a whole, individual cells can be insulin resistant or insulin sensitive. Many people can have a lot of fat tissue whose cells are in a healthy, insulin-sensitive state. These people are referred to as "metabolically healthy obese." They can remain insulin sensitive throughout their bodies, and they have relatively low risk for disease.

Conversely, there are countless people who appear slim but whose fat tissue is unhealthy, insulin resistant and inflamed. This leads to whole-body insulin resistance. These people are referred to as "metabolically unhealthy normal weight," or "thin outside, fat inside."

Your whole-body insulin sensitivity depends hugely upon the health and sensitivity of your fat tissue. We'll talk about this more on page 360.

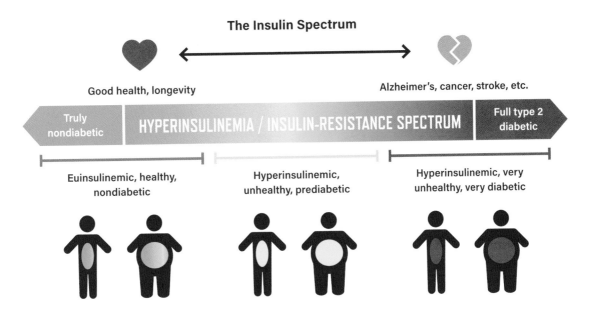

The Insulin Spectrum

Good health, longevity

Alzheimer's, cancer, stroke, etc.

Truly nondiabetic

HYPERINSULINEMIA / INSULIN-RESISTANCE SPECTRUM

Full type 2 diabetic

Euinsulinemic, healthy, nondiabetic

Hyperinsulinemic, unhealthy, prediabetic

Hyperinsulinemic, very unhealthy, very diabetic

THE GENIUS OF DR. JOSEPH R. KRAFT

If you wish to resolve insulin issues and move to the safe end of the insulin spectrum, you need to appreciate the incredible work of Dr. Joseph R. Kraft. Kraft was an expert pathologist and a doctor of nuclear medicine (one of only a few in the US). Over his career, he managed to generate some of the most important data ever gathered in medical history. He decoded the puzzle of insulin resistance and disease well before Reaven. What's more, he verified his hypothesis with five-hour insulin tests he conducted on nearly fifteen thousand people.

In the 1960s, Kraft pioneered the glucose tolerance with insulin assay method of showing insulin status. His work spanned three decades of investigation and looked at 14,308 individuals ages eight to eighty-eight. Crucially, Kraft recorded the *pattern* of insulin response for all of his patients—how their insulin rose and fell after eating. Kraft discovered that there were only five types of patterns. The first four patterns are of most interest for our purposes (the fifth pattern relates more to type 1 diabetes).

Figure 10.3 on the following page shows these patterns of insulin response after eating. The green line is the pattern seen in someone who is healthy and truly nondiabetic. Kraft called this *euinsulinemia* (*eu*, Greek for "good," + *insulin* + *emia*, Greek for "blood"). This response means there is a normal (appropriate) insulin response to carbohydrate.

Kraft Patterns: The Earliest Diagnosis of Diabetes

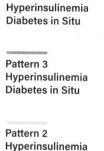

Pattern 4
Hyperinsulinemia
Diabetes in Situ

Pattern 3
Hyperinsulinemia
Diabetes in Situ

Pattern 2
Hyperinsulinemia
Diabetes in Situ

Pattern 1
Euinsulinemia
Nondiabetic

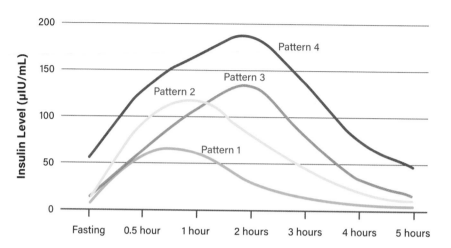

Figure 10.3. Kraft patterns: to truly tell if you are diabetic or healthy. Source: J. R. Kraft, "Detection of Diabetes Mellitus *In Situ* (Occult Diabetes)," *Laboratory Medicine* 6, no. 2 (1975): 10–22.

The red, orange, and yellow lines show varying degrees of dysfunctional insulin response. People with these patterns essentially have a diabetic physiology, even though the vast majority Kraft identified with these patterns had apparently normal blood glucose measures. Kraft called their disease state "diabetes in situ," and he saw that only 10 percent of his diabetes-in-situ patients failed the standard fasting glucose test. In spite of passing these tests, they were "secret diabetics." Their dysfunctional insulin response would never be seen by the standard diabetes tests—but they would continue to suffer the vascular damage of diabetes regardless.

From his research and pathology expertise, Kraft knew that these people's arteries were burning up with atherosclerosis, which is fundamentally an inflammatory disease. He realized that diabetes was everywhere. And this was back in the 1970s. Huge proportions of the population that did not register as diabetic under the standard criteria were nonetheless diabetic. And they would suffer all the vascular disease that goes with it.

Kraft rightly called his pattern test the earliest laboratory diagnosis for diabetes. It remains so to this day, but pretty much no one is using it. The majority of diabetics remain undiagnosed. Kraft stated in his 2008 book, "Those with cardiovascular disease not identified with diabetes are simply undiagnosed."[10]

Coronary Disease Victims, Ages 18–80, Across All of Europe

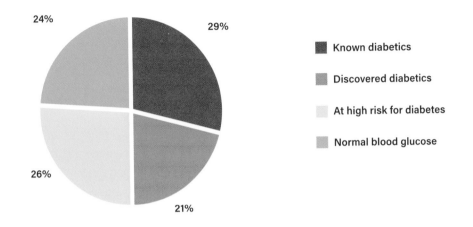

- Known diabetics
- Discovered diabetics
- At high risk for diabetes
- Normal blood glucose

Are most or even all of cardiovascular disease victims really secret diabetics? Let's look at the EuroAspire study results from page 226 again—shown once more above, in Figure 10.4.

We see from these results that Kraft was at least 76 percent correct—76 percent of CAD patients turned out to have some level of diabetes according to blood glucose tests. The remaining 24 percent were not tested using insulin measures, which might have revealed that they, too, had diabetes.

It is important to remember that these insulin measures reflect the presence of a wide range of disease root causes. Many disease-causing factors—such as bad diets, overeating, smoking, an imbalance of gut bacteria, infections, and more—lead to elevated insulin and insulin resistance. The state of hyperinsulinemia itself is a causal driver for disease, too. So without quantifying every cause-and-effect loop, we can rest assured of the importance of Kraft's test.

In short, all bad roads lead directly to both disease and the near-universal evil of insulin dysregulation—which also drives disease risk. There is a seething hive of cause-and-effect loops at the center of this mess. That is why insulin metrics are so crucial in the world of heart disease and other diseases of modernity.

Figure 10.4. Kraft was mostly correct: the majority of CAD victims are essentially diabetic. Source: V. Gyberg et al., "Screening for Dysglycaemia in Patients with Coronary Artery Disease as Reflected by Fasting Glucose, Oral Glucose Tolerance Test, and HbA1c: A Report from EUROASPIRE IV—a Survey from the European Society of Cardiology," *European Heart Journal* 36, no. 19 (2015): 1171–77.

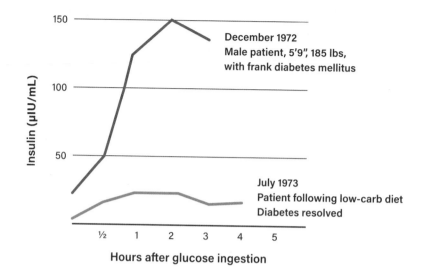

Managing Diabetes with a Low-Carb Diet

December 1972
Male patient, 5'9", 185 lbs,
with frank diabetes mellitus

July 1973
Patient following low-carb diet
Diabetes resolved

Hours after glucose ingestion

Figure 10.5. Dr. Kraft was fixing diabetes with low-carb diets—in 1972. Source: J. R. Kraft, "Detection of Diabetes Mellitus *In Situ* (Occult Diabetes)," *Laboratory Medicine* 6, no. 2 (1975): 10–22.

Dr. Kraft had extraordinary success healing his diabetic patients with low-carb diets. Take a look at Figure 10.5 above.

Both lines of this graph show the insulin response of one patient. The upper curve shows results from December 1972, and you can see it fits the nasty hyperinsulinemic pattern 3. The lower curve represents the same patient's response in July 1973, after eight months on Kraft's low-carb dietary management, and shows a lovely low-insulin response.

If you are interested in finding out where you are on the insulin spectrum, one excellent way is to use a simplified form of Kraft's five-hour test, a two-hour insulin reading. This is achieved by drinking 75 grams of glucose solution and then getting a blood insulin test two hours later. If your insulin is below 30 μIU/mL, you would very likely pass a full Kraft test. If it is above 40 μIU/mL, however, you would very likely fail the full test.

BLOOD GLUCOSE AND A1C

Having high insulin levels is part of what causes damage to your organs, for sure. But if you're in the bad zone of the insulin spectrum, to varying degrees, high blood glucose also wreaks havoc in your body, especially in the period following your meals.

Fasting glucose is a weak measure to judge health by, as we've said. Your arteries will have paid a heavy price by the time this goes out of control. The main value of a blood glucose measure is that if you take it after you have eaten a meal, it will at least flag a problem earlier than a fasting glucose measure would, giving you more time to fix it. But neither post-meal glucose nor insulin are regularly tested as part of a routine checkup.

Glucose is a biologically active molecule that can chemically damage many elements in your body. Your body controls blood glucose in an extremely tight range. Moving above this range is seriously damaging to all organ systems, and your arteries particularly feel the pain. The higher your glucose level, the more damage that occurs. The majority of American adults have experienced the negative effects of excess glucose in their system. This is the price we have to pay for using the stuff to fuel our bodies. It is a very small price for healthy people, but it is a terrible price for the diabetic majority.

Glucose is a sticky molecule that interacts badly with other molecules in your body. The process of glucose-driven damage is called *glycation*. Too much of this phenomenon is very bad news. Testing your red blood cells is a great way to estimate your glycation damage. Over their life cycles—approximately three to four months—red blood cells are constantly exposed to glucose in the bloodstream. They steadily become glycated. The measure of this glycation is called HbA1c, or, more simply, A1C.

You can think of A1C as a pretty good indication of your average blood glucose levels for the past three months. It will generally reveal significant problems with post-meal glucose spikes—not always, but generally. This test is usually only done for people who have already been diagnosed with diabetes. The vast majority of secret diabetics don't get tested. A pity, but that's the way our health system rolls. If you ask your doctor to measure your A1C level, you will get to see how bad your diet is. Your A1C level can also indicate if early mortality is in your future.

A very revealing and well-executed study provides data linking A1C and heart disease and mortality rates. The Norfolk Cancer Study focused on cancer, as the name suggests, but the researchers were taken aback at what elevated A1C meant for the risk of other diseases.[11] They were particularly impressed with the connection to "all-cause death rate." This, of course, is the most important metric of all.

The research team corrected for as many "confounding factors" as they could. These are factors that changed along with the factor being examined and may have contributed to the increased risks observed. But after correction, they still identified A1C as an *independent* risk factor for cardiovascu-

Coronary Vascular Disease Rates (per 100 people)						
Women	3.3	3.8	5.4	9.8	13.7	36.8
Men	6.7	9	12.1	15.2	25	34.8
HbA1C	< 5.0%	5.0% to 5.4%	5.5% to 5.9%	6.0% to 6.4%	6.5% to 6.9%	> 7.0%

Figure 10.6. Coronary disease risk and risk of early mortality both ramp up with higher HbA1C. Source: K. Khaw et al., "Association of Hemoglobin A1c with Cardiovascular Disease and Mortality in Adults: The European Prospective Investigation into Cancer in Norfolk," *Annals of Internal Medicine* 141, no. 6 (2004): 413–20.

lar disease (CVD)—it was associated with the higher risk all by itself. (Note that CVD is largely just another term for coronary heart disease, but it also includes the damage caused by the same vascular issues across the whole body.)

As the A1C measurement increases, the associated risk of CVD rises powerfully. As you can see in Figure 10.6, for both men and women, the lowest rates of CVD were associated with a healthy A1C of 5 percent or lower. For men, an A1C above 6.5 percent gave subjects 3.5 times the risk of CVD, while being above 7 percent gave them nearly 5 times the risk. For women, an A1C above 7 percent gave the subjects ten times the risk of CVD.

Those figures are powerful associational evidence. The scientific literature is packed with papers describing the mechanisms whereby elevated blood sugar causes dysfunction—in other words, there's plenty of mechanism evidence, one of the three pillars of proof from Chapter 2. Researchers are not ethically allowed to acquire experimental evidence—to drive up A1C and see what happens. They would not knowingly feed a subject with a high-carb diet for ten years in order to raise his A1C and see what happens over time. This experiment, however, is being carried out by millions of people every day. The primary way to drive up blood sugar is to indulge in excessive carb consumption. In huge numbers of people, we've seen this drive chronic disease and early death.

One problem with A1C is that it is a late-stage indicator of problems. By the time this metric is high, you will have been essentially diabetic for many years. That said, you may find it interesting that no one really talks much about A1C outside of diabetes management. What a shamefully wasted opportunity to improve our collective health.

All-Cause Death Rates (per 100 people)						
Women	2	2.7	4.4	6.4	6.8	25
Men	3.8	5.5	7.5	9.9	19	18.5
HbA1C	< 5.0%	5.0% to 5.4%	5.5% to 5.9%	6.0 %to 6.4%	6.5% to 6.9%	> 7.0%

Let's now ponder the "all-cause death rate" linkages to A1C level, as shown in Figure 10.7. These are simply mortality rates, from all causes (heart disease, cancer, diabetes, respiratory disorders, infectious diseases, etc.), arranged by A1C level. But the association is stunning: if your A1C is high, the reaper is not too far away. You're most probably overweight as well, but not necessarily. Millions are burning up in the insulin spectrum without being overweight.

The good news is that if your A1C is high, you can collapse it down to safe levels in no time by following our plan. Figure 10.8 below shows the dramatic response seen by just a couple of Jeff's many patients who have achieved this.

Figure 10.7. Risk of early mortality ramps up with higher HbA1C. Source: K. Khaw et al., "Association of Hemoglobin A1c with Cardiovascular Disease and Mortality in Adults: The European Prospective Investigation into Cancer in Norfolk," *Annals of Internal Medicine* 141, no. 6 (2004): 413–20.

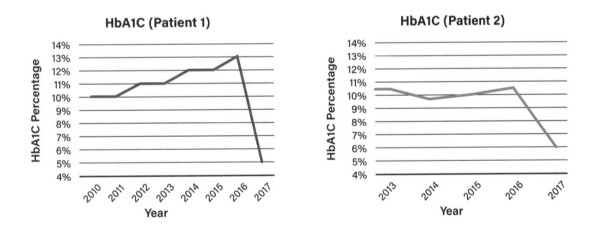

Figure 10.8. What can be achieved through our dietary strategy—and very quickly. The steep drop in 2016 begins with the adoption of a low-carb diet.

ESCAPING TO SAFETY

There is so much more we could say about the link between insulin, glucose, weight loss, health, and longevity. If you're interested in exploring this further, Appendix D (page 356) elaborates on the mechanisms of hyperinsulinemia and how your body can actually degenerate into the insulin-resistant state.

Escaping to the safe end of the insulin spectrum is easy for many people. For these people, simply following a well-formulated low-carbohydrate diet will do the trick. But we would be oversimplifying things and doing you a great disservice if we left it at that. (For instance, as mentioned on page 60, a small minority of people can experience problems with certain types of animal products when taken to excess. These people may need to be more careful in which healthy fats they focus on.) There are many drivers of elevated blood glucose and insulin, and each individual will have to address them as required.

The truth is that longevity is a multifactorial matter, and many important factors vary depending on the individual. We want you to address all the necessary factors in order to assure your long-term health and vitality. We want you to eat rich and live long.

LEANN'S STORY

Leann is a patient of Jeff's who collapsed her A1C easily and was able to drop medications at the same time. Leann is now eating well and set to live a lot longer, having rapidly resolved her diabetic dysfunction.

Leann's family history was riddled with heart disease, obesity, vascular problems, and diabetes. Her father died at fifty-six from congestive heart failure; her mother also had congestive heart failure and bypass surgery; and all four of her grandparents had died from some type of heart or vascular problem. Due to this history, Leann arranged for a full medical exam back in the nineties. She was astounded to learn that not only was she diabetic, but her A1C was nearly three times what was considered normal. She was immediately started on metformin, a medication that lowers blood sugar through different mechanisms than insulin does.

Over the years, her dosage of metformin was increased, until she reached the maximum permitted. Her weight also skyrocketed to 314 pounds. She had tried time and time again to lose weight and failed. It really felt as though she was never going to lose weight, and what's more, she was always hungry.

Leann saw a doctor at a major university medical center for several years, and the doctor regularly wanted her to enter various studies where insulin was the protocol. Lifestyle intervention was hardly discussed. She was simply told to adjust her insulin dosage in line with her carbohydrate consumption. Something didn't feel right about it for Leann—both her parents had ended up on insulin,

and neither ever reached good blood sugar control. Both also gained a scary amount of weight. Her doctors also prescribed multiple other drugs, the last of which was from the class of sulfonylureas, which can have permanent and damaging effects on the pancreas, the very organ that produces insulin. A week after being on the sulfonylurea, Leann was having trouble breathing. She stopped taking it. She really felt defeated and fearful that she would end up like the rest of her family.

With a copy of her bloodwork in hand, Leann sat down with her wife, Sharon, who was working to become a dietitian. Throughout the 2016 holiday season Sharon read study after study on diabetes. When her research was completed, she had closed in on a rather unconventional strategy. Sharon insisted that Leann focus on limiting carbohydrate rather than counting calories or anything else. She wanted her to immediately adopt a ketogenic diet (a *very* low carb, high-fat diet—see page 298). In January 2017, Leann began her ketogenic journey. It had dramatic effects on her health.

Within a week of lowering her carbohydrates significantly, Leann had an amazing burst of energy. She started taking the dog for walks and was starting to look for new activities to do other than sit around waiting for her next meal. She saw 15 pounds come off that first week. It was very encouraging, and she felt great! She lost weight and did not feel hungry or in the least deprived. In mid-February, Leann bought a fitness tracker to monitor her walking. She was walking between twelve thousand and twenty thousand steps per day. Her coworker thought she was a bit nuts as she was now up actively moving and pacing the halls with her wireless headset while waiting to start conference calls.

By mid-March, Sharon and Leann were excited about the weight loss and figured that Leann's A1C must have dropped somewhat. Leann knew she did not want to go back to the university for another visit because, along with pushing her toward insulin studies, they were constantly calling and sending her referrals for a diabetes educator. She had met with the educator once early on, and his suggestion was low-fat dieting—eating things like plain oatmeal and salads and staying away from healthy fats. She had been down that path before, had been constantly hungry, and couldn't maintain the diet.

Leann wanted a doctor who would be keto-friendly and made an appointment to see Jeff in April, just three months into her low-carb lifestyle.

When Leann arrived at the office, she had already lost 50 pounds. Jeff joined her in the exam room, and they talked for roughly twenty minutes before he jumped up and wanted to test her A1C right there in the office. They started to discuss what they thought it would be. She had never had a value below 6.5, so she was thinking it would be somewhere around 8.5, an improvement considering that she'd been at 12 in January. Jeff suggested it might be much lower, based on the details of her successful keto journey to date. He was right—the value came back at 5! Leann was thrilled. In three short months she had lost 50 pounds and reduced her A1C by nearly 60 percent, without injecting any insulin! Based on the Norfolk Study data mentioned on page 239, her risk of coronary heart disease may have dropped by a huge degree.

In another six months Leann lost 50 pounds more, bringing her total weight loss to more than 100 pounds and counting. She also feels more energetic than ever. She is continuing to refine her eating in order to consistently keep her ratio of fat, protein, and carb in the target zone of 70 percent, 20 percent, and 10 percent, respectively. She continues her follow-up appointments with Jeff and is now confident that she can avoid the fate of her disease-ridden relations.

CHAPTER 11

FIXING HEART DISEASE:
CHOLESTEROL IS A WEAPON OF MASS DISTRACTION

> " Stupidity is the same as evil if you judge by the results. "
>
> —Margaret Atwood

In the last chapter we discussed insulin as the primary driver of heart disease, as well as many other chronic diseases. But most doctors continue to focus on cholesterol. The cholesterol narrative has distracted us from the genuine drivers of heart disease. It has also pushed us away from the healthiest diets. It has a lot to answer for. If you don't know the truth about cholesterol, your efforts to achieve longevity will be undermined, as has occurred for the millions who went before you.

Cholesterol has dominated the preventative medicine sphere over the past forty years. Nothing else has even come close. This was partly due to the fact that it was one of the first simple blood measures that seemed to correlate with rates of disease, however weakly. Another major reason was that it was one of the few measures that would directly respond to an available class of drugs.

Cholesterol is carried in the blood in particles called lipoproteins. Current blood tests smash up these lipoprotein particles to get to the cholesterol. They then measure the amount of cholesterol that is carried within each lipoprotein. LDL is one type of lipoprotein particle; it's called "bad cholesterol." HDL is another type, called "good cholesterol." But both LDL and HDL carry the exact same cholesterol molecules inside—there is only one type of cholesterol molecule. We should really say that LDL is a "bad lipoprotein" and HDL is a "good lipoprotein." However, as we'll soon see, even this would be a misleading way to put it. They are simply different kinds of particles with different yet equally important functions.

The truth is that when it's high, LDL is sometimes associated with bad things—but it is a weak and erratic risk factor. When HDL is high, it is almost always associated with good things. It is a consistent and intriguing indicator. HDL has always been a thorn in the cholesterol story because it draws us away from the "cholesterol is bad" ruse and points us toward the genuine root causes of heart disease. Also, while many drugs have had success in lowering LDL, no drugs have successfully raised HDL. So HDL is doubly problematic for the storytellers: it raises awkward questions around true cause of heart disease, and it won't cooperate with saleable drugs. HDL is therefore marginalized and pushed out of the discussion whenever possible.

A CHOLESTEROL FABLE FOR THE AGES

The cholesterol story we have been sold has changed greatly over the past fifty years. It became clear over time that the original cholesterol theory was highly flawed, so the tale had to be twisted into new shapes to fit the desired message. Each time the existing cholesterol measurement was shown to be useless, a new one was found to take its place, so that everyone could maintain some confidence in the fable.

The changes happened roughly as follows:

1. Several decades ago we were all terrified of having a high total cholesterol reading. This number reflected all of the cholesterol transported by lipoprotein particles in the blood. After decades of throwing medications at this number, the focus on total cholesterol quietly dropped from favor. We now know that a higher total cholesterol number generally predicts a *longer, healthier life.* Oops.

2. Total cholesterol was then replaced by LDL, or "bad cholesterol." LDL levels reflect the amount of cholesterol carried in the LDL particles. This was supposedly the proper cholesterol risk factor to use. But after years of throwing meds at LDL, this number has fallen out of favor too, because it doesn't properly predict risk, either. High LDL can be associated with bad things, but so can low LDL—because LDL only hints at the *real* causes. The plot thickens.

3. As more and more researchers realized that LDL was misleading, the advanced lipoprotein test came to the rescue. Remember that the standard LDL metric only gives a measure of the cholesterol quantity inside the LDL particle. However, the advanced lipoprotein test counts

the *number* and *size* of the LDL particles themselves. In a sense, this test measures the *quality* of the LDL particles, rather than simply the cholesterol inside them. As a result, it is a somewhat better predictor of any potential issues. But it is still looking at LDL instead of the real underlying causes, so the test can therefore be misleading.

You could be forgiven for wondering what the hell has been going on here. How did we spend decades prescribing meds based on the wrong measures? What's more, huge numbers of doctors are still taking direction from the thoroughly debunked "total cholesterol" phobia. They are stuck in a cholesterol time warp, worrying about a meaningless number. Many more doctors are stranded in step 2 above, medicating based on LDL. Yet LDL as a direct treatment target has now been removed from the 2013 drug treatment guidelines produced by the American Heart Association and the American College of Cardiology.[1] These folks who are worrying about LDL are still running aimlessly after the old-fashioned "bad cholesterol." A small minority of doctors are at least working with the latest science and using advanced lipoprotein testing—but most of them don't realize that the numbers are still mostly a reflection of something else.

The cholesterol story is both a wonderful and a terrible one: wonderful due to the beautiful elegance of our cholesterol-trafficking systems, terrible because we have misunderstood them for so long. We tragically blamed cholesterol rather than focusing on the real drivers of heart disease. Blinded by associations, we left the real causes off the hook—and we are doing so to this very day.

Dr. William P. Castelli, an expert in cardiology and data analysis, led what is essentially the biggest and longest-running coronary heart disease study in history: the Framingham Heart Study. What he said revealed everything that you need to know about LDL as a risk factor.

Since 1948, the Framingham study has tracked the health and lifestyles of more than five thousand people from Framingham, Massachusetts, looking for causes of cardiovascular disease. Castelli published a detailed paper in 1992 analyzing the data. Here we quote directly from it: "Unless LDL levels are very high (300 mg/dl (7.8 mmol/l) or higher), they have no value, in isolation, in predicting those individuals at risk of CHD."[2]

He was absolutely correct about this, but the world was never allowed to hear this vital message. The outcome from Framingham was instead twisted to fit the required message. Simply put, the message was that LDL had to be the bad cholesterol. Everyone *needed* this message, because decades of official communications had already declared it from the rooftops. And so that's what it was made to become. Castelli also established another extremely important fact: "The [total-to-HDL] ratio was found to be a better predictor of [coronary heart disease] than [total cholesterol], LDL, HDL and triglyceride, not only in the Framingham Study but also in the Physician's Health Study and many other studies."[3]

We will soon explain the importance of the ratios. But first, we'll introduce you to the basic molecules that caused all the fuss.

CHOLESTEROL AND TRIGLYCERIDE

Cholesterol is required for life on this planet. It comes from the sterol family of molecules, which are fat-like in nature. The cholesterol molecule enables the structure of cell walls. It is a vital building block for many hormones that are central in the control systems of our bodies. Cholesterol is a key part of the immune system and is central to the body's tissue repair apparatus. The phenomenal human brain contains around 30 percent of the body's cholesterol, even though the brain is only around 4 percent of our body weight. It is required for much more besides. Without cholesterol there would be no life.

We have around forty trillion cells in our bodies, so you have forty trillion reasons to be glad of cholesterol. With some exceptions, all of these cells are blessed with the ability to manufacture their own cholesterol. Cholesterol is that critical. Cholesterol is arguably the most important substance that evolution has designed to keep you healthy. You may rightly wonder how this fundamental requirement for health became something that scientists claimed was somehow conspiring to kill us.

Evolution is not an idiot. It's not the cholesterol that is the problem but rather the system that manages it in the body, which can become dysfunctional. This is why cholesterol measures can correlate loosely with disease. This association has been hyped and pumped out to us continuously since the 1970s.

Cholesterol

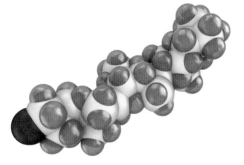

Cholesterol cannot travel around the bloodstream by itself, so nature has evolved some very special "boats" that carry cholesterol molecules safe inside them. These are lipoprotein particles. They are hollow spheres that travel in the bloodstream with the cholesterol packed safely inside. There is also another pivotal molecule that travels with cholesterol inside these lipoprotein particles: triglyceride.

A triglyceride molecule is simply three fat molecules grouped into one glycerol (or sugar-like) molecule. These triglyceride molecules can be consumed through fat-containing food. They can also be created in your liver. Your body assembles, disassembles, and transports triglyceride to fuel your body.

There can, however, be a bad side to triglyceride, if its level in your blood is higher than it should be. Excess fat in your blood is a major issue. Unfortunately this is the case for most people today, and the most common driver of high blood fats is excessive carbohydrate in the diet.

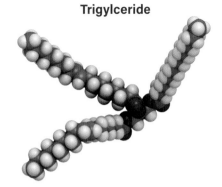

Trigylceride

THE LIPOPROTEINS

In 1928 French biochemist Michel Macheboeuf isolated a water-soluble lipoprotein now known to us as HDL. This complex macromolecule is capable of transporting water-insoluble substances, including cholesterol and triglyceride, in your water-based blood. Following World War II, progress was made in the emerging field of lipidology. In 1949, molecular biologist John Gofman identified a whole family of lipoproteins, including VLDL, LDL, IDL, and others. He was in turn followed by Fredrickson, Gordon, Olson, and Vester, who identified specific lipoprotein patterns associated with atherosclerosis.

All of these discoveries fueled the excitement about "cholesterol" (really lipoproteins) as a causal agent in vascular disease. Advances in measurement continued, and lipid metabolism surged forward as a hot new science. It was the newest kid on the block. By the 1970s, standard lipid testing had become widely available to doctors. Everyone was all over the exciting new tools.

On the right is a simple drawing of a lipoprotein. Basically, the cholesterol and triglyceride molecules are packed safely inside the lipoprotein's shell. Here they are safely stored for delivery to your brain and bodily tissues. Think of lipoproteins as boats with the cargo safely battened down in the hold. These lipoprotein boats can move freely through your bloodstream while keeping the water-insoluble cargo tucked inside. They travel in the millions on their delivery and collection missions. These boats need to clearly identify themselves in order to dock properly in many different harbors. They do this

A Lipoprotein Particle

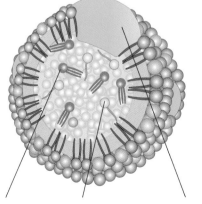

Trigylceride   Cholesterol   An Apolipoprotein

by signaling with a unique protein molecule wrapped around their outer shell: an apolipoprotein.

There are only two classes of lipoprotein particles that you need to know about. Having a grasp of how they work is very important.

WELCOME TO LIPOPROTEIN LAND

LDL and HDL are simply different types of lipoproteins. While the HDL lipoprotein is unique, LDL belongs to a family of LDL-class lipoproteins.

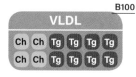

VLDL: Very low density lipoprotein (VLDL) is the mother of LDL—it's where LDL originates. VLDL is the largest of the LDL-class lipoproteins. VLDLs are created by your liver and ferry triglyceride and cholesterol around your body. VLDL's main function is to deliver triglyceride to be used as a healthy fuel in skeletal muscle, heart muscle, and many other tissues (especially if you are a fat-burner!). You can completely screw up your VLDLs by eating the wrong foods. It identifies itself with the B100 apolipoprotein.

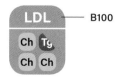

LDL: We now present the most feared lipoprotein in the world. Low-density lipoprotein (LDL) is formed as a VLDL particle gives up its cargo and shrinks in size. LDL still contains cholesterol and triglyceride (with relatively little triglyceride). LDL has many functions, covering both delivery and return trips in the cholesterol transport chain. It's small compared to its mother, VLDL. Like the other LDL-class vessels, it identifies itself using the B100 apolipoprotein. You can *really* screw up your LDLs by eating the wrong foods.

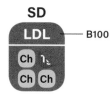

sdLDL: Now we're getting to why little LDL got a bad name. While LDL has been designed by evolution itself, evolution didn't quite plan on people messing up its structure or destroying its functionality, but that is what modern humans have been doing. Small dense LDL (sdLDL) is what results when LDL becomes distorted in an inflammatory environment. Your immune system recognizes a damaged or oxidized sdLDL particle as an unwelcome guest and tries to mop it up, but it often fails to manage this properly. The sdLDL particles may also be less likely to return to the liver, so they stay longer in the blood and have a greater chance of being damaged. The main reason why LDL is associated with so many problems is that it takes the rap for its deranged half brother. There is a time-honored and fully accepted way to make your LDL go bad, and it's remarkably easy. All you need to do is to allow yourself to become insulin resistant. (Note, however, that there are also more benign reasons for having smaller LDL particles, so it can be a fallible marker in many people.[4])

HDL: The most-loved lipoprotein is the celebrated high-density lipoprotein (HDL), which is created mainly in your gut. It has many important functions because it is really the master manager of the whole cholesterol and triglyceride transport system. As with LDLs, you can *really* screw up your HDLs by eating the wrong foods. For good health, you want to avoid a low HDL level at all costs, because low HDL is directly correlated with insulin resistance. HDL is small by design: the little fellow gets to all the places it needs to. It does an amazing job, unless you screw it up with what you put in your mouth. It is unique, and so it identifies itself using an A1 protein tag.

LDL FOR ENERGY AND CHOLESTEROL TRAFFICKING

Now we'll reveal how these lipoproteins play in your bodily orchestra. Most importantly, we will explain how to avoid destroying their evolutionary function.

The VLDL particle is created by the liver. Its cargo hold is packed with fatty goods to meet the body's needs. VLDL must "dock" with muscle and/or fat tissue before releasing its goods. After giving up its triglyceride cargo, the VLDL particle shrinks and transforms into an LDL particle. In spite of LDL's fearsome reputation, there is nothing bad happening here at all. Evolution has given us LDL for a purpose. It works fine if you eat the kind of diet humans evolved eating, high in fat and low in carb.

But for the majority of people, especially as they get older, a high-carb diet tends to make VLDL particles large and triglyceride-rich. This is universally bad news. Large, triglyceride-rich VLDLs turn into smaller and denser LDLs that carry less cholesterol. With less cholesterol carried per particle, you need more LDL particles in circulation.

With more LDL particles in circulation, more particles are exposed to oxidative damage. Also, such dysfunctional systems damage the endothelium (the artery's inner surface)—and this can certainly *cause* LDL to be a problem, too.

Ironically, breaking the rules of a healthy diet not only means more particles are there to be exposed to damage, but it also damages LDL particles itself. Damaged LDLs don't get taken up properly by your liver; instead, your immune system has the thankless task of trying to mop them up. That means they hang around for longer in your blood (approximately four days rather than the ideal two days). You are now really playing with fire.

These damaged particles are a different breed of LDL that may not like going back to the liver. But there is a place where these problematic particles will end up: inside your inflamed arterial walls. This is what ultimately leads to arterial plaque, blockages, and, eventually, heart attacks.

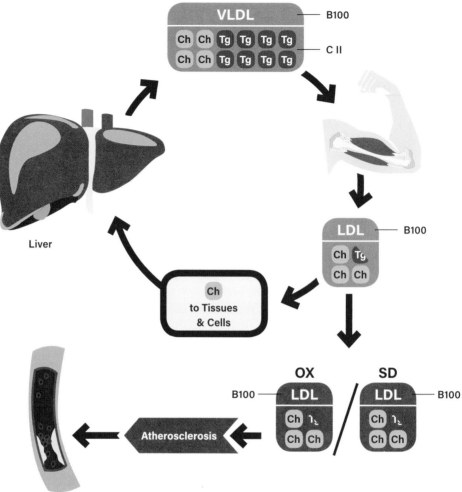

Figure 11.1. VLDL primarily transports triglycerides to muscles for energy purposes; after dropping off these molecules, it becomes LDL, which continues to transport triglycerides and also distributes cholesterol to tissues. Healthy LDL returns to the liver, where the cholesterol is recycled and reused. LDL can also become damaged, turning into sdLDL and oxidized LDL, which contribute to atherosclerosis.

Insulin resistance is a primary driver of sdLDL and oxidized LDL. It is also what helps link a high LDL count to higher disease rates. The amount of undamaged LDL has little relevance to disease for the vast majority of people, as long as they are not driving an inflammatory environment in their bodies.

Insulin resistance also promotes damage and weakness in your arteries through high blood pressure, high blood glucose, and many other mechanisms.[5] Altogether, these effects are why we talk about insulin resistance as the primary factor in heart disease—and why the focus on cholesterol levels is, at best, a distraction from the real problem.

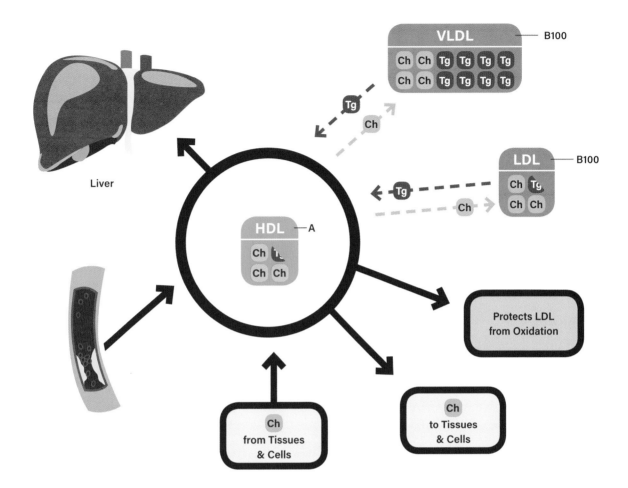

Figure 11.2. HDL is a wonder worker, keeping the LDL-class lipoproteins in healthy working order by managing their triglyceride and cholesterol content. HDL also protects LDL from oxidation damage and delivers vital cholesterol to the few tissues that cannot make their own. HDL even picks up excess cholesterol from tissues and extracts problematic deposits from atherscle-rotic plaques.

HDL FOR SYSTEM TRANSPORT, REPAIR, AND MAINTENANCE

HDL is more than just "good cholesterol." It is something of a miracle worker. It plays multiple instruments in the lipoprotein orchestra. Let's see how it all works—we'll give you the super-short version.

HDL starts off as a simple protein. It then swells as cholesterol and tri-glyceride are added to it. Armed and ready, it carries out its many crucial functions:

► swapping cholesterol and triglyceride molecules in and out of VLDL and LDL particles to balance the system

► extracting excess triglyceride from VLDL and LDL particles to prevent them from becoming dysfunctional

- collecting cholesterol molecules from cells where there is an excess
- delivering cholesterol to the rare types of cells that can't make their own
- supplying the gonads and adrenal glands with cholesterol, which is needed to synthesize important hormones
- carrying antioxidant artillery to protect the LDL lipoproteins from damage
- removing cholesterol from places where it ought not be (like arterial walls)

And a lot more besides. All this HDL does tirelessly. HDL is evolutionary engineering at its best.

But one pivotal function of HDL is truly remarkable. HDL constantly manages the contents of the complete LDL class of lipoproteins, transferring cholesterol and triglyceride molecules in and out of the LDL particles. HDL conducts a complex dance to stop the LDL particles from becoming problematic.

However, HDL can only do so much. Push your system too far with what you eat, and even HDL will break down.

Losing your HDL functionality will cost you dearly. But it is happening all the time, to hundreds of millions of people around the world who are destroying their HDL through what they put in their mouths. A low HDL value is a serious problem. What is the best way to keep your HDL level high and healthy?

You need to keep both your insulin and your insulin resistance low.

ESCAPING THE CHOLESTEROL MASS DISTRACTION

Castelli, the director of the Framingham Heart Study, whom we quoted earlier, rightly declared that LDL level is a useless measurement when taken alone (unless it's absurdly high, which applies only to a fraction of a percent of people). Many studies since have proved Castelli to be absolutely correct, showing that both total cholesterol and LDL level don't have any significant predictive power.

For example, a 2007 study looked closely at the later Framingham data for both men and women.[6] It found that, while total cholesterol and LDL did not predict CHD events at all, the cholesterol *ratios* predicted CHD events very well. This is because the ratios are an excellent indication of your insulin-resistance level! We quoted Castelli on this ratio point earlier. Here's what he said again (yes, it is that important): "The [total-to-HDL] ratio was found to be a better predictor of [coronary heart disease] than [total cholesterol], LDL, HDL and triglyceride, not only in the Framingham Study but also in the Physician's Health Study and many other studies."[7] What Castelli did not understand at the time was that the ratio reflected insulin-resistance status rather than "cholesterol" issues per se.

A standard cholesterol panel is often provided in routine blood tests. This test method breaks apart all of the lipoprotein particles—smashes them open, if you will. What's left behind is then analyzed. In this way you get the total amount of cholesterol and triglyceride that was carried within the lipoproteins. Therefore, all of these traditional tests quantify the amounts of triglyceride and cholesterol in your blood. It doesn't look at the amount of each kind of lipoprotein at all, even though it's only lipoproteins of a certain kind and size that you need to be concerned about. This is one of the many reasons why standard cholesterol panels are so misleading.

THE DANGEROUSLY MISLEADING LDL LEVEL

Your LDL number is the total, summed-up quantity of cholesterol carried by all your LDL-class particles. It should really be called the "LDL concentration," and in fact in the scientific literature it is more properly denoted as "LDLc" or "LDL-C."

If your LDL value is well above 200 mg/dL, it is more likely to have some meaning—that's fairly high, and it can indicate that your blood is full of damaged LDL particles that contribute to arterial inflammation. But it still may not mean this at all—you must examine all the other values we've discussed (including HDL, triglyceride, insulin, and blood glucose) to make a call. Castelli went further and said it had to be above 300 mg/dL before it would be predictive on its own. Yet most doctors still draw meaning from the LDL value alone, regardless of how high or low it is. This is beyond tragic.

Ironically, people with the most serious issues can often have a *lower* LDL than healthy people, especially as they get closer to a heart attack. These unhealthy people have insulin-resistance problems, which means they have excessive triglyceride in their lipoproteins, which crowds out cholesterol. So these unfortunate people end up with a lower LDL value in the test even though they are on fire inside. Also, their HDL desperately tries to remove the excess triglyceride and becomes poisoned with it, driving down their HDL levels—blood tests reveal the problem elegantly. But the message to doctors has been to focus on LDL, not HDL, so the clues to what is going on are mostly missed.

This absurdity of using LDL as a measure of health was highlighted recently. In 2009, there was a massive study of nearly 137,000 people who presented in hospitals with vascular disease.[8] More than 75 percent of these atherosclerosis-afflicted people had LDL levels well below the average. And the reason was not because they were taking lipid-lowering drugs, either. Only 20 percent of these people were on those drugs. LDL can also drop following trauma—but again, this did not account for the results. The outcome was rather due to insulin resistance—a *real* factor in heart disease. This was also flagged in the results, as the patients' HDL levels were markedly lower than average. This same reality has been seen in many other studies, too.

In standard cholesterol tests, the LDL number is not even directly measured. It is estimated using an old and unreliable formula. This makes it even more undependable and misleading.[9]

We'll now move to a far more useful metric: your HDL level.

THE RATHER USEFUL HDL AND TRIGLYCERIDE

Your HDL number is the total, summed-up quantity of cholesterol carried by your HDL particles.

Your HDL number does indeed have utility in assessing risk. There is genuine risk if the HDL value is below 40 mg/dL for men or 50 mg/dL for women (though ideally, HDL should be quite a bit higher than these targets). Low HDL consistently highlights genuinely problematic mechanisms in your body. It is a genuinely valuable flag that relates directly to the true root causes of disease.

One key problem with HDL occurs when HDL particles are forced to accept excessive triglyceride. This damages the HDL particle's ability to function properly. Another is that excess insulin can damage HDL's ability to remove problematic material from atherosclerosis-afflicted arteries.[10] There are so many other important functions of HDL that interact intimately with insulin dynamics that we cannot even begin to detail them here.

In the 2009 study of nearly 137,000 people, the average HDL level was below 40. In comparison, the population average is approximately 50.

But HDL is not an infallible marker—no marker really is. You can have a high HDL and still have some disease risk—HDL functionality can be problematic even when the HDL level appears good. That is why it is very important to look at ratios, as we'll discuss in a moment.

Your triglyceride number also has utility in assessing risk. Triglyceride is most useful as an indicator of insulin-signaling status—high triglyceride indicates that high insulin and insulin resistance are disrupting your system. Many guidelines suggest that triglyceride should be below 150 mg/dL, and this is fair. From extensive research, however, we would say that an ideal level would be below 100 mg/dL.

A high triglyceride value means that your LDL-class particles are carrying a heavier load than they're designed to. As HDL attempts to manage this overload, the HDL value will be driven lower.

Triglyceride is a statistically noisy risk factor—its relationship to disease risk is quite erratic and variable, unless it is particularly high in value—for many mechanistic reasons. Its level can vary greatly, even among people who are at similar risk for atherosclerosis progression. If it's below 100 mg/dL, however, it is highly likely that your insulin signaling is in a reasonably good state. If it's above 200 mg/dL, your insulin signaling is pretty certain to be impaired.

It's best to get your triglyceride measure from a nonfasting test. Many studies show that nonfasting triglyceride links very closely to heart attacks and risk of early mortality.[11] This makes absolute sense because people who have a spike in their post-meal triglycerides are—you guessed it—insulin resistant.

FOCUS ON THE RATIOS

Cholesterol ratios reign supreme in assessing real risk. You can easily calculate the crucial cholesterol ratios from the numbers on standard cholesterol tests. These ratios are a true indicator of metabolic health. They truly show how well your cholesterol transport system is functioning and genuinely reflect the underlying causes of vascular disease.

TRIGLYCERIDE/HDL

The shorthand for this ratio is "trig/HDL," and it's the best one from the cholesterol panel for assessing real risk.

A study as far back as 1997 came to the conclusion that this ratio is vastly more predictive than the LDL value.[12] Nothing has since changed—for both heart disease and death risk, the trig/HDL ratio reigns supreme. Recent recommendations say that the value should ideally be below 2.0. Based on the science, the clear mechanisms at work, and all of the published risk data, we would aim lower: below 1.2, or even below 1.0.

The 1997 study we just mentioned showed that the 25 percent of people with the highest trig/HDL ratio values had nearly *sixteen times the risk for heart attacks* as those with low ratios. This risk barely changed when correcting statistically for a large range of variables. Trig/HDL even beats the latest advanced lipoprotein ratios much of the time. Other studies point to the extraordinary predictive power of trig/HDL for deaths from any cause.[13] Yet more studies show that trig/HDL predicts atherosclerosis severity in patients—whereas LDL completely fails to do so.[14] So why didn't trig/HDL become the primary number used from the lipid panel? We can think of a few reasons for this:

1. It greatly undermines the theory that "high cholesterol" causes heart disease.

2. It particularly wreaks havoc with the simplistic "LDL = bad cholesterol" message.

3. Since high triglyceride and low HDL levels are closely associated with and directly caused by insulin problems, it focuses the spotlight on insulin signaling as overwhelmingly the primary problem in heart disease.

4. No patented drugs work properly to reduce this ratio. The trials on HDL drugs have bombed spectacularly. This is because low HDL reflects the underlying causes—shoving HDL up with chemical cattle prods doesn't address these causes.

The predictive power of trig/HDL is to be expected. It is self-evident once we understand how the lipoprotein system interacts with insulin signaling. The mechanisms actually make evolutionary and technical sense (which is not the case with LDL). Trig/HDL is essentially a magnified measure of the insulin dysfunction that we discussed in Chapter 10.

When you have pushed your insulin signaling into a bad place, triglyceride levels tend to increase and HDL simultaneously drops. When this occurs, the trig/HDL ratio changes much more rapidly than these individual measures change. It is therefore a fantastic indicator of a system gone to hell.

So has your doctor been working to reduce your trig/HDL ratio to safe levels? He or she can of course do this by advising you to lower your ingestion of carbohydrate and increase your healthy fat intake. If he or she has been advising this, you are one of the lucky ones.

In addition to the straightforward trig/HDL ratio, you might find it valuable to calculate your AIP, an excellent version of the trig/HDL ratio. Once you know your triglycerides and HDL numbers, you can plug them into an online calculator to find your AIP—a good one is available at www.biomed.cas.cz/fgu/aip/calculator.php.

TOTAL CHOLESTEROL/HDL

The ratio of total cholesterol to HDL (total/HDL) is as easy to calculate as it is to address, and it speaks volumes.

People who have significant insulin resistance often have a "normal" LDL. But they also have low HDL and high triglycerides. The triglyceride value jacks up the total cholesterol number, which means that the ratio of total cholesterol to HDL also gets jacked up. In this way, the total/HDL ratio is closely related to the trig/HDL ratio and has similar usefulness.

The total/HDL ratio cuts a swath through all the noise. It doesn't even require any exotic laboratory tests.

So go ahead and calculate your ratio—the current guideline suggests you should be lower than 5 or even 4.5. Achieving lower than 4 would be the ideal target. We transformed ours many years ago, from about 5 to about 3, by reducing our insulin levels.

The power of the total/HDL ratio has been repeatedly demonstrated again and again across many studies. Let's look briefly at the outcome of just one recent example that carefully measured and tracked more than three thousand people for eight years.[15] This study illustrates the point rather well.

The numbers in the bottom row of Figure 11.3 are hazard ratios, which show the relative risk of heart disease. A hazard ratio above 2 is accepted as being very meaningful indeed—there's a high risk of heart disease that is intimately linked to the ratio value. So what pattern emerges when studies like this are done properly and carefully analyzed?

The total/HDL ratio accounts for pretty much *all* of the increase in risk. LDL is irrelevant in comparison.

In other words, study participants with high LDL still had a low hazard ratio as long as their total/HDL was low. And if they had low LDL but a high total/HDL, their hazard ratio was also high. It is the ratio that drives the CHD bus.

Coronary Heart Disease Hazard Ratios			
LDL < 130 (Average LDL = 107)		LDL > 130 (Average LDL = 175)	
Total/HDL < 5	Total/HDL > 5	Total/HDL < 5	Total/HDL > 5
1.00	2.49	0.97	2.15

Figure 11.3. Only the total/HDL ratio properly predicts risk—just as Castelli noted. Source: T. D. Wang et al., "Efficacy of Cholesterol Levels and Ratios in Predicting Future Coronary Heart Disease in a Chinese Population," *American Journal of Cardiology* 88, no. 7 (2001): 737–43.

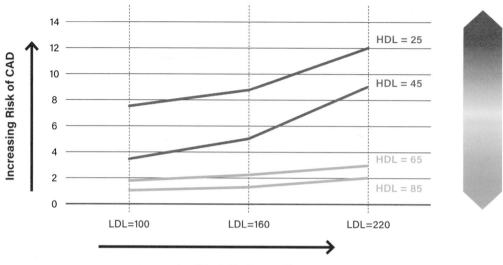

CAD Risk by LDL & HDL

Increasing Risk of CAD

- HDL = 25
- HDL = 45
- HDL = 65
- HDL = 85

LDL=100   LDL=160   LDL=220

Increasing "Bad Cholesterol"

Figure 11.4. Higher LDL cannot tell us anything without looking at HDL also. Source: W. P. Castelli, "Cholesterol and Lipids in the Risk of Coronary Artery Disease—The Framingham Heart Study," *Canadian Journal of Cardiology* 4, suppl. A (1988): 5A–10A.

LDL/HDL

The Framingham Heart Study, one of the largest and longest-running population trials ever conducted, scrutinized LDL and HDL and identified many of the risk factors that are used today to identify probability of heart attacks for people.

Figure 11.4 shows the risk of coronary artery disease (CAD) in fifty- to seventy-year-old men—a rather important group, since it's the group with the most heart attacks. (Note that this data is from 1977, when our population was not yet ravaged by very high rates of insulin resistance—smoking was the big driver of heart disease back then.)

The data showed that people with a lower HDL (upper red lines) were universally at very high risk of CAD—even when their LDL was nice and low.

But the worst-off were those with high LDL and low HDL. Their risk is jacked up because the combination of high LDL and low HDL screams insulin resistance. Ideally your LDL/HDL ratio should be below 3.5 or so.

CHOLESTEROL MASTER CLASS: THE ADVANCED LIPOPROTEIN TESTS

The advanced lipoprotein tests are rarely used compared to the standard ones, but they are now becoming more widely available. These tests actually count the lipoproteins and measure their size. Although these measures are important for all particle types, we will focus on the LDL-class particles, whose size and number are particularly important.

THE SIZE OF YOUR LDL PARTICLES

Advanced testing methods can measure the size of your LDL particles and give you a distribution of their dimensions. If a large percentage of your LDL particles are in the "small, dense" category (sdLDL), it's not a good sign. Having lots of these sdLDL particles is also referred to as being a "pattern B" type person. Smaller LDL particles are more prone to oxidation damage—and being insulin resistant can also drive down LDL particle size. That is mainly why sdLDL is a bad thing to have; the sdLDL measure tracks reasonably well with vascular disease.

THE NUMBER OF YOUR LDL PARTICLES

The advanced testing methods can also count the *number* of your LDL particles. The count of the LDL particles is generally called "ApoB" or "LDL-P." For our purpose here, "ApoB" is essentially just another term for "LDL-P"; the test for ApoB simply uses a different methodology. The value of ApoB is more strongly associated with vascular disease than the standard LDL measure, but it does not track more strongly than the ratios discussed on pages 257 to 260. High ApoB can be a problem mainly because most heart attacks are due to insulin-signaling problems and associated issues, and these also often drive a high ApoB—so a high ApoB flags the risk of insulin resistance. If there are no insulin resistance or inflammatory issues present, then a high ApoB is very likely not an issue.

Remember that all markers are fallible. A high ApoB should be taken as a cue to investigate carefully to see if there are any underlying issues in your system. The investigation should cover the other important markers of underlying dysfunction that we discuss throughout this book—insulin, HDL, triglycerides, and blood glucose (the tests for all these are listed on page 85).

Most importantly, the lipoprotein measure discussed below is a far more powerful metric than ApoB. With a high ApoB, you really need to check the following ratio to verify whether a problem is present or not.

APOB/APOA1: THE MASTER RATIO

We'll close with the most powerful risk indicator by far: the ApoB/ApoA1 ratio. Remember from page 250 that lipoprotein molecules are wrapped in a unique protein called an apolipoprotein. LDL particles have B100 apolipoproteins (ApoB), while HDL particles have A1 apolipoproteins (ApoA1). So the ApoB/ApoA1 ratio tells you the ratio of LDL to HDL.

While this seems similar to the LDL/HDL ratio, it looks at the actual number of the particles themselves—the LDL/HDL ratio looks the quantities of cholesterol contained *within* the particles.

People with insulin resistance tend to have fewer HDL particles and more LDL particles, and the ApoB/ApoA1 ratio reveals this. People without insulin resistance tend to have the opposite—more HDL and less LDL. Hence, the ratio is very revealing and trumps the individual ApoB measure.

The ApoB/ApoA1 ratio obliterates the ApoB measure as a risk factor, just as the LDL/HDL and other traditional cholesterol ratios obliterate the LDL measure.

A good illustration of this comes from an excellent study on cholesterol risk markers.[16] The study included data from 15,632 women between ages forty-eight and fifty-nine—both traditional cholesterol panels and advanced lipoprotein tests. This gave a great comparison between the markers, showing which ones more powerfully predicted risk. In these association studies, any marker that predicts less than a 2x increase in coronary heart disease risk is a *weak* marker—it's unlikely to be a cause of CHD. In Figure 11.5 you can see that LDL comes in as very weak marker (as expected). However, if a marker predicts a 2x or ideally 3x increase in CHD risk, it is dependable marker and is likely linked to causal mechanisms of CHD. In this study, as in all the others, the ApoB/ApoA1 ratio put in a great performance, trumping ApoB alone. Interestingly, the total/HDL ratio did even better, as it sometimes does depending on the study. All of this is normal and expected when you understand the science. The importance of looking at ratios rather than at LDL has also been demonstrated in studies of familial hypercholesterolemics—people with a genetic disorder that gives them high levels of LDL.[17] Even for these high-LDL guys, the ratios always matter more.

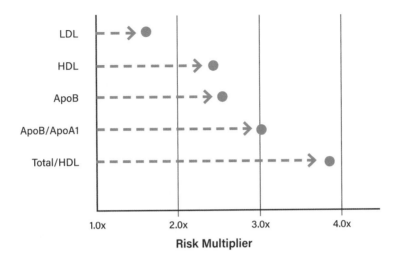

Comparison of Risk Predictors

Figure 11.5. LDL is always blown away by the ratios. Source: P. M. Ridker et al., "Non-HDL Cholesterol, Apolipoproteins A-1 and B100, Standard Lipid Measures, Lipid Ratios, and CRP as Risk Factors for Cardiovascular Disease in Women," *JAMA* 294, no. 3 (2005): 326–33.

THERE'S NO SUCH THING AS A SUDDEN HEART ATTACK

We all fear heart attacks—we worry that they can just happen like a bolt from the blue. But this is a lie. There's nothing sudden about the inflammatory disease sequence leading to that "sudden" heart attack.

Most heart attacks are caused by atherosclerosis, the inflammation of the arterial walls. Atherosclerosis is a progressive disease that's driven by multiple causes. Diabetic physiology (insulin-signaling dysfunction) is the primary factor in progression of heart disease, and tragically, millions of people are riddled with heart disease before they even get their diabetes diagnosis.

If pilots flew by the LDL gauge, we would have aircraft raining down from the sky.

The best way to verify your actual heart disease status is to use the best technology—a technology that can actually *see* this disease in your body. This has been possible to do since the 1980s. There is a simple five-minute scan that can identify heart disease and how bad it is: the coronary artery calcium (CAC) scan.

DECADES BEFORE DISASTER: THE STEADY MARCH OF CALCIFICATION

Before we get to what the CAC scan does and how it works, let's start with some background on heart disease.

The primary cause of cardiac death is damage to your coronary arteries—the blood vessels that feed the heart muscle itself—as a result of sustained inflammation. This damage can lead to a heart attack, and in around 50 percent of cases, this will result in death.

There are a few things that can happen in damaged coronary arteries to cause a heart attack (plaque on the arterial walls can break off and form a blood clot that blocks the flow of blood; the arterial wall itself can rupture or spasm, interrupting the flow of blood)—but no matter what triggers a heart attack, the body's response to damaged coronary arteries is always the same, and that response is what the CAC scan directly observes and quantifies.

Your body tries to repair itself by depositing calcium in the damaged areas of the arterial wall. As the damage continues, these repair processes quicken. They desperately attempt to shore up the arterial walls before a rupture occurs. This growing calcium becomes the telltale sign of imminent danger—the ultimate canary in the coal mine or visible tip of an iceberg, the vital evidence of your real risk of sudden death.

And it can be clearly and easily measured with a CAC scan.

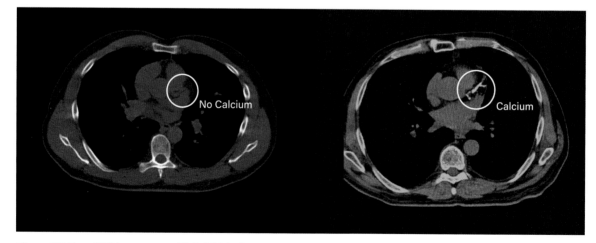

Figure 11.6. Zero CAC is a warranty. High CAC is the master risk marker. In the CAC scan at the right, there's coronary calcium along the left anterior descending artery—the widowmaker.

THE TELLTALE HEART: CORONARY CALCIUM REVEALED

A CAC scan can directly measure the amount of damage in coronary arteries and tell you whether a fatal heart attack is looming or not. It can prompt you to take evasive action. Afterward, it can verify that you have achieved safety. Following decades of misunderstanding, the CAC scan finally made the European Society of Cardiology preventative guidelines in 2013.[18] It is now recommended for the middle-risk people—where most heart attacks occur. Better late than never. But the vast majority of doctors are not aware of the updated recommendation to use the CAC scan. They do not have time to keep up with the guidelines—and so the vast majority do not realize that things have changed.

All astronauts and US presidents *must* take this scan; they are not given a choice in the matter. For about $150 and a few minutes of your time, you can get your CAC score. Crucially, it gives you advance warning so that you can take action to fix your arteries before it's too late.

Figure 11.6 shows a technological wonder: a CAC scan of the heart showing calcium deposits. On the left side is a heart with healthy coronary arteries. It has not been subjected to insults over its lifetime. It is not aflame with disease. No calcium appears in the image, meaning that the body hasn't been attempting to repair damaged arterial walls. Congratulations are in order. A CAC score of 0 is recorded.

The heart on the right is in a very different state. Within the white circle we see the looming iceberg: coronary calcium has formed along the length of a main coronary artery. The bright white is hard to miss, is it not? It's direct evidence of years of emergency repair work carried out on a damaged artery. This person probably never even knew there was a problem, but they have a CAC score of *almost 1,000*. This means they have around ten times the risk of a major heart attack as someone with a score of 0 to 10—regardless of any other risk factor. (Incidentally, the affected artery here is the left anterior descending artery, which is the responsible for the greatest number of deaths from heart attacks. Cardiologists have given a well-earned name to this artery: the widowmaker.)

CAC VERSUS OTHER RISK FACTORS
FOR HEART ATTACK

The CAC scan only costs $150 and takes just a few minutes, but it punches way beyond its weight. There are now many studies examining the CAC's ability to predict heart attack and early mortality. Here we will look through just a representative one.

We'll start with a simple comparison. Pretty much everyone knows that smoking is very bad for your health, and lung cancer is a much-feared consequence of smoking. The smoking-related deaths from cancer don't touch those from heart disease and stroke, though: in some studies, smoking has been shown to be the single greatest risk factor in cases of sudden death from cardiac-related events (SCD).[19] So let's be harsh and compare the predictive value of a CAC score against that of smoking.

In 2006, a large study looked at 10,377 people over the course of five years; 40 percent were smokers.[20] None of these people had a history of coronary heart disease. They were all given CAC scans at the start, and their CAC scores were recorded. Then the investigators waited to see what would happen.

Unsurprisingly, the smokers died at a faster rate than the nonsmokers. On average, the smokers were twice as likely to die before the five years were up as nonsmokers. This "doubling your risk" pattern is quite typical for smokers. But let's look at what a very high CAC score meant for probability of death. Does it bode worse than having a full-time smoking habit?

It does—far worse. For the *nonsmokers* who had a CAC score greater than 1,000, the chances of dying were nearly seven times higher than for a *smoker* with a low CAC score. Thus, having a high CAC score blew away even the crazy mortality risk of a full smoking habit. That illustrates the immense predictive power of CAC.

Let's look at another common way of evaluating risk. When doctors assess your heart attack risk, they use an old system of statistically noisy guesswork based on heart disease data from a few decades back. Included are things like cholesterol level, family history, blood pressure, and the like. Based on this information, you are given a Framingham Risk Score. This is your chance of having a major heart attack within the next ten years—a score of 10 percent means that you have a 10 percent chance. How does this fuzzy lottery system compare to your CAC score? Very badly indeed. All studies of CAC tell the same story. Figure 11.7 summarizes several of these studies.[21]

FRAMINGHAM RISK SCORE	CAC SCORE (which reveals the real risk level)				
10%? Really?	CAC: 0	CAC: 1–80	CAC: 81–400	CAC: 401–600	> 600
	2.4%	5.4%	16%	25%	36%

Chance of heart attack in the next ten years

Figure 11.7. Framingham metrics are weak. CAC tells the real risk story. Source: Matthew J. Budoff and Jerold S. Shinbane, eds., *Cardiac CT Imaging: Diagnosis of Cardiovascular Disease* (New York: Springer, 2010).

The left-hand column shows people who got a Framingham Risk Score of 10 percent. Graveyards have countless residents with good Framingham Risk Scores.

If you look at the CAC scores of all these Framingham 10 percent people, everything changes. We can now directly see the presence or absence of disease—a much more realistic way to evaluate risk. Using the standard Framingham system, we were in fuzzy lottery land—supposedly a 10 percent risk applied to everyone. If CAC is checked, however, we get the reality. Some people are indeed in good shape, but others have a 36 percent, not 10 percent, chance of having a heart attack over the next ten years. The following guide to risk now applies:

▶ A CAC score of 0 is good—you can relax.

▶ Between 1 and 80 is a concern, and you should be reconsidering your lifestyle.

▶ Between 81 and 400 means it's time to take serious action to attend to root causes.

▶ Greater than 400 means it's write-the-will time—or else address all root causes immediately so you can get to safety.

People who have very high CAC scores need to take action fast. Their arteries will likely rupture in the coming years—no nice retirement. Even people with a Framingham Risk of 10 percent can be highly diseased, though some are just fine. Who is who? We simply look at the proper measure—their CAC score. Those who need to can then take action fast.

In the cardiology business, these Framingham 10-percenters are in the "middle-risk" category. Most US adults are in this group. But the majority of heart attacks occur in this middle-risk category, not the high-risk one. What's more, many CAC studies that have looked closely at this middle-risk group and tracked actual heart attack rates have proven that, based on their actual amount of atherosclerosis (shown in a CAC scan), most of them—about 60 percent—were not middle-risk at all.[22] The Framingham system was wrong more than it was right, because 20 percent of the middle-risk people were revealed to actually be low-risk while 40 percent of them were really high-risk. So for this middle-risk majority in particular, it's crucial to know your CAC score—your risk may be much higher than you think.

But what's most important is the rate of increase in the CAC score. If your calcium is growing fast, then you *must* take action immediately to lower your insulin and reduce inflammation—the primary root causes of arterial damage.

To explain, let's look at a 2004 study (see Figure 11.8).[23] When this study was started, the participants had no symptoms, just like the other millions who die from "sudden" heart attacks. But they did all have evidence of calcium in their arteries.

	INITIAL CAC SCORE			
	30–100	101–400	401–1000	> 1000
Heart attacks over 6 years with LESS than 15% annual CAC increase	3%	3%	3%	3%
Heart attacks over 6 years with MORE than 15% annual CAC increase	20%	50%	> 50%	

Figure 11.8. CAC progression of more than 15% per year is the real killer. Source: P. Raggi, T. Q. Callister, and L. J. Shaw, "Progression of Coronary Artery Calcium and Risk of First Myocardial Infarction in Patients Receiving Cholesterol-Lowering Therapy," *Arteriosclerosis, Thrombosis, and Vascular Biology* 24, no. 7 (2004): 1272–77.

All were put on treatment to help with their vascular disease, revealed by their CAC score. But only the people who managed to slow their CAC progression could expect good outcomes. In fact, these people could expect *excellent* outcomes. Having an annual increase of coronary calcium deposits below 15 percent meant only a 3 percent chance of a heart event over the six years of the study. Even those with very high initial scores—as high as 1,000—shared the same low risk of heart attack! These people had managed to quench the fires inside, and their arteries had cooled. They were saved.

In stark contrast, the people whose calcium continued to build at a rate above 15 percent per year showed a much, much higher risk of heart attacks. Even those with lower initial CAC scores had a 20 percent risk for cardiac events within six years. Those who had higher initial scores *and* an increase above 15 percent per year were much worse again: their risk level was around 50 percent. Cardiac carnage, in other words.

This is the power of the CAC score. It can accurately tell if the disease has been burning inside. Crucially, it can tell you over time if you are still alight.

Did the participants' cholesterol levels show any difference between the saved and the doomed? No, they did not. There was no significant difference in cholesterol levels between the ones with excellent chances of escaping a cardiac event and the disaster-bound. As we've covered in this chapter, cholesterol is a highly misleading marker. The ratios (see pages 257 to 262) are the most valuable metrics, as they are quite consistent and dependable.

CAC PREDICTS ALL-CAUSE MORTALITY, TOO

The root causes that drive cardiac disease also drive cancer and many other killers. Therefore, the CAC score has even more power than we revealed above. Many studies have shown that the CAC score predicts death from all causes even better than it predicts death from coronary disease.[24]

Figure 11.9 gives a snapshot of the massive disease difference between a low CAC score and a high CAC score. This study included over 44,000 people averaging in their midfifties. The height of the bars show the actual mortality rates per thousand person-years, a common way of displaying mortality data. So a value of 25 on the y-axis means that 25 percent of these middle-aged people died over a ten-year period—a one-in-four chance of death. That's worse than the odds in Russian roulette. As you can see, the mortality rate for a high CAC score is around *fifteen times greater* than for a low one. That's a

Mortality Rates and CAC Scores

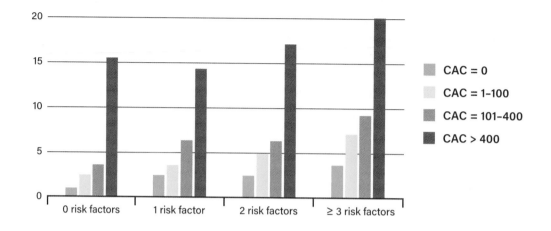

Figure 11.9. CAC blows away the usual risk factors in prediction of mortality. Source: K. Nasir et al., "Interplay of Coronary Artery Calcification and Traditional Risk Factors for the Prediction of All-Cause Mortality in Asymptomatic Individuals," *Cardiovascular Imaging* 5, no. 4 (2012): 467–73.

1,400 percent higher risk! (The figure also takes into account the number of "risk factors," but the CAC predictive power obliterates them.)

In short, a CAC scan is the ultimate test to assess your risk of death from most chronic diseases. It will enable you to take action to ensure longevity and tell you if your efforts are hitting the mark. Here is a quote from one major landmark CAC study: "Participants with elevated CAC were at increased risk of cancer, [chronic kidney disease, chronic obstructive pulmonary disease], and hip fractures. Those with CAC of zero are less likely to develop common age-related comorbid conditions, and represent a unique population of healthy agers."[25]

CAC RISING? TAKE ACTION!

Damage to your coronary arteries will only kill you prematurely if you encourage its growth in your body. It's not simply a consequence of aging. It is not an inevitability based on genetics and risk factors. You can actually do a hell of a lot about it. The damage is driven by a specific disease process: atherosclerosis. You either have this progressive disease or you don't. If you do, you can deal with it *very* effectively. And the best way to know if you have it is to get a CAC scan.

This simple scan was invented decades ago. You may well ask why it only became recommended for the middle-risk millions in 2013. It is a long and fascinating story, best told in the movie *The Widowmaker*, released in 2015. David Bobbett spent millions of dollars of his own money to fund the movie. After saving his own life, he committed to help others save themselves (setting up a charity to help get the message out: Irish Heart Disease Awareness, www.IHDA.ie).

What is the main reason for the delay in recommending the scan? This is best summed up in the words of Dr. Steve Nissen, the leading preventative cardiologist in the US. Here is what he had to say in 2014: "Well, I'm not a fan of the CAC Score. To date, no one's been able to show that knowing how much calcium is in the arteries actually allows you to change the outcome for the patients. So it tells you who's at risk, but it doesn't tell you what to do for them."

False! In this book you are learning which actions to take—actions that deliver. In the next ten years it will become apparent that the progressive disease of atherosclerosis can be slowed to the point of safety and even reversed. You can be one of the first people to take part in this revolution.

There is a notable lack of data in the scientific literature showing CAC regression—not just slowing coronary calcium buildup but actually reducing it. This is partly because the orthodoxy believes that regressing CAC is impossible.[26] But we are now seeing some studies illustrating that it is indeed possible.[27] The only snag: you can't lower your CAC score with the orthodox approach of a low-fat diet and medication. You need to follow the Eat Rich, Live Long plan, especially reducing your insulin by eating a low-carb, high-fat diet.

A final reminder on the meaning of the CAC score: it tells you what was happening in your arteries in the past, up to the time when you got the scan. It is your summed-up history of inflammatory damage. If you get a high score, don't panic. The key is to take action and stop the score from progressing quickly. If progression is stopped, your risk collapses rapidly. It is your choice whether to stop the damage going forward. It is your choice to save your own life.

JEFF P.'S STORY

One of Jeff's patients not only was able to stop his CAC score from rising but actually reduced it. Jeff P. managed to do this for himself by following the Eat Rich, Live Long plan.

As an aerospace engineer, Jeff P. has always been driven by data. His father had a mild heart attack at age fifty-three and Jeff's longtime goal has been to avoid that fate, so he tracked his annual blood work even though doctors kept assuring him his risk of heart disease was very low. From age thirty-two through fifty-four, Jeff's total cholesterol averaged 160 mg/dL while his LDL was around 100. This led his doctors to applaud his excellent health. They even advised him to maintain his dietary habits. They only suggested that he exercise more to raise his HDL above the low to mid-forties. They seemed to be unaware that his triglyceride-to-HDL ratio flagged potential issues. In Jeff's late forties and early fifties, that ratio averaged nearly 3 and even reached 5 at one point. (Recall from page 257 that most recommendations say it should be below 2, and we would say it should be below 1.2.)

Jeff ate a low-fat diet, as recommended by the 1977 Dietary Goals for the United States, which was released his first year of college. He resumed being a vegetarian at age forty-four, after a two-year experiment with it in college, vowing that this time it would be for life—his life, the life of animals, and the life of the planet. His diet was grain-heavy, and he loved "heart-healthy" Raisin Bran with almond or soy milk. Since brown sugar and honey are fat-free, he put them on his morning oatmeal. Not surprisingly, Jeff's weight crept up over the years, peaking at 170 pounds, 20 pounds more than his high school graduation weight. Jeff had a dad bod before it became a meme.

At age fifty, Jeff moved to Boulder, Colorado, and connected with its strong vegetarian and vegan community. At age fifty-three, he became a vegan. Lactose intolerance led Jeff to get tested for additional food sensitivities. He was shocked to learn he was allergic to gluten and angered when he was told to eliminate it from his diet. Jeff tried to be a gluten-free vegan for a few months, but he began craving meat. His profound initial skepticism with the Paleo/primal and low-carb, high-fat lifestyles faded as he appreciated the high-quality meats and fats from pastured animals available in Boulder. His appetite stabilized, his sleep improved, his skin cleared, and he regained and maintained his youthful weight. Jeff's energy level is high: he starts each day with a dip in the pool and bikes or walks for transportation.

A Paleo friend suggested that he get a CAC scan but warned that it would reveal the results of his past lifestyle rather than his current eating. Jeff was shocked when his score of 61 at age fifty-five put him in the worst third of his age group. It made him highly skeptical of his past blood profiles and the diet-heart hypothesis. He also wrote his own calcium-scoring program to independently verify his calcium scores. He devoured the medical literature on the predictive power of the CAC and became Dr. Gerber's patient. Together they decided to work on stabilizing Jeff's CAC score, but privately Jeff made it his ultimate goal to have a score of zero.

A year after Jeff's first CAC scan, his score was down to 38—a remarkable 36 percent reduction. Since eating low-carb, high-fat foods, Jeff's total cholesterol has increased significantly, but his crucial triglyceride-to-HDL ratio is now routinely less than 1. Also, his important HDL value has been as high as 88 mg/dL.

Fortunately, Jeff's cardiologist appreciates the power of the CAC score. At their last appointment, the doctor was astounded and nearly speechless upon seeing Jeff's clear regression in combination with a total cholesterol of 367 mg/dL. As a result, Jeff left the appointment without a statin prescription. Jeff will continue to pay attention to his data. His next scan will be in a couple of months at age fifty-nine, but he already knows that he looks and feels great!

IMPORTANT TAKEAWAYS

Here's a summary of the valuable measures that can be gleaned from the standard cholesterol tests.

► Triglyceride should be safely below 80 to 100 mg/dL.

► HDL should be safely above 40 mg/dL (for men) or 50 mg/dL (for women).

► The ratio of total cholesterol to HDL is crucial and should be below 4.5, preferably below 4.

► The ratio of triglyceride to HDL is also crucial and should be well below 2, preferably around 1.

► A CAC scan will enable you to discover hidden heart disease where the risk factors can fail. Crucially, you can take action and check back later to verify that you have stopped the progression of atherosclerosis.

> **"Growth for the sake of growth is the ideology of the cancer cell."**
>
> —Edward Abbey

CHAPTER 12

CANCER:
WHEN YOUR METABOLIC CONTROL SYSTEM FAILS

If you want to scare people, saying that something causes cancer is about as good as it gets. No one is comfortable with potentially increasing the risk for cancer. People arguably fear this disease even more than they fear heart disease. We believe that the low-carb lifestyle may get a huge boost in the coming years due to growing understanding of the links between high carb intake, hyperinsulinemia, and cancer.

But first, let us be clear: we are not in any way saying that a low-carb, high-fat diet can cure or treat cancer. That's simply not the case, although emerging evidence suggests that it may add support to conventional treatments. But it is very possible that eating a certain kind of diet may help *prevent* cancer.

You may have heard the phrase, "Cancer cells feed on glucose." There is certainly truth in this, and the mechanisms were worked out long ago. That said, your body will maintain glucose concentrations at a certain level no matter how little glucose you eat—the liver will make glucose if necessary. So there will always be some glucose around to feed those killer cancer cells. You can, however, take action to minimize the glucose load that your body has to deal with. We feel that minimizing the glucose you eat is a very sensible strategy to help prevent cancer growth. The ideal situation would be to target a combination of low blood glucose, low insulin, and high ketones. This is the basis of exciting new research that suggests that ketogenic diets can even help in treating existing cancer cases.[1] (We'll talk more about ketogenic diets on page 298.)

But the bigger factor is what we always come back to: insulin.

SAY HELLO TO INSULIN. AGAIN.

Hyperinsulinemia and insulin resistance have long been connected to increases in cancer risk. The insulin axis is particularly associated with cancers of the breast, endometrium, prostate, colon, and lung, among several others. Most of the really serious cancers with the highest mortality rates are right there in that list.

Insulin has anabolic functions, meaning that it promotes the growth of new tissue. Tragically, when you move toward the bad end of the insulin spectrum, your rising insulin levels drive growth like crazy! Thus it is no surprise that insulin dynamics are enormously important in risk for cancer.

Let's take as an example breast cancer, which is one of the most common cancers. First, we'll mention a fact that may surprise you: breast cancer incidence rates have historically been four to seven times higher in the United States than in Far Eastern countries.[2] When these women migrate to the United States, however, their breast cancer rates catch up over several generations, eventually becoming similar to those of Caucasians in the US. This is clearly *not* a genetics-driven issue—it is a nutritional and environmental one. "Genetics" are often blamed for cancer rates, but they account for only a very small percentage of cases.

What nutritional or environmental causes lead to this horrifying risk multiplier for breast cancer? A recent study from South Asia sheds light on this question.[3] South Asian countries are experiencing a rapid rise in cancer rates, and breast cancer is leading the charge.

The researchers carried out a detailed analysis of forty-five cancer patients and fifty-five healthy people and compared the HOMA insulin-resistance metric of the two groups. It turned out that having higher insulin resistance was a 12x multiplier of risk for cancer—that is, those with high insulin resistance had a risk of cancer that was twelve times higher. That blew away all the other factors. Obesity, hypertension, and triglycerides showed up as risk factors, but their risk multipliers were much lower. The key thing to note is that obesity, hypertension, and triglycerides are mainly insulin-resistance issues, so it is not surprising that insulin resistance itself has a stronger linkage to cancer rates.

Everyone in breast cancer research knows that obesity is hugely implicated as a risk factor for breast cancer. But it is not obesity itself that drives the risk—rather, it is insulin-related factors that drive the risk. Insulin-related factors also drive obesity, which is then merely associated with breast cancer. An excellent 2015 study illustrates this point.[4]

This research team compared 497 women with breast cancer to 2,830 women without cancer of any kind. They split the women into two groups: normal weight and overweight. They used the HOMA insulin-resistance metric as well as fasting insulin. Both metrics told the exact same story: breast cancer risk was approximately doubled in those with a high insulin level. This applied to all breast cancer cases, whether the woman was normal weight or overweight. Likewise, a low risk applied to women with low insulin, again whether a woman was normal weight or overweight.

There was, in other words, no extra risk for being overweight as such. The risk was attached to a much more important causal factor in breast cancer—a factor common in overweight women but just as dangerous in normal-weight women. All of the risk was attached to the woman's insulin level.

That is one of many reasons why we suggested that you calculate your HOMA measure (see page 39 for instructions) and work to bring it down. Avoiding most modern chronic diseases depends on avoiding insulin resistance!

RED MEAT, PROTEIN, AND CANCER

The World Health Organization has given carcinogen status to hundreds of modern compounds, tobacco smoke and asbestos being two of the most obvious. Recently, the WHO branded meat as a potential carcinogen, based exclusively on weak associational evidence from flawed studies. Crucially, no human experiments ever explored a connection between meat intake and disease. Once again, weak associational data is being used to create false theories, just as we saw with fat in Chapter 2. Same show trial, different scapegoat.

One of the most inflammatory headlines relating to the concern about protein and cancer was as follows: "Diets High in Meat, Eggs and Dairy Could Be as Harmful to Health as Smoking."[5] This is absurd. Tobacco smoke contains hundreds of known carcinogens. The smoking habit involves inhaling huge quantities of these carcinogens into the body every day. How on earth could the very foods we evolved to eat be as harmful as this? The article was designed to get attention, and it worked rather well.

The truth, of course, is that that meat, eggs, and dairy are not as harmful as smoking. They are not harmful at all—in the context of a healthy, nutrient-dense diet.

The study that this headline referred to concluded that people ages fifty to sixty-five who ate less protein had a lower cancer incidence, and that people older than sixty-five who ate less protein had a higher cancer incidence.[6] When averaged out, the overall protein link to cancer was a wash. On average, protein intake did not affect overall cancer or any other cause of mortality. Therefore, the headline was highly misleading.

Diabetic dysfunction—that is, being anywhere in the bad zone of the insulin spectrum—is accepted as a serious driver of both cancer and mortality rates. This is extensively documented in the scientific literature.[7] The mechanisms include hyperinsulinemia, disruption to the signaling of IGF-1 (an insulin-like hormone), elevated blood glucose, and many other aspects of insulin resistance.[8] In the study that linked lower protein intake to less cancer, the authors mentioned that the incidence of diabetes was much higher in the high-protein group, but they quickly glossed over that anomaly and focused instead on protein. But the whole study is undermined by this fact. While the researchers linked IGF-1 levels to cancer risk, they never mentioned that IGF-1 is intimately linked to hyperinsulinemia and diabetes mechanisms—and the high-protein group in the study was racked with these issues.[9] (We'll talk more about IGF-1 in the coming pages.)

Remember, too, that in this study, protein intake had no influence on all-cause mortality or cancer mortality overall. In fact, it's impossible to draw any useful conclusion from this study. In that respect, it is very similar to the other associational studies that seek to link animal protein intake and cancer.

THE ROLE OF IGF-1

Insulin-like growth factor 1, or IGF-1, is a cell-growth-signaling molecule that is very similar to insulin. Both have common roots in our evolutionary development. Insulin was the original growth signal, while IGF-1 later evolved to take over some functions. Both insulin and IGF-1 have sensors and receptors all over the body. Insulin and IGF-1 work together in a system that is often referred to as the "insulin/IGF-1 axis." In fact, insulin and IGF-1 are so closely related that they can activate each other's receptors, and they are intimately connected on many levels. This interconnectivity extends to their influence on issues like obesity, diabetes, and cancer.[10]

In addition to stimulating tissue growth on its own, insulin also directly influences how cells respond to all the other growth factors, including IGF-1. Importantly, insulin can dictate the quantity of *free* IGF-1 in circulation—this is IGF-1 that's not bound to other molecules, which would make it less active and less effective. Therefore, we must always take insulin's influence into account whenever we look at the effect of a growth factor.

It appears that free IGF-1 has been underinvestigated generally, with most research focus being on standard blood IGF-1 measures. For example, people with cancer-promoting obesity and insulin-resistance issues have been shown to exhibit much higher free IGF-1, but they have little change in their standard blood IGF-1 levels. To make things even more complex, the whole inappropriate-growth symphony is also conducted through other elements like insulin-like growth factor-binding protein and human growth hormone.[11]

The key point is that there has been controversy and scientific debate around IGF-1 links to cancer. As a growth factor, IGF-1 does encourage cell growth, and in cancerous cells, this could lead to the development of tumors. The study mentioned earlier chose to solely blame protein for the high IGF-1 that links to cancer risk. We would take a more complete view. We would say that refined carbohydrate, sugar, and vegetable oils are far, far more important factors in the cancer risk problem. That is in part because these foods are majorly implicated in driving chronic hyperinsulinemia and other problematic pathways. Also, protein increases insulin, which affects IGF-1, so isolating protein's direct effect on IGF-1 is peering at a small part of the picture.

We prefer to look at the whole picture when risk of such serious diseases is involved. We must look at the enormous importance of insulin's action as part of the insulin/IGF-1 axis. We must keep our focus on the big issues. Also, it must be kept in mind that while IGF-1 levels do correlate with disease rates, the relationship has shown inconsistencies. A recent meta-analysis pulled together the data from twenty-one IGF-1 and cancer risk associational studies, and the conclusion was not too surprising: there was "an increased risk of common cancers, but associations [were] modest and [varied] between sites."[12] (Note that "sites" refers to different cancer types.)

In another meta-analysis, high levels of IGF-1 were associated with increased risk for premenopausal but not postmenopausal breast cancer. The relative risk for premenopausal breast cancer was calculated to be around 1.5x—participants who had a high IGF-1 had a 1.5-times greater risk of breast cancer than those who did not. In contrast, studies of insulin and breast cancer risk often find a stronger risk multiplier—one showed a that higher insulin metrics resulted in a 2.9x greater risk of breast cancer.[13] And unlike the IGF-1 study example, the insulin risk multiplier applied equally to premenopausal and postmenopausal breast cancer. This emphasizes that IGF-1 levels can be weak and misleading—a focus on insulin metrics offers much more insight. The best scientific studies of the past decade correctly link insulin, insulin resistance, and IGF-1 together in the analysis, rather than focusing just on IGF-1.[14]

But there is another factor that's become a more popular topic of discussion recently in the world of cancer. It is a complex thing indeed, but we'll give you the lowdown here. The new kid on the cancer block is called mTOR.

THE MTOR FACTOR

We first mentioned mTOR back in Chapter 10—it's one of the nutrient sensors that manages energy utilization and growth signals for living organisms. In many studies, the mTOR pathway has been implicated as being closely linked to cancer initiation and progression. Therefore, any discussion on cancer deserves to include a summary of what may drive mTOR inappropriately in our bodies.

Where insulin primarily works with carbohydrate and leptin primarily works with fat, mTOR (short for the "mammalian target of rapamycin") primarily works with protein. There are two main complexes of mTOR, but to simplify this insanely complicated arena, we will give a general overview of mTOR function, without separating the two variants.

The nutrient-sensing mTOR pathway is essential for the development and growth of a young animal. But later in life, this pathway can drive cellular and general aging effects. So mTOR is a kind of double-edged sword in health and longevity. Unfortunately, it is the most complex double-edged sword you will ever come across! But if you manage to optimize your mTOR, a long, healthy life will likely be the result. So what can you do to optimize it?

mTOR takes inputs from a dizzying array of nutrient and environmental signals, in addition to protein. It integrates inputs such as growth factors, stress, energy status, oxygen, and amino acids. It also receives and integrates signals from many other sensors in the body. Both glucose and insulin can activate the mTOR pathway in different ways. High glucose and hyperinsulinemia will activate mTOR in negative ways. Insulin resistance can both drive and also be caused by mTOR's negative effects. And excessive protein can also activate and drive it in a negative way.

Activating mTOR—whether directly, through eating protein, or through myriad other pathways dependent on carb intake and more—can have positive effects, but when insulin resistance or obesity are present, these positive effects turn negative and can actually make the problems worse. We'll share a short list to illustrate:

► In the hypothalamus, mTOR activation aids in reducing appetite. Insulin resistance blocks this beneficial action, however, and can promote obesity in this way.

► mTOR enables fat tissue expansion, which can help divert excess energy to a safe place that avoids overloading your system. In someone who's overweight and metabolically unhealthy, however, excessive calories and inflammation responses can drive mTOR to induce insulin resistance and other problems.

- mTOR activation promotes glucose uptake into adipose cells with beneficial effects, but with increasing insulin resistance, this does not function properly.

- In muscles, mTOR plays a crucial role in protein synthesis and generating new mitochondria—the parts of a cell that produce energy—to burn energy efficiently. Muscle use through exercise increases mTOR activity for all the right reasons, so in this case higher mTOR is good.

- In the liver, mTOR is overactivated in obesity/overeating through the action of insulin and other mechanisms. It then blocks ketone production and promotes the accumulation of fat in the liver. This in turn promotes liver insulin resistance, unrestrained glucose production, and hyperglycemia (high blood sugar).

- In the pancreas, mTOR promotes the health of beta cells, which produce insulin. Sustained overactivation of mTOR, however, can lead to beta-cell death and thereby promote diabetes.

So the problem is that mTOR can have both positive and negative effects, depending on countless factors. We hope you also noticed the intimate links between mTOR and insulin signaling. One of the primary strategies for keeping mTOR function healthy is to lower insulin and remain insulin sensitive, whatever your protein intake.

Where does cancer come in? Like insulin, mTOR can adjust various stimuli to encourage the growth of your body's tissues. If mTOR is provoked excessively, this could lead to greater risk of cancerous growths. But mTOR can be judged only in the context of all the other growth pathways and how these are being driven through overall nutrition and lifestyle choices.

Our closing comment on cancer is simple. A science-based strategy to lower the risk of cancer would be to keep your carb intake, and therefore insulin, low. The other action steps also incorporate the most important healthy lifestyle strategies to lower cancer risk, from eliminating processed foods to exercising.

" And take your father and your households, and come unto me: and I will give you the good of the land of Egypt, and ye shall eat the fat of the land. **"**

—Genesis 45:18

CHAPTER 13

HEALTHY FAT:
THE FUEL FOR LONGEVITY

In Chapter 11 we clarified what cholesterol levels really mean. This misleading marker managed to single-handedly launch the war on fat. Tragically, it still serves to maintain it. We are now breaking free of the bad science, but progress has been glacial. Countless authorities and enormous global businesses are deeply invested in the mistaken theories; they refuse to yield in spite of the conflicting evidence. In recent years they have been resurrecting the data from old associational studies on dietary fat. In their last stand, this is what they have been reduced to.

THE DESPERATION OF THE ANTIFAT CAMP

A general guideline with associational studies is you should generally demand a 2x multiplier of risk to get excited—that is, the risk should be doubled when a particular factor is in play. This goes for any possible risk factor. Smoking is a significant causal driver in heart disease rates; it is associated with at least a doubled risk of coronary heart disease, as you might expect. Smoking is also a really serious driver of lung cancer—the risk multiplier here exceeds 10x. The studies that look at saturated fat and heart disease, on the other hand, don't come anywhere close to a 2x multiplier. In fact, many show *lower* risk of heart disease with a higher-fat diet. Let's look at the outcome of a recent antifat study that grasped at yet more associational straws.

In this study, the average risk multiplier they squeezed out against saturated fat was trivial—around 1.2x.[1] In other words, eating the most fat was associated with 20 percent higher risk of events compared to eating the least. But the healthy-user bias effect blows this away like a feather. The healthy-user bias phenomenon happens because the people who most strictly follow the official advice on nutrition are those who are most health-focused, and therefore they also deploy a whole range of healthy behaviors that are largely unaccounted for in any particular study. Regardless of the focus of the study, they achieve better health outcomes because they engage in healthier behavior overall.

The official advice for decades has been to lower saturated fat and replace it with polyunsaturated fat. The most health-focused people on the planet are the ones who best followed this advice. These participants therefore grant the low-fat diets with unearned credit. In many ways the studies are therefore highly misleading, creating dodgy data that helps to support bad science.

Figure 13.1 illustrates how big the statistical adjustments can get when the study methods are unusual. On the left side is the original relationship between natural saturated fat and heart events (based on raw baseline data acquired from an earlier paper, where only small age differences were at play between groups). It appeared that a diet higher in saturated fat resulted in fewer heart events. But the authors of a later paper adjusted for changing dietary patterns over time, which led to huge age differences appearing between the groups (the older people were more health-focused, actively pursuing the "official" advice). On the right side we see that now saturated fat looks bad. (Note that "hazard ratio" is just a way of saying "risk multiplier.") The message became "Guzzle industrial oils instead of natural fats."

Figure 13.1. Saturated fat appears good (left), but major adjustments mean major changes. Source: D. D. Wang et al., "Specific Dietary Fats in Relation to Total and All-Cause Mortality," *JAMA Internal Medicine* 176, no. 8 (2016): 1134–45; G. Zong et al., "Intake of Individual Saturated Fatty Acids and Risk of Coronary Heart Disease in US Men and Women: Two Prospective Longitudinal Cohort Studies," *BMJ* 355 (2016): i5796.

Saturated Fat and Heart Events

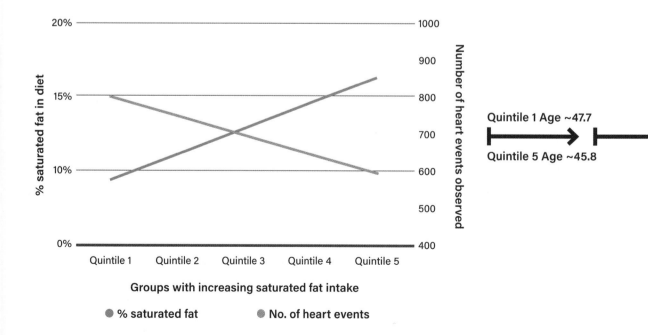

In the later study, the team fully deployed an unusual technique. They incorporated how the subjects' diets changed over the years using input from later questionnaires, and this led to the massive fifteen-year age difference between the lowest and highest groups. Unlike common age correction, this study dynamically created age differences between groups nearly as large as the study duration. This is where the healthy-user bias distortion could go into overdrive, as methods depart from established norms. The healthiest people during the period of this study were constantly being told that they should reduce saturated fat and replace it with polyunsaturated oils—and the older ones were listening more. Their later questionnaires then beautifully reflected these dietary changes. Even if their other healthy habits were responsible for their better health outcomes, reduced saturated fat gets the credit. Great for the desired message—but not for scientific accuracy.

We don't need to look at any more associational studies that seek to implicate natural fats as harmful. They all limp in with risk multipliers around 1.2x (or even lower). But let's look at some similar studies from the opposing camp. Can these associational studies debunk the fat-bashers? It appears that they can.

Saturated Fat and Age-Adjusted Hazard Ratios

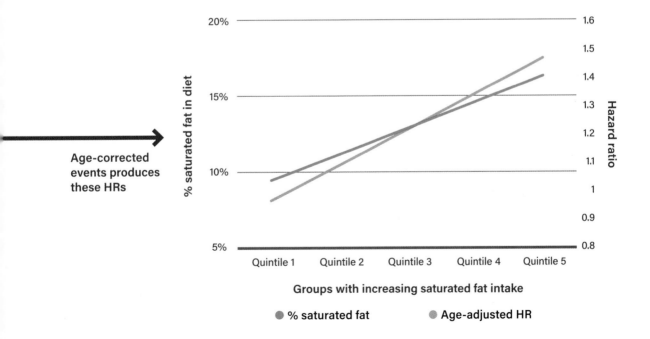

Age-corrected events produces these HRs

Groups with increasing saturated fat intake

● % saturated fat   ● Age-adjusted HR

STUDIES DEFENDING SATURATED FAT

The conclusion of a recent large, well-conducted study says it all: "Saturated fats are not associated with all-cause mortality, [cardiovascular disease], [coronary heart disease], ischemic stroke, or type 2 diabetes."[2]

There are many more studies like this from recent years. Some suggest that replacing saturated fat with polyunsaturated oils can actually increase the risk of heart disease. One of them recorded the following conclusion: "Substituting SFAs with … polyunsaturated fatty acids (PUFAs) or carbohydrates was significantly associated with higher [coronary heart disease] risks."[3]

For the 35,597 Europeans who participated in this study, saturated fat appeared to be the safest fat. The risk multiplier reached 1.3x for each 5 percent of saturated fat that was replaced by other ingredients. As with many of these studies, the risk multiplier was too low to mean a whole lot. Yet saturated fat in this study appeared to be safer than other foods examined.

Here's the conclusion of yet another study, from September 2016: "Our results do not support the association between CVD [cardiovascular disease] and saturated fat, which is still contained in official dietary guidelines. Instead, they agree with data accumulated from recent studies that link CVD risk with the high glycemic index/load of carbohydrate-based diets. In the absence of any scientific evidence connecting saturated fat with CVD, these findings show that current dietary recommendations regarding CVD should be seriously reconsidered."[4]

And finally, the most revealing study of the bunch was published in August 2017. Called the Prospective Urban Rural Epidemiology (PURE) study, it tracked 135,335 men and women in eighteen different countries for 7.4 years.[5] The PURE study found that neither coronary heart disease mortality nor mortality in general was associated with intake of fat in general or saturated fat specifically. In fact, a higher saturated fat intake was associated with lower stroke rates. Unsurprisingly (to us), it did show that increasing carbohydrate intake tracked with increasing mortality. In a separate PURE analysis of participants' cholesterol metrics, the findings agreed with what we have been saying: ratios are far more predictive of problems than the misleading LDL, and higher carbohydrate intake is strongly linked to a higher ApoB/ApoA1 ratio.[6]

True, these are all associational studies, and as we've said before, associational evidence only points to an association between two things; it doesn't prove that one thing causes another. However, associational evidence is good for *disproving* a theory: if two things aren't even associated with each other, then no causal relationship can even be suggested. And if there's an *anti*-correlation—the more you have of one thing, the less you have of another—you can be sure that the thing you have more of (in these studies, saturated fat) isn't causing the thing you have less of (heart disease and overall mortality). The most well-executed associational studies certainly indicate that natural dietary fats should never have been demonized and that higher carbohydrate intakes are far more concerning.

CLOSING ON THE TRIALS

We will not waste your time trudging through all the low-fat trials and experiments. When you roll them up, you are left with confusion. Billions of dollars have been spent with nothing worthwhile to show for it.

Two of the biggest studies were particularly embarrassing: the Multiple Risk Factor Intervention Trial (MRFIT) and the Women's Health Study, each of which cost hundreds of millions of dollars to complete. Participants decreased their intake of overall and saturated fat and increased their intake of polyunsaturated fat. The researchers threw their best possible shot at proving that saturated fat causes heart disease, and the shot failed spectacularly. Some of media reported quite honestly on the disaster. The *Wall Street Journal* ran a story on the MRFIT study entitled "Heart Attacks—A Test Collapses."

There were also many trials that showed significantly worse outcomes when replacing saturated fat with vegetable oils.[7] These negative-outcome trials were not publicized truthfully, nor were they included properly in many meta-analyses (studies that pool together many other inconclusive studies).

In 2015, a very large meta-analysis examined many of these experimental results. It was a final desperate effort to implicate saturated fat as a cause of heart disease. The key findings overall were that reducing or replacing saturated fat in the diet resulted in:

▶ no significant effect on all-cause mortality

▶ no significant effect on cardiovascular mortality

▶ no significant effect on heart attack mortality or the rate of heart attacks

▶ no significant effect on stroke incidence or mortality

There was a slight reduction seen in cardiovascular events, which just nudged into the statistically significant zone. However, this limited effect—mainly a reduction in the incidence of angina—was solely restricted to studies where polyunsaturated fat replaced saturated fat. The selection process also resulted in several negative cardiovascular trials not being included, so even this is open to debate.

Amusingly, the only trial that showed a slight effect on cardiovascular mortality was one where the intervention did not reduce cholesterol levels. Also, a later analysis showed that the reduction in cardiovascular mortality was cancelled out by an increase in cancer mortality.[8] Go figure. The remaining fourteen of the fifteen studies in the meta-analysis did not show any reduction in cardiovascular mortality at all, which speaks volumes.

The real reason these trials failed is that *the wrong hypothesis was being tested.* They all assumed that saturated fat was independently bad for heart health—harmful all by itself. This in turn rested solely on the idea that it raised LDL levels. Presuming that LDL was universally bad completed the deception. As we explained in Chapter 11 and as countless studies have found, there was never sound science supporting this idea in the first place.

Saturated fat will only have meaningful negative effects if you eat too much carbohydrate, are too high in omega-6, or are too low in omega-3. This was not appreciated by the experimenters, and that is the main reason why the experiments failed.

These experiments were playing with saturated fat changes while not controlling for the interactions. When dietary carbohydrate is too high, there may be a slight advantage gained by replacing saturated fat with polyunsaturated. But this slight advantage at best only tweaks cardiovascular events downward slightly. Some of the experiments just barely picked up on this, but they sold this quirk like there was no tomorrow, even though any gains made are offset by other issues from polyunsaturated fats.

The most valuable experiment would center on reducing insulin and insulin resistance, not the misleading LDL cholesterol. It would focus on reducing trig/HDL or total/HDL ratios. These reflect healthy insulin signaling and low inflammation very well. This experiment would also be informed by insulin metrics. The results of this experiment would address real root causes of heart disease, rather than playing around the edges of statistical noise.

A high-fat and low-carbohydrate combination should have been tested in large experiments. The detrimental potential for excessive omega-6 oils should have been accounted for. And with so much supportive science behind the ratio of omega-6 to omega-3 (see page 53), this factor should also have been included.[9] Several other important factors should have been controlled for, too. Sadly, there's no large human trial that looks at all these factors. The controllers of the funding squandered it on desperate efforts to rescue the low-fat theory.

We do, however, have many experiments that reveal the reality of what fat can do for us in the right ratios.

ADVANCING YOUR HEALTH WITH HEALTHY NATURAL FATS

In Chapter 4 we showed that the majority of American adults now have some level of metabolic insulin resistance syndrome (MIRS), which is at the root of heart disease and many other modern diseases. Everyone is at a different level—we are all on a spectrum when it comes to this disease process. We called this the hyperinsulinemia/insulin-resistance spectrum in Chapter 10, but it is essentially the MIRS spectrum also. Now we need to get into the core of why dietary fat is so important. It is crucial in fighting the real root causes of this disease. It enables us to address the biggest health problems in the world. It helps us to move people to the safe end of the insulin spectrum— where slimness is achievable and longevity is within grasp.

This is all possible because reducing the amount of carb and getting most of our calories from healthy fats resolves insulin resistance and hyperinsulinemia. These are the problems at the core of MIRS and many chronic diseases, especially heart disease and obesity, and resolving them has enormous implications for health and longevity.

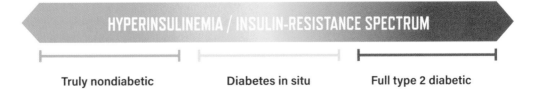

HYPERINSULINEMIA / INSULIN-RESISTANCE SPECTRUM

Truly nondiabetic   Diabetes in situ   Full type 2 diabetic

As we explained in Chapter 5, a properly formulated low-carb, high-healthy-fat diet:

▸ is hugely effective in resolving prediabetes and diabetes

▸ improves appetite control

▸ optimizes the absorption of vitamins A, D, E, and K

▸ strengthens the immune system

▸ minimizes systemic inflammation

▸ enhances rapid recovery after sustained vigorous exercise

▸ lowers the important risk markers for heart disease

▸ slows aging and improves energy

▸ promotes healthy skin, hair, nails, and many other outward signs of health

A fascinating 2006 experiment revealed exactly why reducing carb and increasing healthy fat is the key to health.[10] It specifically investigated a range of people affected by the MIRS epidemic. This was a perfect group to focus on. Engineers love looking at the parts that have the problem. You can learn so much from scrutinizing these "failed parts."

The researchers split the participants into four randomized groups. They wanted to test differing ratios of carb to fat in their diets; they also wanted to try out something rather special.

First, each group was put on a different dietary regimen for three weeks, without having to reduce their calories. This simulated what would happen with a dietary regimen in a real-life situation. The high-carb diets had complex carbs but also simple sugars—mimicking a typical high-carb diet. The highest-fat diets were broadly similar to the ratios we would recommend. In summary, the four diets were low fat (54 percent carb), moderate fat (39 percent carb), high fat (26 percent carb), and high saturated fat (again 26 percent carb, but here the fat was mostly saturated). (We would generally recommend 20 percent carb or less.)

The next step after the three-week diet was ingenious. They kept the four groups on their diets, but they also *starved* them for the following nine weeks. One thousand calories per day was taken away from everyone. This would not happen in real life. But it revealed something really interesting.

Crucially, the researchers went far beyond measuring the misleading LDL metric. They recorded all the powerful metrics we talked about in Chapter 10: trig/HDL ratio, total/HDL ratio, and all the advanced lipoprotein measures. So what happened to the different groups? Let's look first at the nonstarvation period.

The lowest-carb, highest-fat diets achieved *superb* improvements in just three weeks—with no reduction in calories. The lowest-carb diet that emphasized saturated fat was the best performer of all. This diet reduced trig/HDL by 44 percent in three weeks flat. That's right: the high-fat diet nearly halved the most important cholesterol health metric of all.

It also increased HDL by 5 mg/dl, lowered triglyceride by 37 percent, and substantially shifted the important total/HDL down by 13 percent. It also improved the metrics on the number and size of LDL particles.

In contrast, the high-carb, low-fat diets achieved almost nothing without calorie restriction. There was only a 10 percent drop in triglyceride and trig/HDL, with the other metrics not shifting at all.

So a big win here for a low-carb, high-fat diet, and a dunce's hat for a low-fat diet.

But this experiment then got even more interesting. What do you think happened during the starvation period? Let's take a look.

After nine weeks' starvation, the highest-fat diets had improved the key markers even more. Not too surprising to us. The highest-carb diets also finally began to see improvements in the key markers. But what is most interesting is that *even after nine weeks of starvation, the highest-carb diet had only achieved half of what the highest-fat one had achieved with no starvation.*

You can stick with a typical high-carb, low-fat diet and cut your calories in half, and you'll start to see some improvement in health metrics. Or you can try a low-carb, high-fat diet, stop obsessing about calories, and eat delicious low-carb food, and you'll see *twice* the improvement.

THE MIXTURE MATTERS

The world may be still wedded to the misleading, noisy marker of LDL. But many pioneers of sound science are forging ahead. They are carefully monitoring *proper* health markers. This enables them to focus on real root causes of disease—and, of course, to formulate the best diets to prevent it.

Professors Steve Phinney and Jeff Volek are two such pioneers. Phinney realized in the 1970s that vilifying natural healthy fats had been an enormous mistake. His early experiments proved something of immense importance: that the healthfulness of natural saturated fats was hugely dependent on keeping carbohydrate low.

Volek has carried out a series of fascinating human experiments that demonstrate the importance of lowering carb.[11] His subjects were typical examples of what our population has become: overweight people with

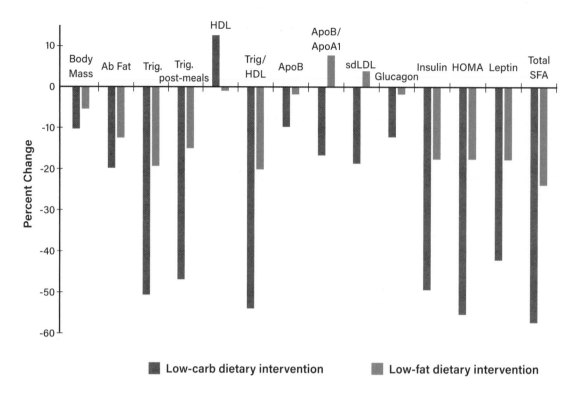

Figure 13.2. All cholesterol and inflammatory markers improve much more with low carb. Source: J. S. Volek et al., "Dietary Carbohydrate Restriction Induces a Unique Metabolic State Positively Affecting Atherogenic Dyslipidemia, Fatty Acid Partitioning, and Metabolic Syndrome," *Progress in Lipid Research* 47, no. 5 (2008): 307–18.

"cholesterol issues"—perfect people to test the power of different diets on. In these experiments, half of the participants were put on "healthy" low-fat fare—not junk food by any means but genuine food-pyramid fare—and the other half were put on a very low carb (keto) diet. Figure 13.2 shows how the low-carb diet obliterated the low-fat one.

On the low-carb diet, at the end of the twelve-week experiment, HDL had risen and, more importantly, trig/HDL had collapsed by more than 50 percent. This is a halving of the most important "cholesterol" measure. The subjects' insulin and triglyceride responses after a meal were greatly improved. The team also carried out human experiments examining the dietary effects on the most dependable markers of inflammation.[12] Again, it was seen that the low-carb diet dramatically improved these, where the low-fat diet, if anything, worsened them.

Note that the low-fat diet, while trounced by the low-carb one, still managed to achieve some improvements. This is because most overweight people are on a really bad diet, a high-carb and high-fat combo, so even a low-fat diet was an improvement. But why settle for mediocre improvements using an unappetizing diet? It is much better to achieve massive improvements using a delicious diet.

Remember that the body weight is not really a *cause* of issues. The health of fat cells is much more important. How do you dramatically improve the health of your fat cells? You could technically do it with a combination of a very low fat diet, calorie restriction, and very careful monitoring and supplementation to ensure nutrient sufficiency. Or you can do it the way we do—by eating a well-formulated low-carb diet. The low-carb diet naturally targets all those delicious and nutrient-dense ancestral foods. It is an easier, more effective, and vastly more enjoyable way to eat yourself into excellent health.

MASS EXPERIMENTS LEAD TO MASS APPEAL

In recent years, low-carb science has been really breaking into the mainstream, though there are of course regular reports in the media trying to undermine it. After all, huge businesses and massive reputations are at stake. If low-carb becomes the default, countless organizations and individuals have a lot to lose.

In 2016, we saw one of the most impressive mass experiments yet. The leaders of the Diabetes.co.uk charity are not establishment medical professionals—they are technical experts from the IT world who have set up what has become the biggest type 2 diabetes resource group in the world with the goal of joining together all of the world's diabetics to share what works best to improve their condition. They started off by supporting the standard high-carb advice for diabetics.

But then the team researched the science and realized that low-carb was a basic requirement for managing diabetes. They launched a live experiment for their members to deploy a simplified low-carb diet.[13] Guidelines for what to eat and a tracking app were provided for free. More than 120,000 people signed up for the experiment.

Even though this was not a randomized controlled trial, the results were dramatic. Within ten weeks, 80 percent of the self-experimenters reported significant weight loss—more than 10 percent reported losing at least 20 pounds. More than 70 percent experienced improvements in blood glucose. And around 20 percent were able to get off all blood glucose medications.

All of this in ten weeks—through applying the opposite of what the official dietary guidelines dictate.

LOSING MASS THROUGH EATING FAT

A huge element of why low-carb, high-fat diets work is the appetite-control factor, but this factor is expressly excluded from most diet-experiment designs. Many experiments fix calorie intake at a set value, thus hiding the appetite factor completely (participants don't have the option of eating when they're hungry, as would happen in the real world). Others pit a calorie-restricted high-carb diet against an "eat all you want" low-carb one. (In many of these experiments, the low-carb diet still beat the calorie-restricted high-carb diet!) Other shenanigans include calling something a low-carb diet if it is below 45 percent energy from carbs. This makes a comparison between low- and high-carb meaningless, since it essentially compares high-carb to very high carb. This behavior ends up kicking the results into the statistical noise. A true low-carb diet is around 20 percent energy from carbs—or even lower.

We saw in the last section that 80 percent of 120,000 people in one experiment had a good weight-loss experience when moving to low-carb—even though they had already been striving to follow a "good" diet to lose weight. The low-carb approach gave them a super boost in success: it dropped their weight and lowered their medication needs. So why does the establishment keep claiming that human studies don't show an advantage for low-carb?

Figure 13.3. The trials have concluded that low-carb performs the best. Source: Public Health Collaboration, "A Summary Table of 53 Randomised Controlled Trials of Low-Carb-High-Fat Diets of Less Than 130g Per Day of Total Carbohydrate and Greater Than 35% Total Fat, Compared to Low-Fat Diets of Less Than 35% Total Fat Compiled by the Public Health Collaboration," n.d., https://phcuk.org/wp-content/uploads/2016/04/Summary-Table-53-RCTs-Low-Carb-v-Low-Fat.pdf.

Low-Carb vs. Low-Fat Weight Loss in Randomized Controlled Trials (RCTs)

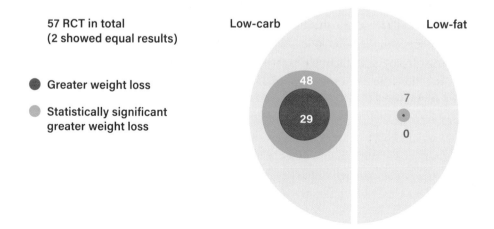

57 RCT in total
(2 showed equal results)

● Greater weight loss

○ Statistically significant greater weight loss

Low-carb

48
29

Low-fat

7
0

Sam Feltham of the Public Health Collaboration UK researched the matter quite thoroughly in 2016.[14] He gathered together fifty-seven human weight-loss trials. All of them tested low-carb, high-fat diets against low-fat diets. The trials ranged from short six-week interventions to two-year-long experiments.

The result was unequivocal. The low-carb approach beat low-fat in forty-eight out of the fifty-seven trials—with clear statistical significance in twenty-nine. The low-fat diet edged ahead in only seven out of fifty-seven, and none of these were statistically significant. This means that the low-fat diets *failed* in all fifty-seven trials.

Case closed, even when some trials are weakly designed or even biased toward defending the low-fat establishment. Also, keep in mind that many of the low-carb groups in these trials did not get proper advice, so they were exposed to many pitfalls. But still the low-carb approach overwhelmingly won out.

ABSORBING VITAL NUTRIENTS THROUGH FAT

The low-fat fad of the past few decades not only has contributed to our obesity problem, but it has also promoted many more serious health issues. This is partly because the incorrect fat-lowering advice has a negative effect on the consumption of many vitamins required for optimum health. The most significant downside here is that on a low-fat diet, we can end up deficient in the fat-soluble vitamins, which are required for optimal health.

The four important fat-soluble vitamins are A, D, E, and K. In order for your body to absorb these, they need to be consumed with plenty of fat. Being low in any of these contribute to a dizzying array of health issues. Sadly, the chances of a doctor tracking these health problems back to an inadequate vitamin intake is extremely unlikely—the current medical system is overwhelmingly focused on using medications to resolve problems. Your best strategy, therefore, is to eat a diet that will keep you well into the sufficiency zone on these and other vital nutrients. A well-formulated low-carb, high-fat diet is a superb way to do this.

Another important point to note is that vitamins A, D, and K interact with each other to a great degree. They also interact synergistically with minerals, including magnesium and zinc. Modern populations tend to be deficient in these and many other minerals. There are more reasons for this than simply the damaging lunacy of the low-fat guidelines. Depletion of minerals from the soil due to modern agricultural practices is just one other issue we all face.

Your first strategy is to get onto a high-fat real-foods diet and make great choices. The most nutritious foods should be targeted in order to get these vitamins and more. Luckily, the most nutritious fatty foods are also the most delicious—pastured eggs, wild-caught fish, and grass-fed meats.

You can also leverage the power of fats to boost your absorption of vitamins from the plant foods you eat. Consuming tasty fat with plant foods will enhance nutrient transport into your body. For this reason you should always eat vegetables and salads with some olive oil or grass-fed butter. Coconut oil is another excellent choice for this purpose—it has been found to improve absorption of antioxidants and other nutrients even more than other fats.

It won't take long for your skin, hair, and general well-being to improve when benefiting from a regimen high in healthy fats.

HIGH-FAT AND FASTING

One of the most important benefits of a low-carb, high-healthy-fat diet is an indirect one: it enables much better control of your appetite. This means that it greatly enables you to habitually space out your meals—in other words, it helps you incorporate fasting into your daily life. (Another term for this is *intermittent fasting*.) Properly implemented fasting habits will help with weight loss, for sure, but the fasted state is also a health-promoting one that works its magic on many levels.

Pretty much all religions and spiritual groups throughout history have had a place for the practice of fasting. It was not just about self-denial, either. Fasting encourages mental clarity and enhances the thought processes. They may also have had an inkling that fasting in a sense cleanses the body. Hippocrates, Paracelsus, and Galen, the three fathers of modern medicine, all believed fasting to be a powerful medical intervention. In fact, Paracelsus said, "Fasting is the greatest remedy—the physician within." These old guys were entirely correct, long before modern science could prove it.

The health benefits of fasting have been recognized increasingly in the past decades, particularly among medical researchers. Studies have shown that fasting:

► promotes insulin sensitivity in all people[15]

► reduces insulin resistance in people with prediabetes[16]

► reduces inflammation[17]

► helps reverse type 2 diabetes[18]

► reduces blood pressure[19]

► improves the health of fat cells and improves fat-burning[20]

► improves weight loss while retaining muscle better than calorie restriction[21]

► improves mood and mental clarity[22]

► enhances autophagy (cellular regeneration and repair)[23]

► protects against damage from radiation in cancer patients[24]

► may protect against damage from chemotherapy in cancer patients[25]

► promotes longevity[26]

None of this surprises us in the least. Sadly, there is a dearth of human studies in this arena; the reality is that funding is extremely difficult to obtain for studies on interventions that will negatively impact many industries. However, adding together all the available studies and deeper mechanisms, one can come to a solid scientific conclusion that fasting is beneficial.

We've been skipping meals as part of our weight-maintenance and health-optimization plans for many years. We don't restrict our calories in the way that the jaded "eat less, move more" advice would suggest—by counting calories or peering at portion sizes. We simply skip meals occasionally because our low-carb diet has turned us into excellent fat-burners. If it's easy to do something that's very good for you, then why not do it? We would never go back to the habit of eating meals at every allotted time slot. It's so restrictive, really—the days of responding mindlessly to the mealtime bell are thankfully over.

Freedom is another key benefit of fasting lifestyles: Freedom from excessive appetite. Freedom from hunger that drags you back to the table or pantry. Freedom from the concept that you need to eat frequently. Freedom to use the enormous energy stores our bodies carry. Freedom that feels real good.

KETOGENIC DIETING

There has been a lot of talk about ketogenic diets in recent years. As we briefly discussed in Chapter 5, a ketogenic diet is the ultimate version of a fat-burning diet and maximizes the advantages of that diet. It's called "ketogenic" because fat-burning creates molecules called ketones, which are used for energy. People on a ketogenic diet are in a state of nutritional ketosis: they have a certain amount of ketones in their blood.

Some people confuse the healthy state of nutritional ketosis with a very dangerous condition called *diabetic ketoacidosis.* With diabetic ketoacidosis, the body has no insulin available (as in untreated type 1 diabetes) and blood glucose spirals upward out of control. Simultaneously, the lack of insulin allows ketone production to go out of control. Double trouble—and it's likely to end in a coma or death if insulin is not made available quickly. It's virtually impossible for someone who does not have type 1 diabetes to have diabetic ketoacidosis.

In stark contrast, the state of nutritional ketosis is a beautifully regulated natural state for humans. Some indigenous peoples are very rarely out of ketosis for most of their lives. It occurs naturally when you are low on carb or sugary foods. Fat and ketones smoothly take over fueling the body where glucose was previously used.

Deep ketosis is a state in which your body's use of glucose is minimal and your ketone levels are very high. It can be highly therapeutic in the treatment of many diseases, including epilepsy and obesity. But we do not all need to pursue the state of deep ketosis. Most people already live somewhere on a keto spectrum, which goes from the heavy glucose-burner (very low ketone use) on one end all the way to super fat-burner (very high ketone use) on the other end.

You can choose where on this spectrum you want to be. We find it best to live in the mild ketosis end of the spectrum. We do, however, move in and out of deep ketosis regularly through a combination of food choice and fasting strategies. This way, we intermittently receive the extra benefits of fasting, including enhanced mental acuity and autophagy (the breaking down of unhealthy old cells and creation of healthy new ones).[27] We like tapping into excellent benefits and the many other advantages of fat-burning and ketone use without becoming obsessed with ketone levels. Let's now look at how you can navigate the keto spectrum.

First, remember that a high-carb diet pumps glucose into your body. With a lot of glucose available, there will be no fat-burning or keto action in sight. On this diet, you're also very unlikely to be slim or healthy.

If you greatly reduce your carbohydrate intake, however, your body starts getting ready to move along the keto spectrum. This way of eating depletes your glycogen stores quite quickly, and as those stores fall, your body begins to produce increasing levels of ketones to meet your energy requirements. It also begins to fabricate a small, steady stream of glucose for the few tissues that need it (most tissues can run on fat and ketones alone). This process of creating glucose from stored fat and protein is called *gluconeogenesis*.

Your body can create this required glucose with ease. Your liver could pump out many times the level required. Glucose is easy to make out of fat and protein stores—it's having too much glucose that is the common problem!

As you go deeper into ketosis, your body increasingly switches to relying on nonglucose fuel sources. Fat is burned directly by many tissues while ketones supply the rest. In this state, the brain's use of glucose drops from 100 percent to as low as 30 percent—with those crucial ketones providing the remaining 70 percent.

Nutritional ketosis is an entirely normal human state. It is arguably healthier than any other nutritional state.

GETTING INTO KETOSIS

If you're interested in getting into ketosis—and, actually, on any low-carb, high-fat diet—be careful not to overeat polyunsaturated fats. In the past, doctors who believed that saturated fats were problematic overloaded their keto-following patients with epilepsy with large quantities of omega-6-rich polyunsaturates. But eating high quantities of polyunsaturated fat actually works against many of the benefits of keto (see Appendix E for details). It is important to ensure that most of your fat calories come from saturated or monounsaturated fat—or, indeed, your own body fat.

Many keto adherents measure the amount of ketones in their blood regularly. This can be very useful because it lets you know if you're actually in ketosis. It can also help flag foods that push you out of ketosis. If your ketone level is above 0.5 mmol/L, you're in a state of nutritional ketosis; a level of 2–4 mmol/L means you're in deep ketosis. You can use a blood ketone meter to test the ketones in your blood—in fact, the glucose meter we recommended on page 84 will also measure ketones in your blood. But for measuring ketones alone, we recommend the Ketonix system, which measures ketones from the breath, with no blood sample required. The Ketonix system is very capable and inexpensive to order online. It is also arguably more accurate, since the ketones on the breath reflect what you are actually producing, whereas the ketones in your blood may appear low because you are constantly burning them up to fuel your body.

As we mentioned in Chapter 5, to achieve ketosis, aim to get approximately 70 percent of your daily calories from fat, 20 percent from protein, and less than 10 percent from carb. In contrast, a standard low-carb diet is approximately 60 percent fat, 20 percent protein, and 20 percent carb. For comparison, the traditional Paleo diet is generally 50 percent fat, 20 percent protein, and 30 percent carb. Volek and Phinney have produced a useful diagram to illustrate the differences, Figure 13.4.

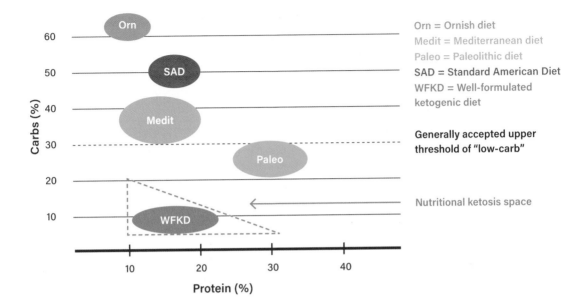

Dietary Protein and Carbs by Diet Type

Orn = Ornish diet
Medit = Mediterranean diet
Paleo = Paleolithic diet
SAD = Standard American Diet
WFKD = Well-formulated ketogenic diet

Generally accepted upper threshold of "low-carb"

Nutritional ketosis space

Figure 13.4. Different macronutrient ratios for different dietary strategies. Used with permission from Jeff Volek and Steve Phinney, Beyond Obesity LLC.

THE BENEFITS OF KETO

Pushing far into the keto spectrum has effectively no downsides and huge potential benefits. These are just a few of them:

▶ Moving toward deep keto can have major advantages for the very overweight and those who are on the wrong end of the insulin spectrum. It promotes fat-burning, enhances appetite control, and helps resolve insulin resistance.

▶ Emerging science is indicating that keto diets may be helpful in the management of certain cancers. There are no miracle cures, but adding a well-formulated keto diet to traditional treatments could improve outcomes considerably.

▶ Many neurological conditions respond very well to the keto diet. Keto has been used for nearly a century to successfully manage epilepsy. Even in people for whom the drugs fail entirely, extraordinary control of the disease has been achieved with keto.

The ability of ketosis to improve many disease risk factors is beginning to be realized in the orthodox medical world. A tipping point is expected in the coming decade, and we believe keto will become an accepted approach for managing appetite and achieving optimal health.

The fear of cancer is perhaps the greatest subliminal health worry that most of us have. The huge and increasing number of people living with cancer strongly desire actions that they can take to increase their chances of survival.

The scientific data supporting the anticancer effects of keto has been ramping up in the past decade. An increasing number of researchers are working in this area. Cancer research expert Dominic D'Agostino told us: "When I got into this line of research five years ago, there was nothing on www.clinicaltrials.gov [i.e., no keto/cancer human trials]. Now, as evidence that this is a very promising, compelling approach, there are no less than ten registered clinical trials from institutes which are doing this."[28]

Orthodox experts in the cancer world are also increasingly waking up to the issues with high-carb, particularly when people are overeating (a very common issue for people on high-carb diets). Dr. Craig B. Thompson, the head of Memorial Sloan Kettering, a renowned cancer research center, had the following to say in a 2011 lecture to medical students: "We now have good evidence in model organisms...that if you overfeed someone with fat, you don't increase their cancer risk at all—good? You overfeed someone with carbohydrates and you dramatically increase their cancer risk. And protein is halfway in between."[29]

As Richard Feinman, a professor of biochemistry, observed recently: "Where Atkins and weight-loss desires drove the first low-carb revolution in the 1980s, it will be cancer fears that drive the second. And this time it will succeed."

With ketogenic diets being the ultimate low-carb weapon against carcinogenesis, the keto trend will continue to grow around the world.

JOE'S STORY

Joe is a classic case of someone who had to fully embrace the Eat Rich, Live Long prescription to be healthy and happy.

For most of his life, Joe struggled with his weight. Although he was a very active person—biking, hiking, and rock climbing—he tended to be between 10 and 20 pounds overweight. No matter how hard he worked out, Joe could never seem to get down to the lean body he desired.

Growing up, Joe's family was mostly vegetarian, though they ate some fish on occasion. They didn't eat a lot of processed sugar or sodas, as they had a strong "healthy living" focus. Joe grew up eating mostly beans, rice, pasta, cheese, and bread.

By high school, Joe had started eating hamburgers and chicken at restaurants. Once he moved out of his parents' house, he expanded his diet to include a range of meats and styles of cuisine—mostly Asian and Indian dishes. But even these largely revolved around noodles, rice, and beans or lentils.

By the time he was thirty-two, Joe was on the medication fenofibrate to treat high cholesterol and triglyceride levels. By thirty-five, he realized that biking, climbing, and doing all the sports he normally did was getting harder. It was then he admitted to himself that he was unhealthy and on a path to more severe health problems. Joe weighed himself and realized he was at his heaviest weight ever. He tipped the scale at 210 pounds on a five-foot-nine frame.

That was when he decided to try something new. After some research and reading, he thought he would try a real-food approach based on Paleo and keto. He started with a modified Whole30 based on Mark Sisson's Primal Blueprint recommendation. He immediately dropped 10 pounds, felt better, and had far less gas and irritability. He decided he needed to learn more and go for even greater health and weight improvements.

After consulting with Jeff, Joe realized the importance of eliminating all processed carbs. He also drastically reduced starchy vegetables like white potatoes. He now eats and craves nutrient-dense foods, including lots of avocado, leafy greens, kale, Swiss chard, broccoli, Brussels sprouts, asparagus, and roasted root vegetables. He still eats a fair amount of meat: burgers, steaks, chicken, lamb, and some bacon and sausage. He also eats a good amount of raw mixed nuts and seeds.

It's been a little over a year, and Joe is now at 168 pounds. He feels absolutely fantastic. He is performing better than ever in sports and activities, and he sleeps much better, too. He had to go out and buy new clothes because all his old clothes were falling off his body. Several salespeople suggested he try slimmer-fitting styles because he was such a "skinny guy." His waist size has dropped three inches, and for the first time in a long time, Joe is not trying to cover up his body with hoodies or oversized shirts.

Joe can't say enough good things about this diet and way of life. He feels as if he has finally found the way he should have been eating his whole life. It is not a diet to Joe; it is a new way of living.

"Livestock take inedible and untasty grains and convert them into a protein-packed food most humans love to eat."

—Jayson Lusk

CHAPTER 14

PROTEIN:
BENEFITS AND PITFALLS

The dietary requirement for carbohydrate is effectively zero—humans do not need to consume any carbohydrate. Fat, on the other hand, is essential for health. The other essential macronutrient is protein. The average person must consume 60 to 100 grams of protein a day. Eating too little protein has serious consequences for health and vitality.

The highest-quality protein comes from animal foods—meat, fish, and eggs. That's not to say you can't get adequate protein from vegetable sources—you just have to be much more careful about what you eat. You can be a vegetarian and have robust health, but that's not our focus in this book.[1]

The best protein sources tend to be foods that are also high in natural fats, especially animal foods. These also are rich in the fat-soluble vitamins, and eating them enables you to absorb vitamins and minerals properly.

You need to get the right amount of protein to match your muscle mass and activity level; then you can play with carbs and fat. The generally accepted required protein quantity is 0.4 to 0.6 gram per pound of lean body mass. The figure applies for an average, relatively sedentary human. More protein is necessary when activity levels increase.

Muscles are largely made up of protein and are constantly being broken down and rebuilt. People who exercise a lot and want to build muscle need to eat more protein. The exact amount is disputed, but the most common guideline is to ingest around 0.8 to 1.0 gram per pound of lean body mass. This is approximately double the accepted requirement for sedentary people.

It is important to note that "grams of protein" refers to exactly that—the amount of pure protein. For example, an egg might weigh 35 grams, but it contains only around 4 grams of protein. A slice of bread might weigh 35 grams, but it contains only around 2 grams of protein (and 16 grams of carbohydrate).

But not all advisers agree on these protein requirements. Some believe that it should be much higher, but recently there has been a push toward much lower. This will cause much confusion in the coming decade. These various influencers can't all be correct!

PROTEIN IN A NUTSHELL

Proteins are complex molecules made up of amino acids. Amino acids are fundamental for life—they make up our very DNA. Some amino acids can be produced by the body. Others must be acquired through our diet. The nine amino acids that we must get from food are called *essential amino acids.*

Amino acids can be linked to form long protein chains. These chains can be folded into complex shapes, which give the proteins new and powerful properties. That is where the magic of amino acids plays out—they enable endless possible proteins for myriad crucial functions.

Proteins also enable you to create enzymes, which are themselves clever proteins that can catalyze other necessary processes. Proteins conduct the billions of processes your body requires. Proteins are used to create all your crucial hormones and signaling molecules. Finally, proteins directly supply the main building blocks for your body tissues.

If your main goal is to remain healthy, maintaining the right type of diet can automatically cover your protein requirements, without your needing to count how much protein you're eating. This is easier to achieve when you include nutrient-dense animal foods in your regimen, because these carry the highest-quality protein.

QUALITY OR QUANTITY?

When we ingest food, the proteins in it are broken down into amino acids. We gather up these amino acids and reuse them. This is especially true for the nine essential amino acids.

In *Eat to Live*, a vegan diet book, some claims were made that broccoli provides more protein per calorie than steak.[2] This is simply not true: 100 calories of broiled top sirloin steak has exactly 11.08 grams of protein, while 100 calories of raw broccoli has exactly 8.29.[3] This is also a great example of the fact that animal foods have not just the most protein but the *highest-quality* protein. Figure 14.1 shows the reality (note that the nine essentials are shown here).

Essential Amino Acids	Daily Requirement for a 155-Pound Adult (g)	Amount (g) in 275 Calories (4 Ounces) of Steak	Amount (g) in 277 Calories (9¼ Cups) of Raw Broccoli
cysteine	0.28	0.394 (+0.114)	0.228 (-0.052)
histidine	0.70	0.975 (+0.275)	0.48 (-0.22)
isoleucine	1.400	1.391 (-0.009)	0.643 (-0.757)
leucine	2.730	2.431 (-0.299)	1.05 (-1.68)
lysine	2.100	2.583 (+0.483)	1.099 (-1.001)
methionine	0.70	0.796 (+0.09)	0.309 (-0.391)
threonine	1.050	1.221 (+0.171)	0.716 (-0.334)
tryptophan	0.280	0.201 (-0.079)	0.269 (-0.011)
valine	1.82	1.516 (-0.304)	1.018 (-0.802)

Figure 14.1. Steak nutritionally beats broccoli, hands down. Source: USDA Food Composition Databases, ndb.nal.usda.gov.

A small 4-ounce serving of steak provides almost all the essential amino acids that an adult requires. A serving of broccoli that has the same number of calories (about 9 cups) does not deliver enough of any of these essential amino acids. Don't get us wrong—we like broccoli. It can be part of a healthy diet, and we eat it regularly. But we are not under any illusions when it comes to the best sources of protein. We focus on quality. You should as well!

In fact, there are many people who eat primarily meat and almost no carbs, and there are websites dedicated to their testimonials of robust health and vitality.[4] We would not recommend this particular diet, but many people seem to thrive on it.

You have choices when it comes to protein intake. You can depend on vegetarian sources like artichokes, quinoa, and various high-protein beans and vegetables, but you must have great knowledge and skill to choose carefully from a wide range of foods to achieve optimal protein and nutrient intake. You will also likely have to eat foods that have been shipped long distances. Supplementation with crucial elements such as vitamin B12 is also required—you will not get this vital nutrient from plant foods.

In contrast, it is easy to optimize your nutrition when you consume nutrient-dense animal foods. Meats, fish, and eggs alone will deliver nearly all the nutrients you need. Vegetables and some fruits can then be added for additional nutritional benefits.

PROTEIN'S WEIGHT-CONTROL ADVANTAGES

Most authorities on weight loss are aligned on one thing: a higher protein intake helps with weight-loss efforts. A simple Google search will fill the page with studies validating this point. A good example is a study that looked at high-protein (25 percent of total daily calories) versus low-protein (14 percent) diets in overweight men.[5] Interestingly, the study also investigated meal frequency, a subject we feel strongly about (see page 79). All the participants were on the same calorie-restricted diet to aid weight loss.

The researchers found that the high-protein diet significantly improved three important aspects of appetite:

► increasing a "full" feeling throughout the day

► reducing the late-night desire to eat

► reducing the preoccupation with food

The high-protein diet was well ahead of the low-protein diet on all three measures. This was expected, based on decades of research. But there was an interesting extra finding from the study: when eating the same number of calories but having fewer meals (three rather than six), the high-protein participants were fuller in the evening and late at night. The researchers concluded that the higher-protein diet not only suppressed appetite but also led to the improved feelings of fullness gained through the strategy of eating fewer meals. (The lower-protein group ate very little protein indeed at 14 percent of daily calories, while the higher-protein group ate a more reasonable 25 percent.) Note that this study only scratched the surface in a way, looking at quite short periods of intervention. We would say that a long-term strategy of correct diet combined with adequate protein and smart meal-separation will produce much more dramatic benefits.

Science has shown that if you don't eat enough protein, you will continue to eat until you get it. The body has important requirements for protein, so our brains' appetite-control systems are wired to drive us to get enough. Higher protein in the diet activates hunger-suppressing hormones, including peptide YY, GLP-1, and others.[6]

When digesting carb and fat, you absorb most of the calories they contain, but with protein, there is a significant waste or loss of calories as you digest it. This phenomenon is called *thermogenesis*. Higher-protein diets result in more losses through thermogenesis, but this effect also increases satiety and energy expenditure. The end effect is that you feel relatively fuller with protein than if you were getting the same number of calories from carb or fat.[7]

Higher-protein diets can also help stimulate muscle growth. This can lead to a preferential retention of lean muscle mass paired with a loss of fat mass. Myriad studies prove that quite small increases in protein intake can result in significant advantages in weight loss. Moreover, keeping protein intake higher can help prevent weight regain.

One recent trial examined men and women who had lost 5 to 10 percent of their body weight over a short period.[8] The experiment increased protein from 15 percent of total calories to 18 percent in half the participants. Both groups were tracked over the following six months. Even with this very small protein tweak, the 18 percent group regained significantly less weight than the 15 percent one. This effect was independent of changes in cognitive restraint, physical activity, resting or total energy expenditure, and hunger scores.

A WEIGHT-CONTROL CAVEAT

Despite its advantages for weight loss, there is a slight drawback to a high-protein diet: while it's not nearly as bad as carb, protein still drives an insulin response. If you are eating a lot of protein, the insulin release can be substantial. This is why our low-carb, high-fat plan recommends that you consume moderate amounts of protein.

For people who are not too insulin resistant, a higher level of protein will not have a detrimental insulin-raising effect. Protein generally produces around half of the insulin response that the same amount of carb does, and it has an even smaller relative effect on blood glucose, which rises very little and tapers off steadily.

For people with significant levels of insulin resistance, this is trickier. Type 2 diabetics in particular can have a magnified insulin response. Because protein takes a relatively long time to digest, insulin stays elevated for many hours, and this, of course, is not ideal. Muscle and other tissues are also constantly being recycled. This releases amino acids into the blood, increasing the pool of available protein. If you're losing weight, the breakdown of excess skin and other tissue can supply a source of protein on top of what you're eating, and this can contribute to an excess of protein at any time.

Much of what happens when we eat protein—or carb—reflects the balance between the hormones insulin and glucagon. Insulin and glucagon are opposing forces. At its simplest, insulin drives fat storage and promotes tissue growth (its "anabolic" or building function). Glucagon, on the other hand, promotes the release of fatty acids from adipose tissue and the release of glucose from glycogen—in the absence of food, these are used for energy. In the fed state, insulin is generally high and glucagon is rightly suppressed. The opposite occurs in the fasted state, with glucagon going high to free up energy from fat or other sources.

High-carb meals drive insulin high, keeping glucagon low. Protein drives insulin also, to help build muscle from the ingested protein. But it also stimulates the release of glucagon—that way, the drop in blood glucose insulin causes is balanced by glucose (and fatty acids) coming into the bloodstream from storage, so overall, blood sugar stays stable. But when someone who's insulin resistant eats a lot of protein with lot of carb, this balancing act is tricky to achieve, and this leads to an unstable hormonal situation and unpredictable blood sugar levels. This kind of situation should of course be avoided—we must always strive for low and stable blood sugar and insulin levels.

This is why our plan centers on low carbohydrate and *moderate* protein. If you are keeping carb in a healthy low range, then there is room for a higher amount of protein, since both stimulate insulin. Eating a higher amount of healthy fat provides energy without provoking insulin or a rise in blood glucose, and this combination is optimal for most people. Whether you are losing weight or maintaining your weight, whether you are insulin sensitive or insulin resistant, this combination of low carb, moderate protein, and high fat should fit. The goal should always be to keep insulin low. And generally this means high glucagon, insofar as it is possible.

PROTEIN AND THE KIDNEYS

One of the most common myths about high protein is that it drives kidney disease. No scientific research supports this notion. The myth probably came about due to the fact that people with existing kidney disease can indeed have problems with a high protein load. But it is wrong to suggest that it is a problem for everyone else.

Another possibility is that the kidney-damaging myth arose from the fact that the kidneys clear the protein-released nitrogen from the body. A presumption may have been made that high-protein diets could, therefore, put excessive demands on the kidneys. This doesn't happen in reality.

As we mentioned, the brain has an intricate control system to manage dietary protein intake. The body's ability to manage protein indeed has an upper limit. But just as it demands that you eat until you get enough protein, the brain will step in and tweak appetite and food selection if too much protein is being consumed. You would have to work hard to fully override this control system.

When tested experimentally, it has been observed that high-protein diets change kidney parameters, including glomular filtration rate, which is simply a measure of kidney activity rate, estimated by the blood flow through it. This is to be expected—it is simply the kidney adapting to changing inputs, just the way any organ does. One of the better summaries of how protein affects the kidneys was included in a 2015 scientific paper: "While protein restriction may be appropriate for treatment of existing kidney disease, we find no significant evidence for a detrimental effect of high protein intakes on kidney function in healthy persons."[9]

PROTEIN ACTION STEPS

► For the average person, target protein intake should be approximately 0.4 to 0.6 gram of protein per pound of lean body mass. This ensures adequacy, and there is no evidence to suggest that it is excessive.

► People who are building muscle through exercise can safely ingest more protein. A good target intake is around 0.8 to 1.0 gram per pound of lean body mass.

► Reducing protein could be a good strategy for someone who has health challenges that connect to insulin and mTOR pathways, such as cancer (see page 281)—lowering protein may prevent excessive insulin signaling and overactivation of mTOR.

At the end of the day, protein is a vital part of a healthy diet. We need to consume the highest-quality protein in adequate amounts. This will contribute greatly to health and longevity. It will also assist weight control through the satiety-inducing effects of protein.

The Eat Rich, Live Long plan addresses protein optimization for weight loss and longevity. The beauty of eating nutrient-dense ancestral foods is that they come ready-formulated with a good ratio of fat and protein.

With protein, the important thing is to neither overeat it nor limit it obsessively. The key is to get the balance right.

HOWARD'S STORY

Howard moved to the Denver area from the West Coast and needed to find a new doctor. He started seeing Jeff. Although quite overweight, Howard had never heard the word *diabetes* applied to him by his previous medical professionals. Jeff, however, suspected from his previous blood tests and weight that he was well along the insulin spectrum. Jeff explained that although Howard's fasting blood glucose and other metrics appeared to be within a normal range, this did not mean that he was safely nondiabetic. While Howard's LDL cholesterol was indeed low, the ratios Jeff calculated from his cholesterol panel spoke of insulin problems. Howard had never had a post-meal glucose reading taken to check his true status. Likewise, he had never had an insulin test. Therefore he could be very diabetic inside, but with his pancreas still healthy enough to pump out enough insulin, keeping his fasting glucose at an okay level. Remember that diabetes is properly identified by elevated insulin and insulin resistance criteria. Focusing on blood glucose is misleading; you can have high insulin—and therefore diabetes—even if your blood glucose is normal.

Jeff arranged for Howard to have an oral glucose tolerance test (OGTT). This is a procedure where you drink 75 grams of glucose and your blood glucose rise is monitored for the next two hours. It is far superior to a simple fasting blood glucose test for revealing health issues. Importantly, Jeff also ensured that Howard's blood insulin levels were monitored during the two hours—this information is even more valuable than the blood glucose measurements. The results came back as rather grim: he had spectacularly failed, with both the insulin and blood glucose levels far above the healthy range, just as Jeff had thought he would.

Howard said he had always suspected that something was seriously wrong with his health in spite of his low cholesterol. He was happy now to find out the truth and wanted to know how best to go about fixing the problem. Jeff sat him down and didn't pull any punches. With Howard's level of insulin resistance, he would need to go on a very low carb diet immediately. This would begin the repair process, moving him toward the safe end of the insulin spectrum. Over time he might have to carry out further measures to optimize his health, but first things first.

Within weeks of following a very low carb diet, Howard's belly had begun receding noticeably and he felt better than he had in years. Jeff verified the improvement by checking that his post-meal glucose levels were way down from the initial test. His fasting insulin was dropping sharply as well, sealing the deal. Howard has now fully embraced the low-carb lifestyle, along with many of the other beneficial strategies espoused in this book. Howard has truly collapsed his risk of chronic disease because he now knows about the most important measures of all—even though his previous doctors did not.

CHAPTER 15

WHICH VITAMINS AND MINERALS DO YOU REALLY NEED?

> " By the proper intakes of vitamins and other nutrients and by following a few other healthful practices from youth or middle age on, you can, I believe, extend your life and years of well-being by twenty-five or even thirty-five years. "
>
> —Linus Pauling

The human body is an enormously complex machine. Every moment of every day, billions of biochemical reactions are underway. These reactions require many different vitamins, minerals, and other nutrients. A healthy diet will supply most of these nutrients, and we strongly recommend that you target foods that can supply all your nutrient needs. That said, modern agricultural practices have left foods less nutritionally dense than they once were. In addition, we strive for *optimal*, not just adequate, health and longevity. Therefore, we need to top up certain key nutrients that may not be easy to get via our diets.

Notwithstanding the reasonableness of that goal, there has been much confusion about nutrient supplements. Experts have been wrangling over vitamins, minerals, and supplements for decades. Every expert has his or her particular angle. Also, multiple interest groups have inappropriately interfered in the discussion to further their own ends.

Pharmaceutical companies also produce supplements, and this means that there's big business—and lots of advertising dollars—behind marketing and selling supplements. Pfizer, the maker of prescription medications Lipitor, Viagra, Celebrex, and many others, also manufactures and distributes Centrum and Caltrate. Bayer, famous for its aspirin and a multitude of over-the-counter medications, including Claritin, Aleve, and Alka-Seltzer, also produces One-a-Day and Flintstones vitamins.

Further complicating the issue is the fact that supplements do not have to be evaluated and approved by the FDA, so they can be sold without proof of effectiveness or safety (though there are manufacturing standards that must be met).

With all these large companies with deep pockets having a vested interest in promoting and selling vitamins, and no need to prove that their supplements actually do what they claim, how do you know what vitamins you really need? How do you push aside all the influences and develop a reasonable supplement strategy?

The answer is to look at the results of scientific research, not the claims of big business. In Chapter 7, we talked about the supplements that are most important when your body is adjusting to the Eat Rich, Live Long plan: potassium, sodium, magnesium, and omega-3. In this chapter, we'll go beyond those to look at the main vitamins and minerals that people tend to be deficient in (though there's some overlap here with those discussed in Chapter 7).

We'll start with one that has received endless attention over the past few decades and has been the subject of countless arguments in the medical and research world: vitamin D. The debate on its importance and the appropriate level to consume is still raging.

VITAMIN D: THE SUNSHINE VITAMIN

Humans evolved in the ubiquitous presence of the sun—we were continuously exposed to sunlight. The action of sunlight on human skin has profound biochemical effects, enabling the synthesis of many key photochemicals that are required for optimal health. One of the most important is known as "vitamin D," but it is not a vitamin as such. It is a prohormone that is critical for use in manufacturing the active forms of vitamin D. There are many body processes for which the active forms of vitamin D are crucial: calcium management, bone health, immune system function, insulin sensitivity, vascular health, cell proliferation control, and many others.

You could rightly ask why vitamin D is inextricably linked with so many mechanisms in the body. One reason is that it became part of the human body's control system very early in the evolutionary game. Several hundred

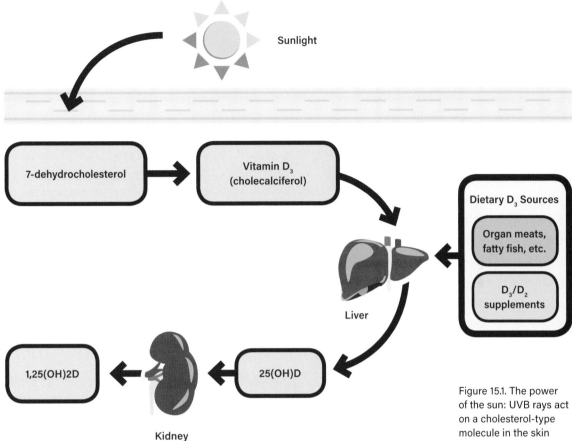

Figure 15.1. The power of the sun: UVB rays act on a cholesterol-type molecule in the skin (7-dehydrocholesterol) and convert it to the crucial vitamin D_3. You can also access D_3 from organ meats, fatty fish, and other rich ancestral sources. The D_3 enters circulation and is used directly by tissues but also gets converted in the liver into 25(OH)D, enabling many more functions and also long-term storage. A final conversion step happens in the kidneys, where the highly active form 1,25(OH)2D is created.

million years ago, aquatic vertebrates had easy access to calcium. Bone synthesis and other important functions were easy to manage, and calcium was readily available in the sea all around them. But when the vertebrates migrated onto land, they faced a major challenge: how would they get calcium? The method that emerged involved the synthesis of vitamin D using ultraviolet (UV) energy from the sun. Vitamin D became linked to many processes besides bone formation. Figure 15.1 shows a simplified diagram of how vitamin D is manufactured in humans.

Sunlight's UV energy acts on a form of cholesterol to create what is called vitamin D_3. This is the primary path humans evolved to get vitamin D. There are also dietary sources, but while ancestral foods were often rich in D_3, modern foods are severely lacking in it. This has led many to take supplements instead.

Vitamin D_3 from any source is processed in the liver and converted to a mildly active version of the hormone called 25-hydroxy D (or calcifediol; in blood test results, this shows up as "25(OH)D"). This is how the body stores vitamin D, and it's what is measured in blood tests to determine vitamin D levels. This 25-hydroxy D is not the final-stage hormone, but it does play an active role in many important processes. Another conversion step is required to produce the more active hormone called calcitriol (in blood test results, this is "1,25(OH)2D"). The kidneys carry out this step. It is precisely regulated to ensure that correct concentrations are always maintained in the bloodstream.

It is important to note that vitamin D has many key interactions with the other fat-soluble vitamins, A and K_2 in particular. Therefore, it is not necessarily a good idea to drive up your D status while neglecting the others. These fat-soluble vitamins as a group also interact synergistically with minerals such as magnesium and zinc. The ideal strategy is to ensure that you are getting adequate amounts of all the key vitamins and minerals—that way, you will be broadly covered for the interactions.

LOW ON D, HIGH ON DISEASE

How does being low in vitamin D associate with disease and mortality? Well, being lower in 25-hydroxy D associates strongly with rates of many modern diseases, as well as with increased mortality from them. Myriad studies consistently bear this out—for heart and arterial disease, colon and other cancers, diabetes, and many other diseases.[1] As we've stressed throughout this book, there is no proof of causation in associational studies. That said, the 2x multiplier threshold, which is the minimum needed to show a strong and meaningful association, is regularly reached.

These studies were carefully executed and corrected for as many confounding factors as possible. They still do not prove causation. There is, however, a massive body of science supporting mechanisms through which vitamin D and its receptors could affect these disease outcomes. There is even experimental proof, but there is a lot of conflicting data in the literature around this. So why are many of these experiments ambiguous?

- Generally, people high in D are more likely to get a lot of sun exposure. The sun has many biochemical effects on humans beyond the production of D. These beneficial effects may partly be driving the better outcomes.

- Having a particular disease or illness can drive down D status, though there is limited data around this. Also, people who are ill may get outside less, thus depriving themselves of healthy sunlight and lowering their D status.

- Some people may take more vacations in sunny locales and sport more of a tan. These people may also look after their overall health better—creating a further confounder.

Modern lifestyles have led to a general collapse in D levels. This is due to sun phobia, the fact that vitamin D is less abundant in food, and that fewer people are eating the ancestral foods that do contain it (e.g., organ meats, fatty fish, and pastured eggs). Another reason for the epidemic of low D levels is that obesity and inflammatory disease can drive down levels in the blood. We certainly have no shortage of these afflictions in our modern world.

We mentioned that vitamin D is primarily stored in the form of 25-hydroxy D. Evolutionary levels of 25-hydroxy D were generally in the 40 to 50 ng/ml range. These levels are observed today in native Africans in their natural environment and in Caucasians who have access to plenty of sun exposure.[2] African natives who move to cities and adopt modern lifestyles end up with D levels around 20 ng/ml. Modern sun-starved Caucasians also tend toward this same lower level.

The implications of the modern drop in D levels is much debated in expert circles. Also, there is much controversy around the right supplementation regimen to maintain healthy levels. D_3 supplements are most commonly measured in international units, or IU. Because this unit was chosen when the science of vitamin D was barely understood, it has an unfortunate drawback: it makes the genuinely required amount of D_3 appear unreasonably high.

We'll put things in perspective here. A minimally clothed Caucasian getting slightly pink from sun exposure will generate 10,000 to 25,000 IU of D_3.[3] The time required will vary greatly depending on latitude, time of day, skin type, and many other variables. In particular, people with darker skin will require much more sun exposure for the same amount of D synthesis. That said, twenty to thirty minutes in a bathing suit between 10 a.m. and 2 p.m. is a good rough guide. Like most natural biological mechanisms, this reaction is self-regulating. Getting a lot more sun will not maintain such high production rates. Evolution is good that way—it leads the body to grab what it needs and then back off when it's happy. Likewise, when the blood level of 25-hydroxy D exceeds around 45 ng/ml, the body tapers off many D-related reactions. It would therefore be reasonable to assume that if you are not getting ancestral levels of sun exposure, you might consider taking several thousand IU daily as a supplement. This would be a reasonable assumption unless compelling evidence indicated otherwise. That is where the controversy lies.

Broadly speaking, there are two significant camps in this sphere:

► Many D experts (including the Endocrine Society, a professional organization of endocrinologists) indicate that for full health, we should have 25-hydroxy D levels above 32 ng/ml.[4] This puts us in the ancestral ballpark. For most adults, getting this level of 25-hydroxy D in the blood would require supplementing with 4,000 to 5,000 IU of D_3 per day.

► Official guidelines from the Institute of Medicine, however, maintain that having above 20 ng/ml of 25-hydroxy D is adequate for bone health. They assume this is good enough for any other beneficial effects and generally recommend supplementation of only 800 IU of D_3 per day. This will have a very weak effect in raising blood levels. Recently, they acknowledged that up to 4,000 IU per day is okay, but they still recommend only 800 IU per day. Before 2013, they recommended only 400 IU per day.

All credible scientific evidence shows that up to 10,000 IU of D_3 per day has no toxicity implications whatsoever. The best evidence suggests that you'd have to get 30,000 IU per day to experience any vitamin D toxicity.[5] The quantity we spontaneously generate during healthy sun exposure bears this out.

LACTATING WOMEN SOLVE THE D_3 RIDDLE

The American Academy of Pediatrics and other authorities currently inform women that their breastmilk is inadequate in D_3; therefore, they recommend that supplements be given to all breastfed babies.[6] How could this have come about? There were no supplements available for babies' benefit as humans evolved. Why should women now have universally inadequate breastmilk? If "breast is best" in every other aspect, then what has gone wrong to make breastmilk inadequate in D_3 today?

Breastmilk needs to have at least 400 IU of D_3 per liter to be deemed adequate and supply the baby with as much D_3 as the recommended infant supplements would achieve. We need to know why women's breastmilk can no longer supply this amount of D_3. Luckily a human experiment explored the enigma and explained it all in 2006.[7] Pediatrician Bruce Hollis led the investigation, and he wanted to demonstrate how utterly obvious the answer was. He knew that women (and men, for that matter) need far more than the miserable 400 IU per day supplement that was recommended before 2013.

Hollis randomly split a large sample of breastfeeding women into two main groups. The first group followed the official recommendations and got a D_3 supplementation of 400 IU per day. The babies were directly supplemented with 400 IU per day also. (When body mass is taken into account, the babies were given around fifteen times what their mothers were—which emphasizes the absurd nature of the guidelines for adults.) The mothers in the second group were given 6,400 IU of D_3 per day.

So did Hollis prove that the correct daily supplement for women is in the 6,000 IU range? You bet he did.

Exactly as Hollis predicted, the mothers on 400 IU per day had breastmilk that was too low in D_3. The breastmilk delivered only 70 IU per liter instead of the required 400. The babies therefore needed the direct D_3 supplementation.

Also exactly as Hollis predicted, the mothers on 6,400 IU per day came through with excellent amounts of D_3 in their milk, more than 600 IU—but only by taking sixteen times the recommended daily supplement quantity themselves.

And so the riddle of the inadequate breastmilk was solved—and with it the riddle of how much D_3 we really need. For adequate D_3 in her breastmilk, a woman needs to get several thousand IU of D_3 a day. During human evolution, women would have gotten this amount through sun exposure and dietary sources. In periods of low sunlight, fish and other D-rich foods would have compensated.

The 25-hydroxy D form of vitamin D stored in the mother's blood does not transfer to breastmilk—it is the vitamin D_3 streaming in daily that transfers directly to the milk. The D_3 form lasts only a couple of days in the body. Therefore, daily access to D_3 through sun, diet, or supplements is required for optimal milk.

When doing experiments involving human subjects, an approval committee must judge on whether safety and ethics are appropriately addressed.

Interestingly, in this case the committee insisted that Hollis include another group: one in which the mothers were given 2,400 IU per day of D_3 (six times the daily recommendation). Hollis told them that this was pointless, as the babies would not get enough D_3 in the milk. But the committee insisted. Exactly as Hollis predicted, this group of women taking six times the recommended amount for adults failed to produce breastmilk that had sufficient D_3. The research team had to stop this group from continuing and immediately began supplementing the babies directly with D_3.

IS THERE SUCH A THING AS A HEALTHY TAN?

Healthy sunlight exposure has a dizzying array of benefits for health, yet we have been told for decades to minimize sun exposure because of the risk of skin cancer.[8] Melanoma is the skin cancer with serious mortality implications, and sun exposure without burning has never been proven to increase the risk of melanoma. In fact, some studies indicate the opposite could even be true—that exposure to sun without burning *decreases* the risk of acquiring or dying from melanoma.[9]

There is good evidence that high sun exposure does increase the risk of the "cosmetic" skin cancers (basal and squamous cell type). But these have very low mortality rates—approximately 1 percent of these cases result in death. Therefore, we believe that sun avoidance will likely lead to far more health problems than it prevents.[10]

Sunlight exposure has more benefits than we can get into here. It enables the release of nitric oxide in the body, which is crucial for vascular health and many other functions.[11] It contributes to vasodilation (artery dilation for improved blood flow) and moderation of blood pressure.[12] It also produces many photochemicals in the skin in addition to D_3—the potential importance of these is only beginning to be explored.[13] The fact that our bodies produce these chemicals when we're exposed to the sun is not an accident. The sun has been with us for all of human evolution, and it has become inextricably bound up with the promotion of health in our bodies.

We do not know how many of the benefits relating to vitamin D levels are actually due to these other advantages gained from healthy sun exposure. There is enough evidence to support supplements as a very important intervention to raise D levels. That said, it is very possible that healthy sun exposure is a far more effective way to raise your levels of vitamin D because of the other benefits it brings in tandem. The jury is still out—and until we decode this area fully, accessing healthy sun exposure or an alternative UV source, such as a vitamin D lamp, is likely the best route to take.[14]

The point is illustrated by an interesting study that looked at sun exposure and its associations with mortality.[15] The team sort of gave away the answer in the actual title of the study: "Avoidance of Sun Exposure Is a Risk Factor for All-Cause Mortality." And that is what they found when they tracked 29,518 women over twenty years. "The mortality rate amongst avoiders of sun exposure was approximately twofold higher compared with the highest sun exposure group."

So, along with many experts in the field, we recommend getting healthy sun exposure wherever possible. Of course, you should never allow yourself to get significantly sunburned—that is when the real damage can occur.

MAGNESIUM

Adequate magnesium is hugely important for a properly functioning body and is arguably one of the most important nutrients to focus on for health and longevity. But our health system largely ignores it.

One major issue is that the blood test for magnesium is a very weak indicator of your true magnesium status. Even if you are terribly deficient, it can come back as "within the normal range." Here's why: Less than 1 percent of the body's magnesium is carried in the bloodstream—most is sequestered in bone and other tissues. If you're low in available magnesium, your body will leach it out of your bones to supply your needs. This will make the blood level appear to be okay—even when a desperate situation is occurring out of sight. Your level of free cellular magnesium is the most important measure, but this is not assessed in standard blood tests.

By 1957, low magnesium was shown in animal experiments to be a co-driver of atherosclerosis.[16] Unfortunately, this was the period when the diet-heart hypothesis—which claimed that saturated fat drives up cholesterol in the blood, and high cholesterol in turn drives up the risk of heart disease—began storming the US. Magnesium didn't have a hope against the growing obsession with cholesterol and fat. The research into magnesium and its connection to heart disease (and other diseases) has quietly continued, but it appears that it is being largely ignored. Again, part of the reason may be that the common blood tests do not properly reflect underlying issues.

Out of 300 People with CHD ...	Low Magnesium (< 1.6 mg/dL)	Medium Magnesium (1.6–2.6 mg/dL)	Higher Magnesium (> 2.6 mg/dL)
	176	102	22
With diabetes	53%	19%	6%
With hypertension	75%	50%	23%
Average HDL	33	47	49
Average Triglycerides	190	145	146

Figure 15.2. Low magnesium strongly tracks with all the CHD risk factors. Source: N. Mahalle, M. V. Kulkarni, and S. S. Naik, "Is Hypomagnesaemia a Coronary Risk Factor Among Indians with Coronary Artery Disease?," *Journal of Cardiovascular Disease Research* 3, no. 4 (2012).

Low magnesium links to nearly all known cardiovascular risk factors, and to a rather impressive extent, as shown in a recent study of three hundred patients with coronary heart disease.[17] The low-magnesium group had a greatly increased rate of nearly all risk factors, with very high statistical significance seen across the board. A selection is shown in Figure 15.2.

In this study, magnesium levels did correlate strongly to the dietary intakes recorded.

It is estimated that 70 to 80 percent of adults are not achieving dietary requirements of magnesium. Because of the blood test's inadequacy, it is hard to estimate what proportion is truly low. Note that diabetes also causes loss of magnesium. So with most adults experiencing some level of diabetes, it is particularly important to ensure a healthy intake of this crucial mineral.

Sudden cardiac death (SCD) accounts for a significant percentage of overall heart-related mortality. These deaths are often attributed to a cardiac arrhythmia—irregularity in the heartbeat—rather than atherosclerosis-triggered events. An interesting associational study on SCD was carried out in 2010.[18] It examined the blood magnesium levels of 88,375 women who were initially free of disease. The women with the highest dietary intake of magnesium had a 34 percent lower risk of SCD. The women with the highest amount of magnesium in their blood had a 77 percent lower risk of SCD. Therefore, the risk multiplier for being low in dietary intake of magnesium was approximately 2x, while the risk multiplier for being low in magnesium in the blood was approximately 4x. The fact that this was an associational study notwithstanding, these are impressive multipliers, and they point to the importance of magnesium in preventing heart disease.

There are also studies showing the effectiveness of magnesium supplementation in reducing heart disease risk. C-reactive protein (CRP), a reliable indicator of inflammation in the body, has always had a strong correlation with heart disease: many studies show a 3x to 4x risk multiplier associated with higher levels of CRP.[19] This is unsurprising, as coronary heart disease is primarily driven by inflammation in the arterial walls, but the relationship between magnesium intake and CRP has attracted little attention. The few studies conducted have mainly been associational ones. In these, CRP usually correlates with low magnesium levels. But there is a 2007 study that was more revealing than the associational ones.[20]

In this study, researchers compared magnesium and CRP levels in heart-failure victims to those in randomly selected patients. As expected, the heart-failure group had lower magnesium levels and higher CRP than the random-patient group (average magnesium was 0.78 versus 0.86 mmol/L, and CRP was 39.8 versus 12.2 mg/dL). After only five weeks of magnesium supplementation, there was a large reduction in CRP in the heart-failure group. It dropped down to roughly the levels of the random-patient group.

Notably, they used only 300 mg/day of magnesium citrate supplementation to achieve this reduction in CRP. This is a modest supplementation for something as vital as magnesium. It is also notable that trials of magnesium supplementation in people low in magnesium have shown remarkable lowering of hypertension.[21]

We recommend targeting foods rich in magnesium. Examples are avocados, full-fat yogurt, and low-carb nuts like Brazil nuts and almonds. Dark chocolate will give you a boost, too. That said, we recommend taking a magnesium supplement to make sure you're getting enough. We use the cheap and cheerful magnesium citrate powder, which can be purchased in bulk online and can be sprinkled on savory dishes without affecting flavor. Note that it can have a laxative effect until you get used to it, so make sure you don't get too large a dose at once by spreading your intake throughout the day and ingest it with or just after a meal. Approximately 300 mg of magnesium in supplement form should suffice, assuming you are also getting reasonable quantities from your healthy food intake.

VITAMIN K$_2$

The "K" in "vitamin K" stands for *koagulation*, the German word for blood clotting. From its discovery in the 1930s through the late 1970s, we knew of no other roles for the vitamin. In recent decades, it has become more appreciated that the two forms of K have very different properties. While K$_1$ is linked mostly to clotting processes, K$_2$ has a unique range of important functions. K$_1$ is important, and we certainly recommend getting plenty of it from green leafy vegetables, spring onions, broccoli, and other K-rich foods. However, K$_2$ is the form today's diets are more likely to be deficient in.

The importance of vitamin K$_2$ for cardiovascular health only began to be appreciated in the last two decades. Of particular interest is its contribution to preventing calcification of the blood vessels and other soft tissues. K$_2$ activates what are called GLA proteins, which inhibit inappropriate soft-tissue calcification. This means that K$_2$ plays an important role in keeping calcium away from tissues where it could be problematic—arterial walls, for example.

K$_2$ is also important for many other health benefits beyond those of the vascular system. It acts synergistically with vitamins A and D: in essence, it enables many reactions that allow A and D to provide their benefits to the human body. K$_2$ is particularly connected to processes that distribute calcium to the parts of the body that require it (primarily bones and teeth).

The Rotterdam Heart Study points to K$_2$'s importance in preventing disease. It followed 4,807 subjects over ten years and found that high intake of vitamin K$_2$ was associated with a 26 percent reduction in all-cause mortality.[22] In the same study, coronary artery disease mortality was 57 percent lower, while severe aortic calcification was reduced by 52 percent. Unfortunately this is an associational study, but still, the risk multipliers seen were very substantial. There are very few experimental interventions.[23] It appears that the interest in K$_2$ has not been high enough to encourage large-scale clinical trials.

In spite of the gap in high-quality trials, we believe that K$_2$ is a very important vitamin to avoid deficiency in. When the associational, mechanistic, and limited trial evidence is combined, a rather compelling case can be made.[24] A final point is that there are variants even within the K$_2$ vitamin itself. On balance, the MK-7 variant would appear to be the best one to focus on.

How much might you benefit from ingesting daily? Generally, it has been estimated that 200 mcg of vitamin K_2 (MK-7) will properly activate the GLA proteins that inhibit calcification.[25] This would be a good ballpark number to aim for. While targeting the foods that deliver K_2 is best, there are many supplements on the market for those who wish to go this route.

K_2 is primarily found in animal fats and fermented foods. We focus on grass-fed butter and cheeses, goose liver pâté, organ meats, and of course a healthy range of grass-fed meats. Occasionally, we also partake of fermented foods rich in K_2, which include sauerkraut and other fermented vegetables. If you really want to hit the K_2 jackpot, you can get ahold of some natto—Japanese fermented bean curd—which is rich in the MK-7 variant.

Unfortunately, most people's diet today is likely very low in K_2. Intakes have suffered greatly during the era of the low-fat fad. With a high-healthy-fat diet, you will be able to buck this sad trend.

IODINE

Iodine is a vital nutrient that is crucial for fetal development and during early childhood. But it is also hugely important to get adequate iodine all throughout life. It is required for proper thyroid function and much else.

The effects of a low dietary intake of iodine are stark. Symptoms can include difficulty losing weight, muscle weakness, lethargy, memory problems, high triglycerides and other cholesterol imbalances, and poor resistance to infections. We'll stop there, but the list goes on and on.

Diet is our sole source of iodine, but the iodine content of the food we eat depends on what is available in the water and soil. The soil gets most of its iodine from the oceans (the primary source of the element), so areas far inland are generally poorly served. It was estimated in 1998 that one-third of the earth's soil is poor in iodine.[26]

The World Health Organization has estimated that over a billion people have inadequate iodine in their diet.[27] Many US experts flagged a growing problem with iodine deficiency in the late 1990s—they found that the number of people who were deficient was growing rapidly.[28] From 1971 to 1974, there were only a few percent of men and women in the "very low" category.

From 1988 to 1994, that figure jumped to nearly 15 percent for middle-aged men and nearly 25 percent for women. The criteria they used were based on absolute minimum perceived levels, and the requirements are arguably much higher for optimal health. So even in the 1990s, it was a rapidly growing problem. It is even worse now, as the soil has become further depleted. The only significant supply of iodine to the world's soil comes from the oceans—seawater evaporates and becomes rainfall over land, transferring iodine to the soil. But with depletion from intensive cropping, alkaline fertilizers, and flooding/leaching/erosion, the supply line from the oceans has been strained.[29] Interestingly, vegetables grown in iodine-deficient soil can have 1/100th of the iodine per pound as those grown in iodine-sufficient soil.

From the early 1970s to the early 1990s, Americans' median iodine concentration decreased by 50 percent, while the numbers of people having levels below the 50 mcg/L minimum increased by 450 percent. The more recent analyses show that the US situation is continuing to worsen, especially for pregnant women. The WHO considers a urinary iodine concentration less than 150 mcg/L insufficient during pregnancy.[30] Yet analyses have shown that median concentrations for pregnant women, which were 181 mcg/L in 2003–2004, reached only 125 mcg/L in 2005–2008.[31] This is essentially a long, slow car crash for human health.

Current estimates also suggest that more than half of Europe's population is iodine deficient.[32] There have been many efforts to raise levels through the promotion of iodized salt and other interventions. These have had positive effects, with Europe's levels now slowly rising. And we have to remember that "deficiency" is measured against the bare minimum requirements. These minimum requirements are what's needed to avoid the most obvious problems, like an enlarged thyroid. But if you only just meet these minimal requirements, the consequences could still be very negative.

Breast cancer is just one area where iodine deficiency may have serious consequences. The breast tissue is particularly dependent on available iodine for healthy function.[33] Quite a few iodine interventions had very positive effects on the common problem of breast pain due to fibrocystic disease and other issues.[34] This would be important in itself, but there is another interesting implication. It appears that the conditions that cause breast pain are quite predictive of breast cancer in the future.

A 2005 study from the Mayo Clinic showed some pretty solid risk multi-pliers.[35] They tracked 9,087 women diagnosed with benign, noncancerous breast disease related to fibrocystic and other symptoms for a total of fifteen years. The intention was to understand if these benign conditions led to higher chances of future breast cancer. They discovered that this group of women did indeed have a 1.56 times greater risk of breast cancer than a control group.

The study also categorized the appearance of cells in the biopsies of breast tissue. They found that 34 percent of the women had "proliferative" type cells, ones that demonstrated a worrying ability to self-replicate. Among these particular women, the risk for breast cancer in the future was approxi-mately twice that of the control group (a pretty notable risk increase). For the 66 percent with "non-proliferative" cells, the risk multiplier was only 1.27x.

We are not aware of any trials testing iodine supplementation against incidence or severity of breast cancer, but because it's well established that iodine supplementation can resolve these more benign diseases that increase the risk of breast cancer, it stands to reason that iodine supplemen-tation may also be beneficial in preventing breast cancer. And there is wide-spread documentation of iodine deficiency in the general population. Scientif-ic investigations have also closely linked iodine's mechanisms in the body to factors involved in the risk of breast cancer.[36]

Because of potential negative effects with excessive dosing, we favor get-ting iodine in your food. Shellfish and seaweed are particularly rich sources, as are eggs, potatoes, and cheese. If supplementing, kelp tablets are a prac-tical and safe way to boost your levels. We would broadly go with the WHO iodine recommendation for lactating women, around 290 mcg/day. But we view this figure as a minimum for most women and men, not just lactating women.

Particularly if you are already deficient, boosting your iodine may give many potent health benefits just by itself. Combined with all the other mea-sures we prescribe, you may not quite believe how good you're going to feel.

OTHER VITAMINS AND MINERALS

A whole book could easily be written on important vitamins and minerals. We've chosen just a few to detail here. In many ways, they are the ones we feel are most in need of addressing. But they're certainly not the only nutrients you need. Below is a short list of other important vitamins and minerals. For each, we'll list some good food sources that are compatible with the Eat Rich, Live Long plan.

Vitamin A: Required particularly to interact with vitamin D, as the two vitamins are very connected in their bodily functions—the ratio of D and A is important to keep in balance. It contributes to many aspects of optimal health. Retinol is the ideal form of vitamin A and is found mainly in animal sources, especially eggs, liver, grass-fed butter, and heavy cream. Cod liver oil is a super supplemental source of retinol. Plant sources provide the less effective carotenoid form of vitamin A. This needs to be converted into retinol in a process that is inefficient in many people. Plant sources include broccoli, spinach, and most dark leafy greens.

Vitamin E: There are actually a range of vitamins under the "E" heading. The E vitamins are carried around the body by the lipoproteins discussed in Chapter 11, and they are important for antioxidant effects. Animal sources are generally not particularly rich in E vitamins, but among these, eggs, liver, grass-fed butter, and heavy cream are the best sources. Plant sources, especially nuts such as hazelnuts, almonds, and walnuts, deliver significant quantities of vitamin E. Green vegetables, including spinach and broccoli, are also useful sources.

B vitamins: The B-complex vitamins comprise vitamin B_{12}, vitamin B_6, thiamine, riboflavin, niacin, folate, pantothenic acid, and biotin. These all have important biological functions; in particular, they help your body turn food into energy. Pantothenic acid and biotin might be less available on a very low carb diet. That said, eggs, cheese, pork, shellfish, fresh vegetables, and organ meats such as liver are all good sources—so you should not skimp on these. In general, it is not a bad idea to take a B-complex multivitamin to cover all the bases. Note that people who are very low in B vitamins can develop profound and debilitating diseases, particularly neurological illnesses. Also, high homocysteine levels (a very significant risk factor for cardiovascular disease) are intimately related to being low on B vitamins, especially B_{12}.[37]

Vitamin C: This important compound was thrust into the limelight through Linus Pauling's work in the mid-twentieth century. It has many functions: helping to repair and regenerate tissues, protecting against heart disease, preventing scurvy, and assisting in lipid or cholesterol metabolism. Pauling and others completed much research that indicated that intensive vitamin C treatment may help protect against a variety of cancers. It may also support healthy immune function.

There is an ongoing debate around whether very high intakes of vitamin C can be instrumental in avoiding heart disease and other chronic diseases, but the jury is still out on this one. There is also some emerging evidence that vitamin C requirements may be much lower while on a well-formulated low-carb dietary regimen.[38]

It is important to note that the complete vitamin C molecule found in foods is very different from the "vitamin C" found in most supplements. The vitamin C molecule in whole foods contains rutin, bioflavonoids, factor K, factor J, factor P, tyrosinase, ascorbinogen, and other components. It also carries an antioxidant called ascorbic acid. In contrast, supplemental vitamin C overwhelmingly consists only of the ascorbic acid component. That is why we target vitamin C intake primarily from low-carb whole foods that are relatively low in digestible carbohydrate. Good sources are asparagus, berries, broccoli, cabbage, cauliflower, citrus fruits (such as lemons, limes, and oranges), kiwis, dark leafy greens (such as kale and spinach), bell peppers, potatoes, and tomatoes.

Zinc and copper: It is key to have an adequate zinc intake. One reason is that zinc interacts with magnesium and the fat-soluble vitamins, helping the latter to function optimally. The good news is that you are very likely to be replete in zinc on a low-carb regimen—lamb, beef, cocoa, yogurt, spinach, and many other recommended foods have plenty. However, being very high in zinc may not be so good if you are very low on copper—and vice versa. The *ratios* are important, rather than individual intakes.[39] The foods richest in copper are organ meats, like beef liver and pâté, and seafood, including lobster, crab, and oysters. Dark chocolate also has impressive quantities, as do hazelnuts and Brazil nuts.

Selenium: Selenium is required for proper functioning of the thyroid gland and many other functions. An excess of selenium can lead to problems, so it's generally best to get it from healthy food choices. Brazil nuts are extremely high in selenium, so a few of these a day will go a long way. Lobster, oysters, shrimp, and other shellfish also contain generous amounts. Meats such as beef, pork, and lamb are also rich sources.

Potassium: It is key to have an adequate potassium intake, particularly on a low-carb diet, when it can help combat the "low-carb flu" phenomenon. (We talked more about this on page 106.) Avocados are especially rich in potassium and also contain plenty of healthy fat, making them a great choice. Spinach and wild salmon are very good, too. If you're not getting plenty of potassium in your food, then potassium salts may be a good addition. See page 101 for more on potassium.

Sodium: It is key to have an adequate sodium intake. The potential issues with excessive sodium intake have been grossly exaggerated during the past decades. It is far more likely that your salt intake is too *low* rather than too high.[40] This is especially true when you're starting out on a low-carb diet. On a grain-based junk-food diet, you may be getting a lot of sodium. When you switch to a real-foods-based low-carb diet, you are likely to require more. (We talked more about this on page 101.) Liberally salting your food and enjoying broths are great measures to take. See page 101 for more details on sodium.

Chromium: Chromium is a metallic element that we require in small amounts. It is an essential part of metabolic processes that regulate blood sugar, and it assists in the many actions of insulin. As with many other elements, modern agricultural practices have depleted the soil's chromium content. Therefore, many people are mildly deficient in chromium, possibly the majority of people on Western diets. Beef, turkey, liver, and other organ meats are good animal sources of chromium. Lobster, oysters, shrimp, and other shellfish also contain generous amounts. Plant sources include tomato, spinach, onion, broccoli, garlic, and green peppers.

Berberine: Berberine exists purely as a supplement. It is extracted from certain types of plants (for example, barberry, Oregon grape, and goldenseal). It has been used for three thousand years in traditional Chinese medicine. Many published studies have shown it to be a moderately helpful treatment for type 2 diabetes and metabolic syndrome. Its beneficial effects can include reducing blood glucose and triglycerides, and improving LDL particle quality. It can also deliver some improvements in overall glucose tolerance. In recent years, the more detailed mechanisms for berberine's action have been studied, and they involve the triggering of many hormonal pathways.[41] In general, we would always favor the proper application of our ten steps to improve these conditions, however.

JIM'S STORY

Jim was a very heavy guy with major health complaints. He was over 350 pounds with 45 percent body fat. His waist size was a whopping 60 inches. Years before, he had had elevated liver enzymes, and his doctor kept asking Jim how much he was drinking. No matter how many times Jim told him that he drank very little, no more than a couple times per month, the doctor kept telling Jim to reduce his alcohol intake. It turned out, the elevated liver enzymes were due to a fatty liver from consuming excessive carbohydrate. Jim was essentially diabetic, though his doctor didn't realize it. It was most frustrating for Jim at the time.

But then he researched a low-carb, high-fat diet and began to follow all the steps of our plan. This enabled him to experience a complete transformation in his weight and health.

He eliminated all sugar, processed food, and vegetable oils, which he feels was crucial to his success. He then went on a whole-foods-based low-carb, high-fat diet. After a week or two, this regimen enabled him to deploy various fasting strategies—one meal per day, some full fast days, and even more extended fasts exceeding twenty-four hours. He also began to focus on always getting a good night's sleep.

After the first six months, when he had lost a lot of weight and was feeling great, he began to take up some exercise. He became an avid runner, and it is now one of his main hobbies.

So what are his body metrics now? Well, in only a year on the plan, his weight has collapsed down to 177 pounds. And his body fat is down to a healthy 18 percent. What's more, he can now comfortably fit into his new 34-inch waist trousers!

> ❝ **Motivation is what gets you started. Habit is what keeps you going.** ❞
>
> —Jim Rohn

CHAPTER 16

THE LONG-TERM EAT RICH, LIVE LONG PLAN

And so, three weeks after you started your new low-carb, high-fat diet, we reach the long-term plan. This is where a new you emerges—securing a brighter, healthier future for you and your loved ones. It is crucial that the transition to long-term success is made properly.

Short-term interventions can often have some success. Almost any diet beats the standard American one. Even the flawed science of the food pyramid can manage that by discouraging consumption of sugar and sweets, even though it leaves in the refined carb of breads and pasta. Other diets that take the simple measure of cutting out these refined carbs will get even better short-term results. But most approaches will not deliver both slimness and optimum longevity for the long term because they do not address the full picture. They leave out a range of crucial elements, like eliminating vegetable oils, maximizing healthy fats, and using your low-insulin fat-burning ability to leverage the power of fasting. This applies especially to people who have developed metabolic issues from their previous lifestyle.

We want to ensure that your success will last permanently. That's what we've achieved with the Eat Rich, Live Long plan, and so have countless others under our guidance.

How do you ensure *permanent* body-weight control and optimal health?

First, internalize the principles outlined in this book and remain guided by them. Knowledge is indeed power. To forget is to drift off the path and back to your old ways.

Second, remember that there is no magical solution to weight maintenance and optimal health—especially as you get older. The ten action steps (page 72) must be applied throughout life. This is not a short-term solution.

Above all, make following the action steps a personal *habit.* By internalizing the principles, you make them part of who you are. While there's no magical solution, the combination of understanding the principles *and then forming habits around them* is as close as you will ever get.

Forming habits is the key, and turning an action into a habit is most successful when the action delivers a reward. This applies both to bad habits and to good ones. Why does a smoker continue with such a destructive habit? It is because he or she has a powerful belief in its supposed rewards. The physical addiction is actually very weak compared to the psychological one. It's the same for good habits like putting aside savings for the future; sure, it would be great to spend all your money, but savers know that greater rewards result from sticking to this habit. This is what sustains habits for a lifetime. You recognize the rewards that the habits deliver.

The Eat Rich, Live Long approach has worked for so many because it is inherently rewarding on many levels. The foods allowed are the wonderful ancestral ones—the very foods that made us human and that leave us feeling nourished and satiated. In the truest sense you are free to eat rich while feeling better every day. In contrast, the foods avoided on the plan may have provided momentary pleasures, but they make you pay the terrible price of sustained hunger. There will be a lasting pleasure and a deep sense of reward in consigning these factory-spawned products to the dustbin.

Of course, even when most outcomes are fantastic, some problems or concerns may arise for any individual. When these crop up, it can raise doubts about the overall plan, and doubts are what undermine and destroy good habits. So let us remind you that you are on a journey in which you are replacing bad science with good. We're surrounded by supporters of the old bad science of low-fat and high-carb, waving confusion and fear in our faces. Sadly, even medical professionals may place barriers to your progress—in some ways the medical profession is the most damaging force of all, steeped as it is in the old flawed science. By parroting that science, it can cause more distraction than the low-carb flu or the effects of mineral deficiencies. Ironically, you may have crossed the bridge to fat-burning with great success only to be knocked off it by an orthodox medical troll. Remember to look at the science and draw your own conclusions.

In this chapter, we'd like to give you some final suggestions that will serve you well in the long term, and we'll troubleshoot some common concerns.

LOVE YOUR GHRELIN!

Ivor applied the ten action steps way back, following a period of intensive research and discovery (as did Jeff). He easily shed over 30 pounds in around eight weeks—without any notable exercise. This ease of success depended utterly on the understanding of physiology and food that we have presented in this book.

But one psychological tool made Ivor's personal journey particularly easy: he learned to love his ghrelin. Ghrelin is the hormone that signals the brain to feel hunger, and Ivor embraced its mild signals *as a mark of his success.* Ghrelin's voice conveys the promise of huge health and other benefits, so Ivor associated the voice of his ghrelin with *reward.* This ensured that the habit of health has remained with him ever since.

Ghrelin is a hormone that raises its voice as your stomach empties. It creates a distinct feeling of hollowness inside you. It can signal you with anything from a whisper to a roar. It can be a friend or a fiend—you decide which. If you don't understand it properly and embrace it, it can make you eat when you should not.

There are two steps to loving your ghrelin:

1. Soften ghrelin's voice in your body. To do this, it is imperative to become fat-adapted. When you are an expert fat-burner, your body will smoothly transition to burning body fat when your stomach empties. This process will quieten your ghrelin. As we've talked about extensively, to become a fat-burner, you must keep your carb intake low—especially refined carb. These foods will raise the ghrelin volume to unreasonable levels.

2. Learn to appreciate what ghrelin is really saying. The message of ghrelin isn't, "Eat something now!" It's actually saying many much more positive things.

   ▶ It says, "Congratulations—you are now burning your body fat, just like your ancestors before you."

   ▶ It says, "You are performing an enormously beneficial metabolic workout as we speak."

   ▶ It says, "You are gaining the huge benefits of fasting for slimness, health, and longevity."

   ▶ It says, "You are lowering your risk of chronic diseases like coronary heart disease and cancer with every passing minute."

   ▶ It says, "You are reliving the experience of what made us human and you will achieve the rightful self-sufficiency of our species, so be very proud."

   ▶ It says, "Congratulations on leaving behind the constant-grazing mentality of our disease-ridden modern society."

   ▶ Most of all, it says, "You are a winner, and you will win."

LEVERAGE THE POWER OF THE CAC SCAN

We talked extensively in Chapter 11 about the value of a CAC scan, a CT scan of the heart that measures coronary artery calcification (CAC). It tells you how much heart disease you have and predicts with eerie precision your future health status, not just for heart-related issues but also for many other forms of chronic disease.

This incredibly effective scan only takes five minutes and usually costs around $150. It will supersede any number of blood tests and will tell you where your real risk level is today. It will also reveal problems that many blood tests may miss, motivate you to stick to your plan, and provide a superb baseline against which to measure your progress. The scan will give you a CAC score, a number that directly indicates the amount of damage your arteries have sustained. But even a high CAC score is not necessarily a problem—*if you take action on it.*

If you get a low score, you need not check back with another scan for five to ten years. If you get a high score, however, you can address the causes using our plan—and check back in a couple of years to verify that disease progression has slowed or stopped.

As always, taking action is the key. It is very important that you read the full detail in Chapter 11. Your life could depend on it!

TROUBLESHOOTING

After three weeks on the Eat Rich, Live Long plan—after following the steps and tips laid out in Part 2—you should be feeling much better than ever. Your belt should certainly be much looser. Your mind should be clearer than it has been in years. Your mood should also be more stable. Hopefully you're looking forward to the long-term healthy lifestyle with gusto.

Some of you, however, may still be experiencing challenges along with the benefits. If so, revisit the beginning of Chapter 8 (page 106), where we talked about potential roadblocks and how you can address them. Remember also that the essence of the Eat Rich, Live Long plan is the ten action steps outlined in Chapter 5. You may need to check the list again and make sure you've addressed *all* of them during your first few weeks.

If you were originally insulin resistant before starting on the Eat Rich, Live Long plan, you should now be much less so. This means you should be feeling much better, although your rate of weight loss may lessen with time. (If you're frustrated with a weight-loss plateau, see below for some suggestions.)

Focus your energy on steps 7 through 10 (pages 79 to 83). Most importantly, make following these steps an ingrained personal habit. They need to be incorporated into your overall lifestyle.

The action steps are all based on science and bring great rewards, including weight control, enhanced vitality, increased productivity, and greatly increased longevity. You will also look better and feel empowered to take on much more. If followed properly, the Eat Rich, Live Long program is a truly life-changing experience. You will never look back.

But that doesn't mean that there aren't some potential pitfalls you may encounter over the long term. In this section, we'll look at these common concerns and how to address them.

I FEEL GREAT, BUT MY WEIGHT LOSS HAS SLOWED

This is the dreaded weight-loss plateau. It happens particularly to insulin-sensitive people who are eating frequent, regular meals. The truth is that your body is rather clever. When it senses that you're in a healthy insulin-sensitive state, it recognizes that there is no health advantage to reducing the current level of body fat, and since a famine could be just around the corner, it decides it's good to have those safely stored calories for future needs. Therefore, it tends to conserve body fat. This generally means that you will have to focus intently on step 7—meal spacing—to start dropping weight again. Yes, that means you will have to step up your fasting routines to shift the weight.

It is important to realize that this is not the clichéd "eat less, move more" routine. Some key distinctions are as follows:

▶ You are not simply restricting calories at each regularly taken meal. Instead, you are skipping meals, which has metabolic benefits that restricting calories doesn't—in particular, it encourages fat-burning and better tackles insulin resistance.

▶ You are leveraging your new low-carb regimen and fat adaptation to manage your hunger between meals. Simply cutting calories with a standard diet is a painful and unsustainable approach. Meal spacing is very different.

▶ The synergy of following all ten steps will translate into an overall sense of well-being and control. You will thus be empowered to effectively apply step 7. This will deliver results.

We talked about this scenario in Chapter 8, but let's now revisit the strategy to get past the plateau: Pull back on the dietary fat you consume while keeping the carb and protein grams per day constant, for an overall drop in calories. This is effective when weight loss has plateaued. Because you are now a fat-burner, you will start burning your body fat smoothly along with the dietary fat in order to compensate for the drop in calories consumed.

Let's look at the numbers to see how this works. Let's say you are in a weight-loss plateau while eating a low-carb diet with the following ratios: 15 percent carb, 20 percent protein, and 65 percent fat. You then keep the carb and protein pretty constant but drop your intake of fat by half while skipping more meals. This will drive your body to supply stored fat (your adipose tissue) for energy. In other words, this stored fat will step in to help provide your energy requirements for the day. So while your dietary intake of fat will drop far below 65 percent of what you eat, your total use of fat for energy will remain close to 65 percent of what is supplying your energy to live. This is the key to breaking out of weight-loss plateaus. You need to keep fat as your dominant energy source—*but use body fat, not dietary fat, to provide this energy.*

Figure 16.1. In fat-burn-ers, a drop in dietary fat means that body fat is burned instead (as long as carb and protein remain constant).

In Figure 16.1, you can see that the drop in dietary fat is compensated for by an increase in body fat, which is now being burned for energy. In reali-ty, your body will conserve energy when it senses reduced food availability. Because of this, the total calories used won't actually stay steady, as shown in the table. We are just simplifying here to avoid getting caught in the weeds. The important point is that you're still getting most of your energy from fat, and it is only the *source* of fat energy that is changing.

Just to be clear, despite the fact that we've talked about reducing calo-ries and using more calories than you consume, we're not subscribing to the

DIETARY FAT PLUS BODY FAT FUEL SUPPLY							
Dietary Carb (g)	Carb %	Dietary Protein (g)	Protein %	Dietary Fat (g)	Body Fat Used (g)	Total Fat Used %	Total Calories
80	15%	110	20%	160	0	65%	2200
80	15%	110	20%	140	20	65%	2200
80	15%	110	20%	120	40	65%	2200
80	15%	110	20%	100	60	65%	2200
80	15%	110	20%	80	80	65%	2200
80	15%	110	20%	60	100	65%	2200

"calories in, calories out" theory of weight loss. This theory is highly misleading, as we discussed in Chapter 3. But that does not mean that calories don't matter. For an insulin-sensitive person caught on a weight-loss plateau, calories do matter. In these cases calories will need to be reduced to drive loss of body fat. But the method by which you reduce calories is the crucial factor. It is the way in which you approach a weight-loss plateau that dictates success or failure in dealing with it.

The crucial step is first converting yourself into a fat-burning machine, which you can achieve by changing your diet as outlined in action steps 1 through 6. Then you will have the power to burn body fat by reducing your fat consumption—without the crippling hunger that would otherwise cause you to fail. This last point is crucially important. You must never forget the synergy that makes it all possible. Remember also to love your ghrelin, as we talked about on page 335. When you feel hungry, let its voice reassure you until your next *planned* meal.

Remembering these things must become a habit for life.

OOPS—MY LDL HAS GONE UP

In Chapter 11 we covered some of the crucial science relating to cholesterol and health risks. We stressed that the ratio of triglycerides to HDL and the ratio of total cholesterol to HDL are overwhelmingly more important than LDL levels when it comes to estimating risk of heart disease. On the Eat Rich, Live Long plan, you are almost certain to improve these pivotal markers. But some people may find that after switching to a healthy low-carb, high-fat diet, their LDL number shifts upwards. This can be due to the way their bodies use the cholesterol-carrying lipoproteins to transport energy, or it may be due to other mechanisms related to the individual's genetic makeup.

As discussed in Chapter 11, LDL is a relatively weak and misleading marker that doesn't predict heart disease well—we strongly urge you to look at trig/HDL and total/HDL instead; as long as those numbers are improving, you're doing well. But we understand if you're concerned about a rise in LDL, and there are things that you can do to lower it while staying on a healthy low-carb diet for all its important benefits. Here are some ways that you can decrease your LDL without undermining a healthy low-carb, high-fat diet:

▶ Consume more plant-based fats from avocados, olive oil, and nuts.
▶ Replace some of your saturated fat intake with monounsaturated fats, without changing your overall fat intake.

- Reduce the animal-based protein in your diet (but keep in mind that protein is important—see Chapter 14).
- Reduce your consumption of cheese, especially if you're eating a lot of it.
- Introduce slightly more carbohydrates—but only the high-fiber, nutrient-dense, slow-digesting kind (see page 75).
- Increase your intake of fish oil, cod liver oil, or other healthy sources of omega-3 (see page 103 for more).
- Get more healthy sun exposure if possible.
- Do more resistance exercise (see page 118).

But keep in mind, it's important not to have a knee-jerk reaction based on a single cholesterol test. The numbers may jump around during a significant lifestyle change. Also, the LDL may be raised for many other reasons besides the change in diet. Losing weight can cause LDL to increase—it's best to reach a stable weight and then establish a new baseline LDL level. Thus a good time to assess LDL is after your weight has remained steady for a period of several weeks. After a follow-up test has verified a sustained high level, you then have the choice of pursuing the dietary changes listed above.

MY ADVANCED LIPOPROTEIN TEST HAS SHIFTED

If you get the advanced lipoprotein tests discussed in Chapter 11, you may observe that your ApoB—the particle count of LDL—has gone up since changing your diet. First, remember that none of these markers are infallible, because their risk multipliers come from associational studies. Second, keep in mind that the ApoB/ApoA1 ratio is a far more powerful marker of potential risk than ApoB (see page 262). Many people can have a supposedly "medium or high risk" ApoB level while the more important ApoB/ApoA1 ratio is okay. Any risk estimation must be judged in the context of the ApoB/ApoA1 ratio. It trumps ApoB importance in the countless studies that compare them. In fact, we both have high ApoB and good ApoB/ApoA1 ratios—and both our CAC scores are a big fat zero, which demonstrates the clear absence of any cardiovascular disease.

If you're concerned about your ApoB and wish to lower it, use the same strategy for lowering LDL we outlined above and retest after three to six months.

The other advanced lipoprotein marker that may go in the wrong direction is the small, dense LDL (sdLDL) number. In particular, this may apply to people with an ApoE4 genetic type—especially if they have sustained metabolic damage (see page 343 for more on ApoE4). In general, the sdLDL readings should ideally remain at a low level as per current guidelines. A higher level is associated with higher rates of coronary heart disease. But there remains a very big question as to whether this has any predictive power for an otherwise healthy, low-insulin person. But we will put aside that for the moment. If you repeatedly have measures of sdLDL in the high range, it may indicate a potential problem. Luckily, just as for ApoB, you can lower your sdLDL using the strategy for lowering LDL on pages 339 to 340; retest after three to six months to check your progress.

Again, it's important to avoid having a knee-jerk reaction based on a single lipoprotein test. The numbers may jump around during a significant lifestyle change. Also, ApoB or sdLDL may be raised for many other reasons, including weight loss—it's best to have reached a stable weight before establishing a new baseline level for both measures. Ideally the tests should be carried out after weight has remained steady for a period of several weeks, and have a follow-up verification test before you take any major actions.

MY FASTING BLOOD GLUCOSE IS CREEPING UP

If you had metabolic issues before starting the Eat Rich, Live Long program, you may see your fasting blood glucose creep up a little. Where readings in the past were maybe 90 to 100 mg/dL, perhaps now you're seeing readings of 100 to 110. The higher-end blood glucose readings may particularly show up in the morning because of the "dawn phenomenon," discussed on page 85. This is not uncommon and is generally not a cause for concern. It's important to look at the bigger picture and examine broader test results before jumping to conclusions.

The situation is often as follows: Many people with underlying prediabetes have normal fasting glucose; in simple terms, their high levels of insulin keep it well down. When they fix their prediabetes with a healthy low-carb diet, their system fundamentally changes. Now their low insulin allows blood glucose to rise a little, even though they're consuming less glucose-spiking foods. The mechanisms involve the interplay between insulin and glucagon hormones, which are constantly undergoing a kind of yin and yang interchange—with the new healthy insulin levels, glucagon may boost glucose manufacture in the body somewhat. This is very different than having a high glucose level *along with* high insulin levels. In fact, the two scenarios are utterly different.

The correct test to use is one that measures both fasting glucose and insulin. With cholesterol, the ratios (triglyceride to HDL, total cholesterol to HDL) are far more important than individual readings. With glucose and insulin, the *product* of the two is far more important than each individual measure. There is a very useful formula that multiplies these to give a standardized measure of insulin sensitivity. It is called the homeostatic model assessment of insulin resistance, or HOMA. The simple formula is as follows: (fasting insulin) x (fasting glucose) / 405 (with insulin in µIU/mL and glucose in mg/dL). This formula gives a great estimate of the health of your glucose/insulin system. It is more important than looking at glucose or insulin alone. (Note: The product is divided by 405 just to standardize the result for international comparisons—it doesn't correlate to any health metric.)

Let's look at one example of a new healthy-diet follower with high-ish blood glucose. Say that before starting the new diet, their fasting glucose was 95 and their fasting insulin was 8.5. Thus, their HOMA was (8.5 x 95) / 405 = 1.99. (Note: When the HOMA is over 1.2 or so, it indicates insulin resistance.)

Now, after being on a healthy low-carb, high-fat diet for at least three weeks, they are seeing a fasting glucose of 105 in the morning and a fasting insulin of 4.5. Thus, their HOMA is (4.5 x 105) / 405 = 1.17. Great job to our healthy-diet follower—they have managed to move from insulin resistant to reasonably insulin sensitive, which is the most important factor for long-term health.

In this case, the slightly high fasting glucose is irrelevant when viewed as part of the bigger picture. Just like with cholesterol, everyone is getting distracted by single measures. The ratios are much more important.

Another good way to check in on rising blood glucose is to get the HbA1c blood test. This assesses the average blood glucose level over the past few months. Jeff has had many patients whose fasting glucose reading did rise slightly but whose HbA1c had actually dropped since they embarked on the low-carb, high-fat diet. This shows that the slightly elevated fasting glucose levels have no real relevance when compared to better measures of health.

If you remain concerned about your blood glucose level, there are some strategies for lowering it:

▶   Fast for extended periods of time (24 to 36 hours) once or twice a week.

▶   Add some more healthy carb (nutrient-dense, slow-digesting whole foods) to your diet (see page 75).

▶   Do more resistance exercise (see page 118).

We do not consider any of these necessary as long as your HOMA and HbA1c levels are good, but some people like to play with their metrics!

Note: If your fasting glucose level is regularly rising above 120 mg/dL, the above discussion no longer applies. In this case, there may be an underlying condition to investigate—talk with your doctor.

SPECIAL CONSIDERATIONS

PEOPLE WITH APOE4

Around 20 percent of the population has the ApoE4 genetic type. By nature, ApoE4 people tend to have higher cholesterol levels along with slightly higher rates of coronary heart disease (approximately 1.4 times the risk in one study, but almost no extra risk in another).[1] You can find out your ApoE genetic type using inexpensive genetic tests that can be ordered online.[2]

There has been much discussion in low-carb circles on how ApoE4 people respond to low-carb, high-fat diets. In general, they have excellent improvements in health and blood test markers, just like everyone else on this dietary regimen. However, some appear to have increased ApoB and/or increased sdLDL. If they do have this response, it may indicate a problem—or possibly not; it's impossible to be sure from these tests alone. Instead, it's essential to triangulate all the risk markers to estimate the need for concern. By all means, if you have ApoE4 and see an increase in ApoB or sdLDL, explore this with your doctor. But if all physical signs and most test results clearly demonstrate that overall health has improved, what should ApoE4s do about an isolated elevation of ApoB or sdLDL?

There are approaches that can lower these metrics—and they're the same ones anyone can follow to reduce LDL:

▶ Consume more plant-based fats from avocados, olive oil, and nuts.

▶ Swap some of your saturated fat intake for monounsaturated fats, without changing your overall fat intake.

▶ Eat less animal-based protein and focus more on fatty fish and eggs.

▶ Reduce your consumption of cheese.

▶ Eat more high-fiber, nutrient-dense, real-food-based carbohydrates (see page 75).

▶ Increase your healthy sources of omega-3 (see page 102).

▶ Get more healthy sun exposure if possible.

▶ Do more resistance exercise (see page 118).

One researcher who has focused much effort on understanding the effect of a high-fat diet on people with ApoE4 is Dr. Steven Gundry. He has many talks and other material freely available online.[3] His advice largely agrees with our suggestions above; he is far less focused on ApoB and is much more focused on sdLDL and various markers of inflammation. We perceive that an overreliance on these isolated "cholesterol" markers could exaggerate the true relevance of the ApoE4 situation. Instead, we believe that these markers are concerning only if they are flagging another underlying problem, particularly a decrease in insulin sensitivity.

One fascinating study reveals the crucial thing that people with ApoE4 should watch for.[4] The study scrutinized a group of 384 hypertensive patients that included all genotypes (including ApoE4). Their analysis revealed that:

▶ ApoE4 people *with insulin resistance* had much higher risk of cardiovascular disease than non-ApoE4 people with insulin resistance— their risk multiplier was 2.42x.

▶ ApoE4 people *without insulin resistance* had much lower risk of cardiovascular disease than non-ApoE4 people without insulin resistance—their risk multiplier was 0.14x, meaning they were six times *less* likely to have cardiovascular disease.

This suggests that the risk of heart disease for people with ApoE4 is overwhelmingly dependent on whether insulin resistance is present or not. We would suggest that ApoE4 types need to be primarily focused on achieving insulin sensitivity—just like everyone else, but even more so. This will protect them from heart disease, and certainly from Alzheimer's, which ApoE4s have *very* increased susceptibility to—as we might expect, since Alzheimer's is an insulin/glucose dysregulation problem in the brain that's also known as "type 3 diabetes."

In closing, people with ApoE4 need to be even more careful to lower their insulin than the average person. They also need to be more diligent about tackling the other root causes of chronic disease (excessive intake of carbohydrate and vegetable oils, lack of sun exposure, etc.). A really good metric for people with ApoE4 to focus on is their ApoB/ApoA1 ratio. Far more predictive of heart disease risk than ApoB or sdLDL, it should be prioritized over both. Using this ratio will give the very best guidance for any diet tweaking that is being experimented with. It goes without saying that the insulin, blood glucose, and other crucial metrics are also prioritized here. It would be a mistake to get sidetracked by individual associative risk factors at the expense of the big picture.

ATHLETES

If you're a competitive athlete, you're likely not looking for help with weight loss or insulin resistance and its accompanying problems, as so many other readers are. Instead, you're probably wondering how the Eat Rich, Live Long program will affect your performance.

The good news is that for endurance sports, performance improves over time on a low-carb, high-fat diet because your body can perform better when burning fat—as long as you're fat-adapted, of course. With fat-adaptation comes the enhanced ability to burn body fat as an optimal fuel. Athletes who have gone through the process of adaptation can double the fat grams they burn per minute.[5] Relatively lower inflammation, which accompanies fat adaptation, can enable a more rapid recovery following large events. The reliance on constant top-ups from unhealthy carb snacks is also greatly reduced. We believe that the low-carb, high-fat athlete will experience much improved health and longevity in the long run.

However, for delivering intense bursts of activity like short sprints, your body still requires glucose as a flash fuel. Therefore, you may see a drop in performance for this type of sport when moving to a healthy low-carb or keto diet. A workaround can be to "carb-up" before events, but this will have negative impacts on the beneficial effects of the diet. At some point you'll need to decide which is more important: performance or health and longevity?

Optimizing sporting performance in certain types of activity is not really within the scope of this book. If this is your goal, we recommend *The Art and Science of Low Carbohydrate Performance* by Dr. Jeff Volek and Dr. Stephen Phinney. These guys are pioneers in the application of low-carb and ketogenic diets, and their book reveals all of the best strategies to achieve both performance and optimum health.

STEPHEN'S STORY

Stephen is one of many people who discovered Ivor's blog (www.thefatemperor.com/blog) and YouTube videos (@fatemperor), which talk about the science and strategies covered in this book. They enabled him to finally understand why he was so unhealthy—and empowered him to turn his life around.

Stephen was in his midforties and had a sedentary lifestyle that included many indulgences, such as Danish pastries. His A1C was 6.2 and his blood pressure was constantly high. He had also developed sleep apnea and weighed in at 330 pounds. He had massive inflammation in his joints and could not walk without pain; he even had to regularly take days off work because of it. Like so many desperate people on high-carb diets, he yo-yo dieted for years, spending a fortune on every fad and more personal trainers than you could count. But he could never overcome the constant hunger. This remorselessly drove him not only to overeat food in general but to specifically crave carb-heavy and sugary foods.

After his doctor told him he was well into prediabetes, he finally went to a top-end clinic to speak to a bariatric surgeon. Afterward, Stephen went home and thought to himself, "There has to be a better way—cutting out healthy body parts cannot be the best thing to do."

That's when he found the information about low-carb and keto diets through Ivor's online resources. That very week he went straight to a keto strategy and never varied from it!

He lost 70 pounds in less than five months. After just a couple of weeks, all the pain in his joints was gone and his blood pressure was dropping fast towards healthy levels. After eleven weeks his A1C came in at a safe 5.3 and his blood pressure was normal every day. He had never felt better. He now understands that he had been high on the insulin spectrum, which was causing the imbalance that drove him to eat in spite of his best efforts at restraint.

He now eats two meals a day and stays under 20 grams of carb every day. And the most amazing thing of all? *He is never hungry!* In fact, he cannot believe that he can now truthfully state that fact—it is a wondrous thing for him to be free from cravings at last.

Stephen has joined the growing legions of people who are discovering the correct science of low-carb, keto, and the crucial need for low insulin.

AFTERWORD

We have really enjoyed putting this book together. It debunks the bad science that has led the Western world into an obesity and diabetes disaster. It replaces it with sound science resulting from years of research and collaboration with some of the best minds in medicine and nutrition. Most importantly, it captures the best strategies to control your body weight and minimize your risk of chronic disease.

We and countless others are thriving as we apply the Eat Rich, Live Long plan's ten steps to achieve optimal health. The plan delivers exceptional vitality, productivity, and robust health, and we are delighted to apply it every day. (Well...almost every day—we all cheat on rare occasions!)

Choosing real food over junk carbs and fake fat—it just feels so good. May you and your family eat rich and live long!

ACKNOWLEDGMENTS

First and foremost, we thank our wives, Eilís and Nicole, who have enabled our dedicated research with such grace and patience over the years. Likewise our extended families, who understand what it takes to get the work done. Pivotal has been the direct assistance of David Bobbett and Irish Heart Disease Awareness (www.IHDA.ie), without which this book would never have been produced. We also owe a great debt of gratitude to our editor Tom Miller—the structure, flow, and readability of this book is largely due to his editing excellence. In his other role as literary agent with the Carol Mann Agency, Tom also placed this book with the wonderful team at Victory Belt Publishing, including Erich Krauss, Lance Freimuth, Pam Mourouzis, Holly Jennings, Erin Granville, and Justin-Aaron Velasco.

We have enjoyed excellent collaboration with countless individuals over the past years. The following list includes just some of those who have enabled us on our journey of discovery:

Robert Atkins, Peter Ballerstedt, Amy Berger, Richard Bernstein, Douglas Boyd, Kenneth Brookler, Bruce Brundage, Matthew J. Budoff, Rangan Chatterjee, Catherine Crofts, Mark Cuccuzella, Marianne Demasi, RD Dikeman, James DiNicolantonio, Petra (Peter) Dobromylskyj, Michael and Mary Dan Eades, Andreas Eenfeldt, Gabor Erdosi, Richard Feinman, Dave Feldman, Sam Feltham, Gary Fettke, Glen and Yael Finkel, Jason Fung, Tucker Goodrich, Sarah Hallberg, Zoe Harcombe, Harvey Hecht, George Henderson,

Steve Horvitz, Guðmundur F. Jóhannsson, Marty Kendall, Malcolm Kendrick, Joseph R. Kraft, Kevin Kraft, Ronald Krauss, David Ludwig, Nick Mailer, Aseem Malhotra, Antonio Martinez, Amy Moore, Jimmy Moore, Scott Murray, Ted Naiman, Timothy Noakes, Gearoid O'Laoi, Donal O'Neill, Rakash Patel, Jeff Pedalty, Steve Phinney, Uffe Ravnskov, Gerald Reaven, Ron Rosedale, Simon Saunders, Amy Savagian, Grant Schofield, Cate Shanahan, Axel F. Sigurðsson, Raphi Sirt, Marika Sobros, Gary Taubes, Rod Tayler, Nina Teicholz, Vinnie Tortorich, David Unwin, Jeff Volek, Jan Vyjidak, Eric Westman, Tommy Wood, Jay Wortman, June Sang Yang, and John Yudkin.

It is impossible to list all whom we have positively networked with over the past several years. The following is an attempt to capture just some of these great people:

Pedro Aceves-Casillas, Chris Armstrong, Shawn Baker, Ashvy Bhardwaj, Ben Bikman, Murray Braithwaite, John Briffa, Bob Briggs, Iain Campbell-Brown, Rodney Cartocci, Pat Caslin, Colin Champ, Kailash Chand, Ann Childers, Jerry Clifford, William Cromwell, Christine Cronau, Daragh and Jean Cronin, Jeff Cyr, Dominic D'Agostino, Annika Dahlqvist, Patricia Daly, Trudi Deacon, Isabela Dengani-Schmidt, Larry Diamond, Emma Dunne, Georgia Ede, Darryl Edwards, Chris Enright, Carl Franklin, Heather Fritz, Deborah Gordon, Pauline Grace, Sarah Hallberg, Rick Henriksen, Adele Hite, Erynn Kay, Charlie Keegan, Christopher Kelly, Domini Kemp, Nigel Kinbrum, Jill and Alex Knopoff, Bill Lagakos, Trevor Land, Kevin Lee, Carol Lofferman, Kjartan and Tekla Hrafn Loftsson, Michel Lundell, Aishe Malick, Joanne McCormack, Emily Mcguire, Robert Miller, Denise Minger, Jasmine Mogassi, Francis Moore, Richard Morris, Dorrit Moussaieff, Adam Nally, Tom Naughton, Paula Nedved, George Newman, Anthony Nolan, Mick O'Connell, L. Robert Oh, Amber O'Hearn, Declan O'Neill, Arjun Singh Panesar, Kevin Rourke, Keith Runyan, Kesar Sadhra, Simon Saunders, Polina Sayess, Andrew Scarborough, John Schoonbee, Ken Sikaris, Eric Sodicoff, Jose Carlos Souto, Franziska Spritzler, Troy Stapleton, Charlotte Summers, Karen Thompson, Eric Thorn, Jen Unwin, Priyanka Wali, Lynn Walsh, Robb Wolf, Nicolai Worm, and David Wyant.

APPENDIX A: RESOURCES

BOOKS

Protein Power, by Michael R. Eades, MD, and Mary Dan Eades, MD (1996)

Lights Out: Sleep, Sugar, and Survival, by T. S. Wiley with Bent Formby (2001)

Carb Conscious Vegetarian, by Robin Robertson (2005)

Diabetes Epidemic and You, by Joseph Kraft (2008)

Good Calories, Bad Calories, by Gary Taubes (2008)

Vitamin D and Cholesterol: The Importance of the Sun, by Dr. David Grimes (2009)

The Paleo Diet, rev. ed., by Loren Cordain (2010)

The Art and Science of Low Carbohydrate Living, by Stephen D. Phinney and Jeff S. Volek (2011)

Dr. Bernstein's Diabetes Solution, by Richard K. Bernstein (2011)

Grain Brain, by David Perlmutter (2013)

Keto Clarity, by Jimmy Moore and Eric C. Westman, MD (2014)

The Big Fat Surprise, by Nina Teicholz (2014)

The Vegetarian and Vegan Guide: The Blood Sugar Solution 10-Day Detox Diet by Mark Hyman, MD (http://10daydetox.com/resources/_downloads/10DDVegetarianVegan.pdf)

The World Turned Upside Down: The Second Low-Carbohydrate Revolution, by Richard David Feinman (2014)

Wheat Belly, by William Davis, MD (2014)

The Ketogenic Cookbook, by Jimmy Moore and Maria Emmerich (2015)

The Ketogenic Kitchen, by Domini Kemp and Patricia Daly (2015)

What the Fat?, by Grant Schofield, Caryn Zinn, and Craig Rodger (2015)

Eat Fat, Get Thin, by Mark Hyman, MD (2016)

The Complete Guide to Fasting, by Jason Fung, MD, with Jimmy Moore (2016)

Real Meal Revolution, by Tim Noakes, Jonno Proudfoot, and Sally-Ann Creed (2016)

The Plant Paradox, by Steven R. Gundry (2017)

Diabetes Unpacked, by Tim Noakes et al. (2017)

Wired to Eat, by Robb Wolf (2017)

Fat for Fuel, by Joseph Mercola, MD (2017)

Deep Nutrition: Why Your Genes Need Traditional Food, by Catherine Shanahan, MD (2017)

Boundless: A Fresh Approach to Real Food Freedom, by Ryan Turner (2017)

The Salt Fix, by Dr. James DiNicolantonio (2017)

INFORMATIVE WEBSITES

Burn Fat Not Sugar (Ted Naiman, MD), burnfatnotsugar.com

Chris Masterjohn, PhD, chrismasterjohnphd.com

Denver's Diet Doctor (Jeffry Gerber, MD), denversdietdoctor.com

Diet Doctor (Andreas Eenfeldt, MD), dietdoctor.com

Dr. Malcolm Kendrick, drmalcolmkendrick.org

The Fat Emperor (Ivor Cummins), thefatemperor.com

FoodMed.Net (Marika Sboros), foodmed.net

Intensive Dietary Management (Jason Fung, MD), intensivedietarymanagement.com

Ketogains (blog), ketogains.com

Livin' la Vida Low-Carb (Jimmy Moore), livinlavidalowcarb.com

Low Carb Down Under (Rod Tayler, MD, and Jamie Hayes), lowcarbdownunder.com.au

Mark's Daily Apple (Mark Sisson), marksdailyapple.com

Nina Teicholz (blog), ninateicholz.com/blog

Optimising Nutrition (Marty Kendall), optimisingnutrition.com

Protein Power (Michael Eades, MD, and Mary Dan Eades, MD), proteinpower.com

Real Meal Revolution (Tim Noakes), realmealrevolution.com

Richard David Feinman, feinmantheother.com

Robb Wolf, robbwolf.com

The Science of Human Potential (Grant Schofield), profgrant.com

Tuit Nutrition (Amy Berger), tuitnutrition.com

2 Keto Dudes (Carl Franklin and Richard Morris), 2ketodudes.com

The Weston A. Price Foundation, westonaprice.org

Zoë Harcombe, PhD, zoeharcombe.com

DEEPER SCIENCE WEBSITES

Break Nutrition (Raphi Sirt), breaknutrition.com

Cholesterol Code (Dave Feldman), cholesterolcode.com

The High-Fat Hep C Diet (George Henderson), hopefulgeranium.blogspot.com

Hyperlipid (Petro Dobromylskyj), high-fat-nutrition.blogspot.com

ORGANIZATIONS

Diabetes UK, diabetes.co.uk

Group of Concerned Canadian Physicians and Allied Health Care Providers, changethefoodguide.ca

Irish Heart Disease Awareness, ihda.ie

The Noakes Foundation, thenoakesfoundation.org

Nutrition Coalition, nutrition-coalition.org

Physicians for Ancestral Health, ancestraldoctors.org

Public Health Collaboration, phcuk.org

MOVIES

Fat Head, fathead-movie.com (2013)

Cereal Killers, cerealkillersmovie.com (2013)

Carb-Loaded: A Culture Dying to Eat, imdb.com/title/tt3558546/ (2014)

Cereal Killers 2: Run on Fat, runonfatmovie.com (2015)

The Widowmaker, vimeo.com/ondemand/thewidowmakermovie2015 (2015)

The Magic Pill, imdb.com/title/tt6035294/ (2016)

The Big Fat Fix, thebigfatfix.com (2016)

APPENDIX B: THE EAT RICH, LIVE LONG GUIDE TO SWEETENERS

We almost never eat sweetened foods ourselves. Nor do we recommend that people in the Eat Rich, Live Long program eat sweetened foods over the long term—except for occasional, exceptional situations. For your long-term health, it's best to wean your taste buds off sweet and on to savory! That said, many people in the early weeks of our program miss sweet foods, so we've included several low-carb, high-fat sweet dishes in Chapter 9.

Table sugar is an absolute no-no at any time on our plan, as are honey, agave, maple syrup, molasses, corn syrup, and all other glucose- and fructose-filled sweeteners. Those sugary poisons have helped create the health problems we need to overcome.

This appendix is a guide to natural sugar-free sweeteners that work on our plan, for those exceptional times when you want something sweet. With many more natural options having become available recently, people are moving away from artificial sweeteners such as aspartame and sucralose, so the recommendations here are for sweeteners made from naturally occurring ingredients.

For reference, nutrition facts for all the sweet recipes in this book have been analyzed using Sola, a sweetener that combines erythritol, stevia, and monk fruit and measures like sugar. See page 352 for more.

STEVIA AND MONK FRUIT

Stevia and monk fruit are excellent options for calorie-free low-carb sweetening when no cooking is involved, such as sweetening a glass of iced tea or a smoothie.

Pure stevia and monk fruit extracts are approximately two hundred times sweeter than sugar, which means that when using an extract to replace the sugar in a recipe, you use a fraction of the amount of sugar called for. It can be difficult to calculate the right amount of pure extract needed, though you will quickly figure out through experimentation how much stevia or monk fruit is right for you.

ERYTHRITOL AND XYLITOL

In addition to stevia and monk fruit, you might want to check out two sweeteners made with pure sugar alcohols: erythritol and xylitol. (Don't worry, they do not contain actual alcohol!) Both are granulated, making them great choices for cooking.

Erythritol is found in small amounts in fruits and vegetables and is approximately 70 percent as sweet as sugar. Erythritol has just 0.2 calorie per gram and is clinically proven not to cause a rise in blood sugar, but it is slightly less sweet than sugar. It's typically well tolerated by the digestive system. The only real drawback to using a 100 percent erythritol-based sweetener is that it sometimes has a cooling effect on the mouth. (This works well in warm or refrigerated desserts, as the cooling effect is much less noticeable, but in room-temperature cakes and pastries, the cooling can be quite apparent.)

Many low-carbers also like xylitol. Like erythritol, it's found in fruits and vegetables, but it has slightly more calories—2.4 per gram—and it will raise blood sugar slightly. Xylitol is as sweet as sugar.

Here are two brands of erythritol and xylitol to try:

- Wholesome All Natural Zero Erythritol (www.wholesomesweet.com/product/all-natural-zero)
- Xyla Xylitol (www.xylabrands.com)

BLENDED GRANULATED SWEET-ENERS

Blended granulated low-carb sweeteners combine two or more of the sweeteners listed above: stevia, monk fruit, erythritol, and xylitol. Erythritol in particular is often blended with stevia or monk fruit extract to increase the sweetness.

These blended sweeteners add texture, viscosity, browning, and structure to baked goods and desserts. They measure closer to the same proportions as granulated sugar—though you should experiment to see what works best for your recipes.

The recipes in this book were developed using Sola brand sweetener, which contains erythritol, stevia, and monk fruit. It measures like sugar, so if you're planning to use another sweetener, adjust the amount of sweetener accordingly.

Here are three recommended brands of blended granulated low-carb sweeteners:

- Sola (solasweet.com)
- Lakanto (lakanto.com)
- Swerve (swervesweetener.com)

APPENDIX C: HIGH CHOLESTEROL CONCERNS

For those who are interested in learning more about the lipoprotein tests, ApoE4, and familial hypercholesterolemia, we'll explore them in more detail here. The truth is that the science around the last two conditions is not nearly the slam-dunk that has been suggested. The risks associated with having the ApoE4 gene or familial hypercholesterolemia are heavily dependent on things other than "cholesterol." We'll pick up where we finished in Chapter 11—the LDL particle count metrics.

CHOLESTEROL MASTER CLASS: ADVANCED LIPOPROTEIN MECHANISMS

We talked about LDL particles and small, dense LDL (sdLDL) in Chapter 11 and noted there that high counts of both may indicate an underlying problem—specifically, they may simply flag that a state of insulin resistance is present and should be addressed. It's possible, however, that these particles may also have a causal, contributory role in and of themselves. The theory is that LDL particles or sdLDL particles—which have been oxidized by inflammatory issues—can more easily enter the artery wall than other lipoproteins, so higher numbers of these would cause more damage to the arteries. But the evidence suggests that this only happens in cases where the artery wall is *already* damaged. LDL-P—the count of LDL particles—especially may have little or no relevance if there is no arterial damage or inflammation present. If your system is already fireproofed, then extra boats ferrying around fuel will not have any impact.

There is also a lot of evidence that damage to the particles causes arterial disease by triggering immune reactions in the arterial wall.[1] There are even scientific studies that suggest that oxidative stress damage to the particles is one of the many causes of hyperinsulinemia and insulin resistance.[2] Therefore, damaged particles can both *cause* and also *be caused by* a state of insulin resistance.

When an inflammatory state exists (due to elevated glucose and/or insulin), your LDLs tend to become oxidized and damaged. Related processes also tend to drive up the quantity of sdLDL particles along with the total number of particles (LDL-P). Therefore, the LDL-P will tend to track with disease, certainly—but because it's indicating an increase in *damaged* particles, not just because of the mere number of extra particles around.

The current orthodox view is that the LDL particles themselves are toxic by their nature. We probably don't need to stress how inherently absurd this really is. There are many studies where the LDL-P was disconnected entirely from the rates of disease.[3] It is at best a fallible indicator of other problems.

Let's look at one study of many where LDL-P showed no relevance for heart attack patients. A large number of recent heart attack patients were compared with a carefully well-matched set of people of the same age and sex who were apparently heart-healthy, with no history of coronary heart disease.[4] What did the analysis show? *All* of the measures that relate to glucose metabolism and insulin resistance were different between the groups, with very high statistical significance. But the measure of LDL-P wasn't different at all.

In this study they also measured an excellent indicator of insulin problems: proinsulin levels. As its name suggests, proinsulin is used to create insulin molecules. Thus, when proinsulin is high, it is highly probable that there is insulin dysregulation. Measuring proinsulin here showed that insulin resistance utterly dominated as an indicator of heart disease. The LDL-P didn't show up as relevant at all (see Figure C.1).

Measure	Heart Attack Patients	Healthy Matched People
LDL-P	1.08	1.06
Proinsulin	6.2	2.5

Figure C.1. Again and again, insulin measures blow away "cholesterol" ones. Source: M. Bartnik, et al., "Abnormal Glucose Tolerance—A Common Risk Factor in Patients with Acute Myocardial Infarction in Comparison with Population-Based Controls," *Journal of Internal Medicine* 256, no. 4 (2004): 288–97.

And there was more. Even though the researchers chose heart attack victims who were not known diabetics, a full 33 percent of them were found to have type 2 diabetes when tested. On further investigation, a full 67 percent of the heart attack patients had major glucose and insulin dysregulation issues (i.e., they were essentially diabetic). We talked about the 2015 EuroAspire study in Chapter 10, and we see here exactly what was demonstrated there: the huge factor in heart disease attacks is the diabetic phenomenon of hyperinsulinemia and insulin resistance. If Kraft's glucose tolerance with insulin assay method of showing insulin status (see page 235) had been deployed, it's likely that most of the remaining 33 percent would have shown glucose/insulin issues also. So what part is really left for LDL-P to play here?

More evidence of the ubiquity of insulin-resistance issues showed up in an unexpected place. The "healthy" group that the heart attack patients were compared to had specifically been chosen because they had no prior health issues at all. But upon testing, it turned out that 11 percent had type 2 diabetes, and an additional 24 percent were well on their way! If they were tested with Kraft's method, we would guess that more than 50 percent of the "healthy" controls were not healthy at all. They would have occult diabetes or "diabetes in situ" simmering inside. We are at the point now where the majority of adults have some degree of diabetic dysfunction—whether they have a higher LDL-P or not. This is where the lion's share of heart disease and other tragedies originate.

So is LDL-P mainly just a good marker for underlying insulin-signaling issues? It would appear to be a very reasonable explanation.

That's why the ratios of triglycerides to HDL and total cholesterol to HDL, which you can get from the traditional lipid panel, are so powerful, especially if you don't have access to the advanced lipoprotein test. The ratios trump the LDL-P in terms of predicting heart disease risk in most studies—so they are really the best cholesterol markers of all. The ratios indicate the level of hyperinsulinemia / insulin resistance, which is what both drives up the level of LDL-P and causes the heart disease that's associated with it. When used properly, these cholesterol ratios win at the cholesterol guessing game.

However, you do not want to be guessing when it comes to your life. That's why we recommend the CAC scan, which directly measures arterial damage (see page 265).

CHOLESTEROL CONFUSION: THE FAMILIAL HYPERCHOLESTER-OLEMIACS

Familial hypercholesterolemia (FH) is a genetic trait where lipoprotein receptors are less active, leading to more lipoproteins and cholesterol circulating in the system. This condition appears to have been mercilessly mined since the 1970s. One reason is that it lends vital support to the "cholesterol is bad" theory. As we mentioned earlier, LDL level only properly predicts coronary heart disease when it's really, really high. Although not publicized, this was nonetheless clear from the Framingham Heart Study, which began in 1948 and is still ongoing. But then it was discovered that approximately one in four hundred people have a genetic tendency to run elevated LDL numbers. These people were recruited to bolster the LDL-is-bad dogma.

Something that affects less than three people in a thousand would normally get little attention. But in the 1970s, the country was convinced that cholesterol was the cause of heart disease. Cholesterol simply *had* to be bad, come hell or high water. So the spotlight was turned on this tiny minority of people, who were enlisted to provide much-needed support for a weak and sickly hypothesis.

These rare and special people with FH are not easy to define. There have been endless efforts to identify genetic markers for the condition; some have been found over time, and some of these are established as accurate. But many medical people still assume that FH may be present based only on an unusually high cholesterol reading.

People with FH have a higher rate of premature heart disease; just how much higher their risk is varies greatly. A risk multiplier of roughly 2.5x is cited by some authorities.[5] But people with FH are not *consistently* at higher risk. Some get heart attacks early in life, but many live long healthy lives. And now the bombshell: *the ones who have heart attacks have the same LDL levels as those who remain healthy.*[6]

You see the massive problem here: If LDL drives the disease, then more LDL should track strongly with more disease. But even for people with FH, who universally have high LDL levels, it simply does not. Therefore, the prevailing theory that LDL directly causes heart disease is again revealed as simplistic and misleading.

So what *does* drive premature coronary heart disease in some people with FH?

A 2001 study on FH looked a little closer at what was driving the risk of coronary heart disease.[7] Here are some of the really high risk multipliers they found:

▶ lower HDL

▶ higher sdLDL (a proxy for oxidation damage—see page 250)

▶ insulin and glucose dysregulation (i.e., insulin-resistance issues)

▶ smoking

What's missing from that list? That's right: LDL-P or ApoB, the measures of how many LDL particles are in the blood. Here's one more study from 2001.[8] The researchers scrutinized a group of men with known FH. Some had had heart attacks at a young age (around forty-one on average). Some were fine and had had no heart attacks. What made the difference here? Let's take a look.

Compared to the FH men who hadn't had heart attacks, the FH men who'd suffered heart attacks had:

▶ significantly higher levels of insulin

▶ significantly higher levels of insulin resistance

▶ significantly higher levels of triglycerides

▶ significantly higher levels of PAI-1 activity (blood-clotting factors driven by high levels of insulin)

▶ significantly lower values of HDL

Again, what's missing from this list and made no difference in whether they had an early heart attack or not? You guessed it: LDL level.

The last study we'll look at is from 2014.[9] This study looked at a relatively large number of FH people from 1994 through to 2013. What were the factors most linked to atherosclerotic events and heart attacks? You guessed it—all the factors that flag insulin-related dysfunction:

▶ hypertension (8x risk multiplier)

▶ type 2 diabetes (6x risk multiplier)

▶ low HDL (2x risk multiplier)

▶ high triglycerides (1.8x risk multiplier)

LDL managed to barely scrape over the line in this one with a 1.16x multiplier, but that's vanishingly small compared to the risk caused by diabetes.

There are many studies that repeatedly show this reality.[10] One from 2000 showed that total/HDL ratio was a crucial measure for risk of heart events in people with FH.[11] One from 2005 placed insulin signaling at the center of FH and familial combined hyperlipidemia, a similar condition.[12]

Unfortunately, the general perception, even in the medical community, is still that FH is about "high cholesterol." In reality, people with FH appear to be simply more susceptible to the various causes of coronary heart disease. Thus, they need to be particularly careful in eliminating them. If you have FH, you need to be especially careful to lower your insulin. You also need to avoid smoking, prevent high blood pressure from developing, and strive to achieve low inflammation (measured by C-reactive protein). You also need to be very diligent in tackling the other root causes of chronic disease: excessive carbohydrate, vegetable oils, lack of sun exposure, a sedentary lifestyle, and other concerns addressed in the ten action steps.

If you have FH and would like to push your LDL levels lower, this is absolutely fine, especially if you are not addressing all of the really important factors named above. For instance, if you're happy to eat according to the carb-heavy food pyramid, avoid healthy fasting behaviors, smoke cigarettes, and never leave the couch, then lowering LDL is quite important.

In contrast, if you're applying all the action steps and achieving excellent results in all markers but the cholesterol ones (insulin, blood glucose, blood pressure, waist size, trig/HDL, total/HDL), then you have more choice in the matter.

It is especially helpful for people in this situation to get a CAC scan. If your CAC score is low and/or not progressing over time, it can be greatly reassuring—especially because the CAC scan actually measures heart disease rather than a fallible surrogate like "cholesterol." Combined with all the crucial measures of insulin regulation and inflammation, the CAC score will settle the matter more decisively than any cholesterol measurements can.

Because genuine FH is a rare and specific condition, some people may have exposure to risk in spite of taking all the appropriate precautions. For that reason, people with verified FH should discuss preventative treatment options with a specialist in the field. It may help to raise the points covered in this section, to ensure that the full picture is discussed between doctor and patient.

APPENDIX D: THE INSULIN SPECTRUM

In earlier chapters, we talked about the insulin spectrum, with an unhealthy insulin resistance (which leads to diabetes, heart disease, and a host of other health problems) on one end and healthy insulin sensitivity on the other end.

Where you fall on this spectrum can determine every element of your health—how heavy you are, how damaged your arteries are, whether you have type 2 diabetes, and much more. So here we'll lay out how insulin resistance develops, and we'll start the story by revisiting the basics: glucose and the role of insulin.

GLUCOSE: HIGH-OCTANE FUEL FOR HUMANS

Glucose—sugar—is a tricky fuel. As we explained in Chapter 3, it must be managed carefully or it will damage your body in myriad ways. Carbohydrate is essentially made up of glucose: in fibrous carb foods, such as vegetables, glucose molecules are arranged in stiff chains. The chains are difficult to break down into individual molecules, which means it takes longer for the glucose from these foods to hit your bloodstream. In contrast, nonfibrous, starchy, and sugary carbohydrates—such as pastas, breads, honey, table sugar, baked goods, and fruit juices—can be broken down rapidly into glucose molecules, so they hit your system rapidly. When this occurs, you could suffer dangerous concentrations of glucose in your bloodstream. Thankfully for most people, the body has mechanisms to prevent this.

The standard glucose quantity in an adult's total blood supply is only 1.5 teaspoons' worth. Carrying significantly more than this amount would cause serious damage to blood vessels, which over time can damage your internal organs, particularly the heart and kidneys. (Damage to the blood vessels from high blood sugar is also why diabetes is associated with nerve damage and poor circulation.) But blood sugar doesn't rise this way unless the insulin-signaling system is damaged. Over the short term, at least, healthy people can handle high-carb foods. Here's how.

Glucose molecules are first sensed in your upper gut, triggering an explosive release of a hormone called glucose-dependent insulinotropic polypeptide (GIP). It is the master glucose sensor. It is also the master switch to trigger insulin release—as GIP surges, it causes a surge in insulin. GIP also primes your fat cells for expansion.

Insulin attempts to safely mop up the incoming glucose by moving it into cells that will use it for energy. It also tells your muscles to stop burning fat—you can't be burning fat when a risky fuel like glucose is flooding in. Insulin also helps to convert glucose to glycogen, a form of glucose that can be stored in your liver, and to fat—both glycogen and fat cells are safe ways to store glucose energy. Insulin also tells your liver to stop all glucose production until further notice and signals the brain to alter appetite response, too. (While insulin can act to suppress appetite in healthy people, it generally fails to perform this function in insulin-resistant people.)

Insulin does all of this and much, much more. It is the master hormone of metabolism.

All of the above processes should work pretty well in a healthy person. After all, our bodies evolved to manage carbohydrate intake. But in anyone who is even partially diabetic—anyone who has insulin resistance—it doesn't work so well. Therefore, it does not work so well for the majority of adults.

Sustained high levels of insulin contribute to the buildup of insulin resistance through many mechanisms. In the simplest sense, the body reacts much as it does to sustained levels of a pharmaceutical drug. Cellular receptors that respond to insulin are downregulated in the face of excessive stimulation over time. This is a protective response intended to prevent overloading cells with glucose energy. However, it backfires badly when you continue to consume high amounts of glucose.

Most of us should not be putting lots of glucose into our bodies. We should be getting the bulk of our energy from healthy fats instead, so we can lower our insulin and improve its signaling. As our glucose and insulin levels drop, we move toward the healthy end of the insulin spectrum, with all the benefits that accrue.

REFINED CARB: THE BEST FOOD FOR THE WORST HEALTH

We've said this repeatedly, but it bears repeating: the best strategy for good health and longevity is to keep your insulin very low, safely away from the insulin-resistance zone on the insulin spectrum. There are other factors, of course, but this is a central pillar—if you're highly insulin resistant, nothing you do is going to have a significant impact on your health until you fix that. So how do we go about keeping insulin low?

For the answer, let's look a little closer at GIP. It is the master switch for insulin release and is triggered by glucose in the foods we eat; it does not appreciably respond to dietary fat. But there is a crucial caveat that must be highlighted: dietary fat *potentiates* the GIP response to glucose. When it's eaten along with carb (glucose), dietary fat, no matter how healthy in itself, has a magnifying effect on GIP release.[13] The combination of dietary fat and glucose is thus to be avoided. In fact, in terms of insulin resistance, this is arguably the worst combination of all.

And of course, even without the addition of dietary fat, high-carb foods are packed with glucose and will send your GIP and insulin skyrocketing. Refined carbohydrates are the very worst offenders. They are true disaster foods.

There are many studies that illustrate this point, but let's look at just one that shows up the problem elegantly. In this experiment, mice were fed three different types of diet.[14] One was standard high-carb chow pellets (the correct evolutionary diet for a mouse). Their weight gain was steady and appropriate, as can be seen in Figure D.1.

The other two diets were nasty indeed. They were made up of high amounts of fat *plus* high amounts of carb. Ouch. You can see the nasty weight gain that occurred with the fat-plus-carb diets in the top two lines of Figure D.1. These were very fat mice indeed—with fatty livers to boot.

But then the researchers took all three of these unrefined pellet diets and did something very clever. They simply ground down the pellets to a powder. Nothing else was changed in the composition of the pellets—they were just mechanically refined. This broke up the "whole food" cellular structure of the pellets and made the glucose much more accessible.

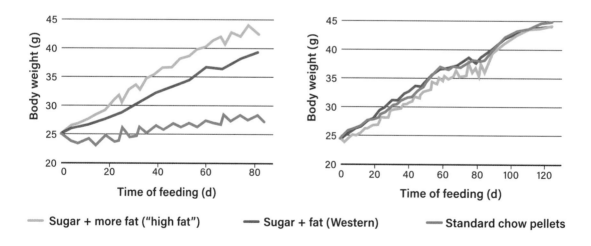

Figure D.1. A sugar-and-fat combo diet destroys those poor mice, and refining the carb makes the "healthy" chow act like a sugar-and-fat combo. Source: C. Desmarchelier et al., "Diet-Induced Obesity in Ad Libitum–Fed Mice: Food Texture Overrides the Effect of Macronutrient Composition," *British Journal of Nutrition* 109, no. 8 (April 2013): 1518–27.

Once it was refined, the previously healthy chow became just as bad for weight gain as the worst junk-food diet, as you can see in the right-hand graph in Figure D.1. We now see the catastrophic implications of refining. And this is just *mechanical* refining—grinding down the original carby chow. Imagine how bad our refined foods are when chemicals and industrially refined oils are added to the mix.

The same kind of effect can be seen in human experiments.

One study that illustrates just one of the many problems with bread and other refined carbs scrutinized the effects of both refining and fiber content on GIP and insulin.[15] Remember, raising GIP also raises insulin, and the higher GIP goes, the higher insulin goes. As you can see in Figure D.2, white bread—the most refined bread—is the biggest offender, triggering the biggest release of GIP. Ouch. The rye bread with added fiber (glu-

can) wasn't much better. The unprocessed whole-kernel rye bread was the best of the lot.

Unsurprisingly, the insulin response corresponds with the GIP levels, as we can see in Figure D.2. Again, processing whole ingredients results in much higher insulin provocation. But the most interesting result from the study was in the detailed analysis. The authors found that the insulin response was not improved by adding fiber (one hypothesis had suggested that speedier "gastric emptying"—moving food out of the stomach faster—would reduce insulin).

What did make a difference? Just one thing: the cellular structure of the grains in the bread. Keeping the grains in their original form helped reduce the insulin response (though it's still too high for us). Yet again, it was mechanical grinding of the grains that transformed the bad into the terrible.

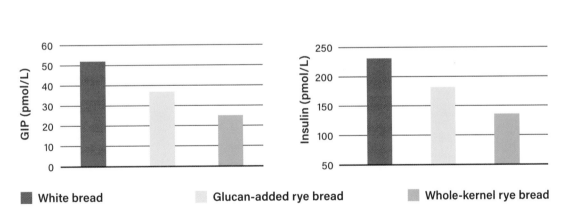

Figure D.2. Unprocessed breads provoke less GIP and insulin. Source: K. S. Juntunen et al., "Postprandial Glucose, Insulin, and Incretin Responses to Grain Products in Healthy Subjects," *American Journal of Clinical Nutrition* 75, no. 2 (2002): 254–62.

THE ROAD TO RUIN: FAT DYSFUNCTION

When insulin levels are consistently high, fat cells are the first to become insulin resistant.[16] The functionality of fat cells, or adipose tissue, is of enormous importance. They produce many key hormones that signal the liver and other organs.[17] The purpose of this signaling is to optimize overall system control depending on how energy is moving in and out of fat cells. This control system was not designed to deal with our modern food environment, however. Breaking the nutritional rules undermines everything. When adipose tissue becomes more insulin resistant, this signaling is disrupted, which primes your body for systemic, overall insulin resistance—and all the health problems that accompany it.[18]

A great example to illustrate this is lipodystrophy, a medical condition in which the body is unable to create sufficient adipose tissue. People with lipodystrophy appear remarkably skinny, but their lack of adipose makes them highly insulin resistant and diabetic from birth.[19] If healthy adipose tissue were transplanted into them, it would resolve their diabetes.[20] Such is the power of healthy fat cells.

In addition to inducing insulin resistance, driving excessive insulin through a bad diet also enlarges fat cells, a state called *hypertrophy*. When this occurs, your fat cells will no longer act as a buffer between the food you eat and your overall system.[21] In normal circumstances, fat cells are able to take in energy smoothly when you eat and release energy smoothly while you are not eating, thus acting as a perfect buffer to keep the system continually optimized. This important function of fat cells becomes damaged when the cells are compromised. Having unhealthy fat cells is the best way to progress along the spectrum toward insulin resistance.[22]

As more fat cells become enlarged, the consequences mount. The immune system is called in to assist the hurting fat cells.[23] Immune cells called macrophages tackle the larger adipose cells and start breaking them apart. Normally this would help, but as long as insulin is kept high, more fat cells become enlarged. Over time, a vicious cycle results: the immune system attack actually enhances insulin resistance through many pathways and slows the creation of healthy fat cells (which might have helped to absorb the bad food).[24]

This inflammation of adipose tissue doesn't only happen in overweight people. You can have a normal body weight and still have damaged (and damaging) adipose. Conversely, you can be obese and have healthy adipose. One study compared obese people who were insulin sensitive to obese people who were highly insulin resistant.[25] Both groups had an average body mass index of approximately 45 (a BMI over 30 is considered "obese"). They were all supersized guys, for sure. But some were healthy and some were burning up inside. Some were in the safe zone of the insulin spectrum and some were falling off the disastrous end.

So what was the crucial difference between them? It turns out, their insulin sensitivity, or lack thereof, was indicated by the macrophage content of their adipose tissue.

► The insulin-sensitive group had "safe fat": their fat cells were small and there was hardly any macrophage activity.

► The screamingly insulin-resistant group had "sick fat": their fat cells were enlarged and there was seething macrophage activity.

This study discovered that you could almost perfectly predict insulin resistance using just two measurements, the macrophage content of adipose tissue and blood levels of adiponectin, a hormone released by adipose tissue.[26] Healthy fat releases much greater quantities of this crucial hormone.

Inflamed, enlarged fat cells are a key signal—and accelerator—of insulin resistance, and they trigger a range of other problems.

THE ROAD TO RUIN: THE VLDL MERRY-GO-ROUND

In someone with small, healthy fat cells, these cells work as a beautiful battery system, absorbing calories, storing them for later use, and steadily releasing them when you are not eating.

When your adipose tissue is impaired, this doesn't work the way it should. It starts because impaired adipose tissue leads to the creation of more VLDL particles—which, as you'll recall from Chapter 11, deliver cholesterol and triglycerides around the body. Triglycerides are fats that can be used as fuel, so they're basically energy floating around the bloodstream.

In addition to absorbing energy from food, adipose tissue absorbs excess triglycerides. So when the adipose tissue is busy mopping up energy (triglycerides) from the increased amount of VLDL particles in the bloodstream, the liver is left to handle some of the energy from food. This is not good. It promotes fatty liver disease. It also results in the creation of more VLDL particles as the liver attempts to export this energy that the adipose didn't want to take. Do you see the craziness here?

This is the VLDL merry-go-round you suffer from when you move up the spectrum toward insulin resistance. As it spins around and around, it racks up your count of VLDL and LDL particles. It all goes back to high insulin and enlarged, insulin-resistant fat cells.

THE ROAD TO RUIN: ENDGAME

People who move beyond the safe end of the insulin spectrum are essentially diabetic. But most become sick or die without ever getting their type 2 diabetes diagnosis. (If they were administered the insulin-response pattern test created by Kraft, their diabetes would become clear. But doctors rarely use Kraft-type tests, so many people remain secret diabetics and never know what's at the root of their chronic health problems.)

For most people, a diabetes diagnosis doesn't happen until they progress to the endgame and the wheels entirely fall off their insulin wagon. At that point, after years or decades suffering diabetic damage to blood vessels and organs, they reach a point where their blood glucose levels finally spiral out of control and the standard tests reveal they have diabetes.

So what does this final stage of diabetes look like? When you're at the bad end of the insulin spectrum, you have built dangerous levels of fat in many of your organs, whether you appear to be overweight or not.[27] Your liver, your pancreas, your kidneys, even your skeletal muscle will be packing inappropriate levels of fat, called ectopic fat.[28] This fat prevents the proper functioning of your organs.

As high levels of glucose in your bloodstream require high levels of insulin and those high levels of insulin lead your cells to become insulin resistant, your body releases more and more insulin to keep the system working, until eventually, after many years of outrageous insulin demands and a buildup of ectopic fat inside and around it, your pancreas begins to give up. And then you are in serious trouble.

In addition to moving glucose out of the bloodstream, insulin keeps the brakes on adipose tissue, preventing it from releasing fat into the bloodstream inappropriately.[29] As the insulin supply from your abused pancreas peters out, the insulin guard finally loses control of adipose tissue, and the adipose begins its jailbreak. Previously locked-up fat begins a steady escape into your bloodstream.[30] It makes its way quickly to your poor old liver, which has to do something with the fat—it has no choice. And so the liver makes glucose out of the fat in a process called *gluconeogenesis*. Glucose begins to flood out of your liver—precisely when it's the very last thing in the world that your diabetic body needs.

The overload of insulin and fat in your bloodstream is joined by glucose pumping out of your liver. These three things should never be elevated together. Welcome to the endgame. You might now finally receive your official diabetes diagnosis.

But of course there's a better way: Right now, adopt the ten action steps on pages 72 to 83. Whether you're one of the lucky few who are currently insulin sensitive or you're heading down the road to severe insulin resistance, these changes will make you healthier, improve your longevity, and reduce your risk of heart disease, diabetes, and other chronic diseases. Then get your fasting insulin and fasting blood glucose levels tested and calculate your insulin resistance using a HOMA calculator (see page 39). With your new knowledge about your level of insulin resistance in hand, you can start to customize your diet and lifestyle to optimize their effect on your insulin.

WHAT WE CAN LEARN FROM THE KITAVANS

Defenders of a high-carb diet always bring up the Kitavans. These indigenous people of Papua New Guinea have vanishingly low rates of coronary heart disease and cancer, even though they eat quite a high percentage of unprocessed carbohydrate, along with a lot of fish, meat, and saturated fat from coconut. And 75 percent of them smoke!

How do they achieve this excellent health with high carbohydrate? Well, they have an incredible number of other factors in their favor: No processed foods, no wheat, no refined sugars. Very low iron status, which reduces oxidative damage to cells. Very high sun exposure (for excellent vitamin D and many other benefits). Very low stress. A diet based on highly nutritious real foods. An excellent ratio of omega-6 to omega-3. The list goes on and on.

It's true that it is possible to make higher-carb diets work. The surprising solution involves eating bizarrely low levels of fat. A quirk of our biochemistry enables insulin sensitivity for some people on ultralow fat diets. But you need the right combination of genes, and you need every other advantage switched hard to the optimum—like the Kitavans. Regrettably, this is simply impractical to the point of impossible for most people in the Western world. There is no "engineering" solution that can make this combination work for most people—and trying to make this work would be much more difficult (and less satisfying) than following a low-carb, high-fat diet, which has the same benefits.

That said, we can learn something valuable from the Kitavans. Their insulin and glucose levels are, unsurprisingly, incredibly low. With the same activity level and other factors accounted for, the Kitavans' insulin levels were half those of Swedes in the 1970s (and that was before the current epidemic of insulin resistance).[31] Also, essentially none of them had glucose levels above baseline healthy levels. Regardless of their diet, they achieved insulin nirvana. That is one of the primary reasons for their vanishingly low rates of coronary heart disease.

APPENDIX E: THE SCIENCE OF POLYUNSATURATED FATS

We talked about polyunsaturated fats and how it's important to avoid vegetable oils earlier in the book. If you're curious about why we're so emphatic about this—especially given the usual advice from health authorities to seek out polyunsaturated fats—this appendix offers quite a bit more information.

THE FATS WE'RE MADE OF

There are three types of fatty acids: saturated, monounsaturated, and polyunsaturated. The word saturated in all these refers to the molecular structure of the fatty acid: if there's a pair of hydrogen atoms for every carbon atom in the molecule, it's saturated; if one hydrogen pair is missing, it's monounsaturated; and if more than one hydrogen pair is missing, it's polyunsaturated.

To visualize a polyunsaturated fatty acid (PUFA) molecule, think of a centipede whose body is a string of carbon atoms. Two oxygen atoms are incorporated at the head. Hydrogen makes up the legs along each side; wherever a carbon atom is missing its own hydrogen pair, it forms a double bond (depicted by small parallel lines in the diagram) with another hydrogen pair. These double bonds make PUFAs more prone to oxidative damage. PUFAs are delicate, and when oxidized, they become very unstable, which can

Polyunsaturated Fatty Acid

cause much damage in the body. (Saturated fatty acids, by contrast, with no double bonds, are stable, robust, and resistant to damage.)

PUFAs play a key role in the construction of our cell membranes and in our signaling networks throughout the body. That said, our bodies consist of mostly monounsaturated and saturated fat. These make up around 90–95 percent of our total fat content. The remaining 5–10 percent is PUFAs.

Because our bodies cannot make PUFAs, we need to acquire them from our food. Up until the beginning of the twentieth century, our food contained very small amounts of PUFAs (though plenty for our needs). Around the mid-twentieth century, monounsaturated and saturated fats made up over 90 percent of the "sweet fat that sticks to our bones."[32] The percentages may have been much higher before the vegetable oil revolution in the early 1900s. So traditionally, only a very small amount of our body fat was polyunsaturated. This makes a lot of sense for safety—saturated and monounsaturated fats are much more stable than polyunsaturated and less prone to oxidative damage. But the percentage of polyunsaturated fat in our bodies has increased dramatically in the past half century.[33] We believe that the implications of this are profoundly negative, as we'll discuss in more detail in a few pages.

Because PUFAs are prone to oxidization, they need to be balanced with the more stable fats. The main kinds of PUFAs also interact with each other to a huge degree, so they need to remain balanced with each other, too. Think of PUFAs like vitamins and minerals: we need them for what they do in the body, but they should not be eaten to burn as fuel. In short, PUFAs are not something you should eat too much of.

And yet we have all heard that consuming polyunsaturated fats is beneficial for heart health. Does the data back that up? The rate of coronary heart disease explosively increased during the first half of the twentieth century. Were people eating more animal fat (that is, saturated fat) during this period? Or were they eating more PUFAs? According to the USDA, animal fat consumption has been decreasing (especially since about 1950) while PUFA consumption has been increasing.

We'll explore why this is the case in the coming pages. It certainly suggests, however, that the usual advice to eat less saturated fat and more PUFAs should be treated with skepticism.

INTRODUCING OMEGA-6 AND OMEGA-3

There are two primary types of PUFAs: omega-6 and omega-3. Both are termed "essential fats" because the human body cannot make them; they must come from dietary sources. The minimum quantities the body requires are very small. Estimates put the figure at less than 1 percent of total caloric intake.[34]

OMEGA-6

Historically, humans consumed very small amounts of omega-6. In nature, it's abundant in eggs, chicken, beef, butter and other dairy, and nuts and seeds. Today it's also found in refined vegetable oils and the many packaged and processed foods they're used in: fast food, cakes, cookies, crackers, salad dressings, and more.

Early human experiments on the consumption of higher quantities of omega-6 backfired spectacularly: people died in greater numbers than the control group, who just ate their normal fats.[35] The

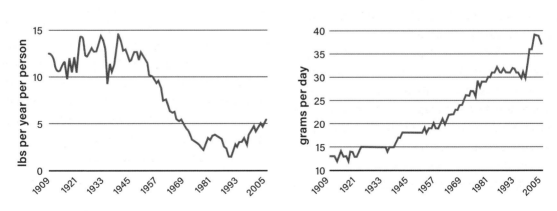

Figure E.1. As saturated fat consumption has fallen greatly and polyunsaturated fat consumption has risen, chronic disease has exploded. Source: USDA.

ınce later indicated that excessive amounts of omega-6 promotes inflammation. Omega-6 fatty acids have been shown to control and regulate the local tissue production of cytokines and chemokines, molecules that are involved in signaling within the immune system and have a direct effect on your body's inflammatory response.[36] There is a very real necessity for inflammation—it's a key part of the body's response to injury or damage. But when inflammation becomes excessive, systemic, and chronic, disease results.[37] The scientific literature is bursting at the seams with mechanisms that link the effects of excessive omega-6 to a vast array of diseases, including our most feared mortality drivers: heart disease and cancer. Billions of dollars have been invested in drug investigations aimed specifically at moderating the excessive actions of omega-6 in inflammation—aspirin, NSAIDs, and many other anti-inflammatory drugs have all been looked at as possible treatments.[38] Increasingly, concerns are being raised about the side effects of some of these drugs. It may in fact make far more sense to tackle these inflammatory pathways with nutritional interventions that positively influence them.

Figure E.2 shows the primary omega-6 fatty acid, linoleic acid. The two sets of parallel lines in the left half show the double bonds between the carbon atoms.

The body converts linoleic acid into arachidonic acid (AA), and from there into yet another fatty acid. AA is a highly unsaturated fatty acid, or HUFA.

OMEGA-3

Historically, like omega-6, omega-3 was consumed in relatively small amounts. It's abundant in fish and shellfish (cod liver oil is an excellent supplement), nuts and seeds, above-ground green leafy vegetables, and pastured eggs.

In contrast to omega-6, omega-3 fatty acids have been shown to have an anti-inflammatory effect in the body, which is beneficial for a wide range of chronic diseases that have inflammation at their root.

Figure E.2 shows the primary omega-3 fatty acid, alpha-linolenic acid. The three sets of parallel lines in the left half show the double bonds between the carbon atoms.

The body converts alpha-linoleic acid into a fatty acid known as eicosapentaenoic acid (EPA). EPA is then converted to docosahexaenoic acid (DHA). Both EPA and DHA are crucial components of a healthy physiology. DHA is central in the healthy functioning of our brain, vision, and reproductive systems. Like arachidonic acid, which is made from omega-6, EPA and DHA are considered highly unsaturated fatty acids, or HUFAs.

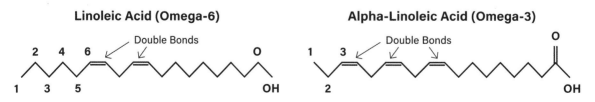

Figure E.2. Linoleic acid, the primary omega-6 fatty acid, and alpha-linoleic acid, the primary omega-3 fatty acid.

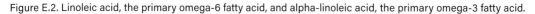

Rather than converting alpha-linoleic acid, we can get EPA directly from grass-fed animals, and both EPA and DHA can be directly accessed from fatty fish and cod liver oil. As a general rule, it is advantageous to get more EPA and DHA from the animals that did such a great job of creating them.

HUFAS

The HUFAs made from omega-6 and omega-3—AA, EPA, and DHA—take up residence in the membranes of your cells and enable their core functionality.

A key point to note is that omega-6 and omega-3 are converted to HUFAs by the same enzymes. They compete, in a sense, over these enzymes. All things being equal, the body slightly favors the omega-3 for conversion. But of course, if you are gorging on omega-6, that slight favoritism won't make a difference. Even if you're trying to take in more omega-3, the amount you're consuming may not be converted to the HUFAs your body needs, because the larger amounts of omega-6 are commandeering the necessary enzymes.

Many of the trials involving increasing omega-3 were of little value. What's key is not necessarily increasing omega-3, although there is some value in that, but in moderating omega-6 intake.

In some the participants were already drowned in omega-6 from their normal diets. In others the people were already quite adequate in omega-3.[39]

THE RATIO REIGNS

In many ways omega-6 and omega-3 are opposing forces. Omega-6 is converted into compounds that enable inflammatory responses. Omega-3, in contrast, tends toward anti-inflammatory effects. They need to remain in balance. The ratios between them thus matter.

Traditionally, humans consumed omega-6 and omega-3 at a ratio of approximately 1:1 to 3:1.[40] But while omega-3 has fallen in our diet over the past century, we are swimming in omega-6. Things have changed beyond recognition in the past century. In the Western diet, the ratio of omega-6 to omega-3 is currently about 20:1. This has significant implications for health.

There is much data linking the ratio of omega-6 to omega-3 to heart disease.[41] (We'll look at omega-6 as a factor on its own shortly.) So let's take a look at how this measure varies across populations with very different rates of heart disease mortality. Figure E.3 shows the percentage of omega-6 HUFAs in their body's cells in several regions and the average number of deaths due to

	MULTI POPULATION STUDIES					
	Greenland	Japan	Quebec Inuit	Quebec Cree	Quebec Overall	USA Overall
Approx. Percentage Omega-6	31%	38%	44%	55%	79%	78%
Approx. Coronary Death Rate per 100,000	20	40	70	90	140	170

Figure E.3. Omega-6 in tissue tracks closely with CHD rates. Source: W. E. M. Lands, "Diets Could Prevent Many Diseases," *Lipids* 38 (May 2003): 317–21.

USA POPULATION MRFIT STUDY				
Lowest Fifth	**Lower Fifth**	**Medium Fifth**	**Higher Fifth**	**Highest Fifth**

	Lowest Fifth	Lower Fifth	Medium Fifth	Higher Fifth	Highest Fifth
Approx. Percentage Omega-6	62%	76%	81%	83%	83%
Approx. Coronary Death Rate per 100,000	100	148	150	150	150

Figure E.4. Omega-6 products in tissue tracked with CHD in MRFIT Study, too. Source: W. E. M. Lands, "Diets Could Prevent Many Diseases," *Lipids* 38 (May 2003): 317–21.

coronary heart disease (CHD).[42] As you can see, the relationship between levels of omega-6 and deaths from CHD holds extremely tightly—as one climbs, so does the other.

Let's take another view and look at this metric within a specific population. The data in Figure E.4 is sourced from the huge MRFIT study conducted in the US.[43] It involved long-term follow-up of 361,662 men with any of multiple risk factors (e.g. elevated blood pressure, high cholesterol, and/or a smoking habit). In this case, the entire population is heavily weighted toward a bad ratio of omega-6 to omega-3—four-fifths have an extremely high percentage of omega-6 HUFAs. Even here, however, the relationship between omega-6 and CHD holds steady: those with the lowest amount of omega-6 HUFAs have markedly lower rates of death from CHD. The death rate here lines up with what we'd expect from Figure E.3: when the percentage of omega-6 is around 60, the death rate is around 100 per 100,000.

Remember that hyperinsulinemia and insulin resistance drive the relationship between cholesterol and CHD, and that is not even being considered here. Imagine the synergistic combo of having high insulin resistance and a high ratio of omega-6 to omega-3. Well, that's the population right there—high in both, and riddled with disease associated with inflammation.

THE DAMAGING EFFECTS OF OMEGA-6

In study after study, omega-6 has been linked to serious health problems, including heart disease, cancer, obesity, and liver disease.

OMEGA-6 AND HEART HEALTH

Polyunsaturated fats have been touted as better for heart health than saturated fats. The belief stemmed from studies showing that additional omega-6 lowered cholesterol levels. Sadly, this data mixed up omega-6 and omega-3 fatty acids entirely. These studies are now being reinterpreted, and evidence suggests that omega-3 (still a polyunsaturated fat, but very different from omega-6) may have an advantage over saturated fat.[44] Likewise, the associational and epidemiological studies often looked at polyunsaturated intakes without properly examining omega-6 versus omega-3 details. There are also review papers being published that highlight this problem.

One of the most influential studies supporting polyunsaturated fats for heart health, the Oslo diet-heart study, looked at people who had already suffered a heart attack. It showed a reduction in heart events with an increase in polyunsaturated fats.[45] But this trial jacked up not just omega-6 but also omega-3 intake, and it reduced trans fats—both of these factors have been shown elsewhere to have significant benefit.

So what about some experiments that focused on increasing omega-6 fatty acids? What did they do for heart events—and, more importantly, all-cause mortality? Let's look at a few examples. One of the earliest of these studies was the anti-coronary club trial, circa 1966.[46] It put 814 men on a diet high in omega-6 while leaving 463 men of similar backgrounds and health on their usual saturated fat regimen. After four years, the rate of new heart events was lower in the omega-6 group. But there were twice as many deaths in the omega-6 group as in the control one, because more people were dying from their heart attacks in the omega-6 group, and more were dying from other causes too. The Sydney diet-heart study of 1966–1973 took 221 coronary heart patients and replaced a proportion of the saturated fat in their diet with safflower oils and margarines, which are high in omega-6.[47] The control group of 237 was encouraged to continue eating their usual amount of saturated fat. After seven years, the omega-6 group had higher all-cause and coronary mortality and higher rates of coronary heart disease.[48]

The Lyon diet-heart study showed dramatic improvements in outcomes by putting people on a "Mediterranean type" diet that was high in vegetables, whole grains, olive oil, and seafood.[49] The control group was kept on a "prudent Western type" diet that was high in red meat, refined grains, and dairy. The differences between the groups in terms of cardiovascular and other mortality was striking. The group on the Mediterranean diet had around 70 percent fewer events over the study period.

Although the saturated fat content was lower in the Mediterranean group (8 grams per day compared to 11 grams per day), it had little relevance: no association was seen for any fat except for omega-3, which was beneficial in reducing coronary heart disease events. It turned out that only omega-3 was statistically linked to the lower rates of death and disease.

These were important studies that flagged massive problems with the idea that saturated fat is a cause of heart disease and polyunsaturated fats are better for the heart. These trials warned us to be very careful with consumption of omega-6 fatty acids. But they were largely ignored amid the war on saturated fat.

OMEGA-6 AND CANCER

There has been a slow-burning controversy around the role of omega-6 fatty acids in carcinogenesis (the development of cancer cells) and tumor progression. We will simplify things here by just looking at breast cancer, but similar results are seen for other cancers.

In one of the early experiments on cancer and dietary fat, researchers induced breast cancer in rats by injecting them with a powerful carcinogenic toxin, then fed one group a diet of 20 percent saturated fat and got a baseline level of toxin-driven tumors.[50] They fed another group 3 percent omega-6 and 17 percent saturated fat, and the number of tumors doubled. A third group was fed 20 percent omega-6 with no saturated fat, and they saw the same doubling in tumor numbers. The study authors observed that most people now have at least 3 percent of total calories from omega-6 in their diets, which was the percentage at which the tumors doubled. Therefore, they suggested that everyone should adhere to an overall lower-fat diet to avoid cancer. What they didn't consider was simply reducing the amount of omega-6 instead.

A good 1997 review paper then pulled together many animal experiments on cancer and omega-6 in a large meta-analysis.[51] This team's statistical analysis was solid. Their high-level conclusions were sound: they saw that omega-6 intake was the strongest driver of breast cancer tumors across all the experiments. But they also found that there was a "threshold effect" of sorts: the most rapid increase in tumors was seen when omega-6 increased from 0.5 percent to around 4 percent of total calories; from 4 percent to 25 percent, there was a slower increase. The conclusion was that once you go above 4 percent omega-6 in the diet, most of the damage may have already been done. Unfortunately, today, the diets of the vast majority of people are above that level.

A very recent review paper also calls out the risks of excessive omega-6 on breast cancer.[52] The authors examined exposure to omega-6 at different stages of life. Interestingly, female rats exposed to high amounts of omega-6 before puberty showed a significantly higher incidence rate of tumors than those who were exposed after puberty. The researchers concluded that the risk of omega-6 may be underestimated due to this factor—no one is investigating omega-6 intake in women at different ages.

The smart approach to lowering cancer risk is to only eat natural sources of fat. Animal sources of fats, including butter, meat, and dairy, are relatively low in omega-6, especially when the animal is grass-fed. In addition, the ratio of omega-6 to omega-3 is more optimal in the grass-fed animals. For instance, in a serving of fatty grass-fed steak, only around 2 percent of the fat is omega-6 (around 1 percent is omega-3).[53] It also comes more loaded with the beneficial conjugated linoleic acid and vaccenic acid, which have been linked to anticancer and antiatherosclerosis effects.[54]

OMEGA-6 AND OBESITY

There are many mechanisms by which omega-6 intake can promote chronic weight gain. One is a loss in insulin sensitivity over time (which is always a bad thing).

Our first insight comes from a research team in 2015 that fed mice a relatively low-sugar, high-fat diet, rather than a high-sugar, high-fat as most other researchers did.[55] As the study authors pointed out, their experiment was the first to properly compare the roles of fructose and omega-6 in the obesity epidemic. They fed one group moderate quantities of fructose, another group levels of soybean oil (which is high in omega-6) that reflect current consumption in the US, and a third group coconut oil instead of soybean oil. This enabled the direct comparison between coconut oil and soybean oil in terms of detrimental effects. This team's primary finding would shock most orthodox dietitians: "PUFA-rich soybean oil is more obesogenic and diabetogenic than coconut oil (which consists of primarily saturated fat)."

The full list of findings is impressive:

▶ Soybean oil induced more weight gain and adiposity (body fat) than fructose.

▶ Soybean oil induced type 2 diabetes, glucose intolerance, and insulin resistance.

▶ Soybean oil caused fatty liver disease and liver-cell damage.

- Soybean oil caused a dysregulation of liver gene expression (i.e., it set the liver on a path to further damage).

- Soybean oil stimulated genetic changes that have been strongly linked to cancer proliferation. (Coconut oil had the opposite effect.)

On the last point, the authors concluded that coconut oil may be protective against liver cancer (and, by extension, saturated fats in general). Worryingly, this protection appeared to be nullified by consuming soybean oil.

Another research team found similar results.[56] In terms of total fat intake, they used both medium- and high-fat diets, with moderate sugar. For each of these diets they kept the total calories from fat constant but varied the contribution from omega-6 fats. They tested different groups on either low levels of omega-6 (1 percent of total calories) or high levels (8 percent of total calories). This allowed them to examine the effects of the lower amount of omega-6 that humans ingested before the obesity epidemic began and compare them to the effects of today's intake.

So what did they find? Let's take a look:

- High amounts of omega-6 significantly increased food intake, body weight, and adiposity (body fat).

- Animals fed the 8 percent omega-6 diet accumulated significantly more body fat than animals fed the 1 percent diet.

- The animals who gained weight on a high-fat and high-sugar diet lost that weight when omega-6 was replaced with saturated fat.

- Adding omega-3 HUFAs (EPA and DHA) reduced the negative effects of the omega-6.

In short, the study showed disastrous weight-driving effects of high intake of omega-6—that is, the amount consumed in a modern diet.

But there were more revelations to come from this team. In the following year they carried out essentially the same experiment, but this time they used low-fat and medium-fat diets. Remember that we have been told to eat a diet low in fat and get most of our fats from PUFAs. So did a high proportion of omega-6 wreak the same havoc in low- and medium-fat diets?

It most certainly did. Let's take a look at what the researchers showed:

- The supposedly ideal low-fat diet can be made highly obesogenic by inclusion of 8 percent omega-6.

- The high omega-6 intake stimulated biochemical pathways in the liver that have been linked to weight gain in other studies.

- The high omega-6 intake caused elevated leptin, increased adipose cell size, and raised immune system infiltration into the adipose tissue (there was no infiltration in 1 percent omega-6 animals). This is important as the scientific literature is now revealing that inflammation of fat tissue is a crucial step in the development of obesity, diabetes, and many, many other chronic diseases.[57]

Both studies make clear that a diet high in omega-6 promotes obesity and increased body fat.

OMEGA-6 AND LIVER HEALTH

The liver conducts the orchestra that delivers system-wide metabolic health. It is downright crucial to keep it in tip-top condition. But omega-6 can greatly expose the liver to damage.

It's well known that people who consume too much alcohol can damage their livers. It's also well established, if not quite as well known, that excessive sugar (specifically fructose) has a similar effect. The liver can be strengthened to help vith these substances—but it can also be weakened and its powers of self-restoration grossly undermined, which means it becomes more vulnerable to damaging substances. Turns out, it's quite easy to ruin your liver's ability to deal with toxins: just consume lots of omega-6.

The mechanisms by which omega-6 harms the liver were verified in a series of fascinating experiments in the 1980s and 1990s. In one of the best, conducted in 1989, the authors looked at large associational population studies that showed a correlation between higher rates of death from cirrhosis and higher intake of omega-6, as well as lower rates of death from cirrhosis in populations consuming more saturated fat, and they hypothesized that omega-6 enables liver damage from alcohol.[58]

To test this hypothesis, the researchers studied rats infused with very high levels of alcohol on different kinds of diets. The results were as follows:

► Rats fed a beef tallow diet (where the tallow contained 0.7 percent omega-6) had absolutely no liver damage. This diet, high in saturated fat, was clearly protective against liver disease due to alcohol.

► Rats fed a lard-based diet (where the lard contained 2.5 percent omega-6 but was primarily high in saturated fat) had minimal to moderate liver disease—so the diet was partially protective against alcohol-induced liver disease.

► Rats fed a corn oil diet (where the oil contained 56.6 percent omega-6) experienced severe liver disease. The diet gave the liver no protection from alcohol-induced disease—if anything, it accelerated the damage.

To really clinch it, the research team designed an experiment that would determine if omega-6 specifically was the offending factor.[59]

Rats were fed three healthy diets, each with 25 percent of calories from fat. They were also fed enough alcohol to inflict substantial liver damage. The diets were as follows:

► Beef tallow (containing 0.7 percent omega-6)

► Lard (containing 2.5 percent omega-6)

► Beef tallow with 2.5 percent omega-6 added in the form of free linoleic acid

The experiment isolated omega-6 as a factor, so the results would therefore be decisive. So what happened?

► The rats on the beef tallow diet with 0.7 percent omega-6 showed no liver damage from the alcohol.

► The rats on a lard diet showed minimal to moderate liver damage.

► The rats on a beef tallow diet with added omega-6 showed extensive liver damage: fatty liver disease, inflammation, and even necrosis (cell death).

The conclusion was clear: higher amounts of omega-6 led to liver damage from alcohol.

There are also more recent scientific papers finally raising this issue.[60] We can only hope that the dots get connected in the coming years.

When authorities instructed people to lower their saturated fat intake and simultaneously increase their intake of PUFAs by consuming more corn oil, soybean oil, and sunflower oil, the intake of omega-6 skyrocketed. And now we have an absolute epidemic of fatty liver disease.[61]

HOW MUCH OMEGA-6 IS ENOUGH?

If we want to avoid the health concerns outlined above and still get enough omega-6 to meet our body's needs (after all, it is an "essential fat"), how much should we aim for? The answer may surprise you. It would appear that we need only around 0.6 percent of total calories from omega-6 in our diet. This was the quantity recommended for human sufficiency many decades ago, and a recent publication in a journal dedicated to the field of these essential fats agreed with the old estimate.[62] It called the evidence behind recommendations for more PUFAs "a house of cards" and concluded that the data supports 0.6 to 1.5 percent of total calories from omega-6 as the optimum range for humans.

Another recent paper on the effects of omega-6 and omega-3 in cancer prevention concludes by recommending that people consume 2.5 percent of total calories from omega-6 while keeping the ratio with omega-3 around 2:1, at most.[63]

These numbers make sense with regard to ancestral intakes and ratios of omega-6 to omega-3. Why would we even consider getting 10 percent of our daily calorie intake from these bioactive molecules? Especially when most of them now come from industrially refined oils—which, as we'll explore in a moment, are uniquely damaging.

Behind these recommendations is the antifat dogma that sprang from the work of Ancel Keys, which we discussed way back in Chapter 2. We now know that those studies never really meant anything, and many experiments flagged major concerns with high intakes of omega-6.

THE PROBLEMS WITH VEGETABLE OILS

During evolution, we had access to small amounts of both omega-6 and omega-3, and a ratio of 1:1 to 3:1 would have been the norm.[64] Things have changed beyond recognition in the past century. Ratios of 20:1 and higher are ingested these days.

The unprecedented rise in omega-6 consumption began in the early 1900s with the advent of industrially fabricated vegetable oils. The original versions of cheap and nasty vegetable oils were used to lubricate machinery. But someone got the bright idea to feed them to people, and the rest is history. In the 1970s, the fear of natural fats propelled the consumption of vegetable oils to yet higher levels. The ultra-low cost of these industrial oils made them hugely attractive for the food industry, and so the industry promoted them as healthy at every turn. The vegetable oil industry was particularly active in supporting the mistaken diet-heart hypothesis, and it in turn financed organizations who actively promoted it.[65] We now ingest twenty times or more of the amount of omega-6 required for health.[66] Thus, a huge human experiment is being conducted even now.

All the health problems of omega-6 discussed above aren't so much related to real, whole foods—foods that aren't chemically processed and refined, as vegetable oils are. The quantities of omega-6 in these are relatively small, and they don't have the oxidation and other chemical damage that comes with processing. The problem is really the consumption of refined vegetable oils, which are high in omega-6.

Most people are now generally aware about the problems with trans fats—fats that, although found in nature in small amounts, are mostly created in the industrial hydrogenation process, which makes vegetable oils solid. With widespread recognition of their contribution to coronary heart disease, trans fats are finally being banned across the world.[67]

But many forms of trans fats still exist in vegetable oils, even before hydrogenation. Though they aren't present in the amounts found in hydrogenated oils, they are an inevitable result of the processing vegetable oils go through. No level of these unnatural molecules is okay. Therefore, no processed vegetable oils should be consumed, ever. Even organic, mechanically pressed canola oils can contain up to 5 percent trans fats and other nasties.[68]

On top of the high amounts of omega-6 and the presence of trans fats, vegetable oils are problematic because polyunsaturated fats are, by nature, unstable. Recall from the beginning of this appendix that PUFAs are fragile and prone to oxidation. In real, whole foods there are relatively low levels of PUFA, and they have antioxidants to help prevent oxidation damage. Not so in the PUFA-rich vegetable oils. Here, the molecules are totally exposed to oxidation, both during their industrial processing and after you ingest them.[69] Cooking heat is also a major offender in oxidizing PUFAs.

Oxidation enables them to create lipid hydroperoxide molecules (LOOHs).[70] Your body can create these naturally and appropriately as a response to injury, which will help to destroy unwanted agents. When cells are injured, the response can go a step further than making these LOOHs. Damaged cells can generate highly active lipid peroxide radicals. These are designed to cause a rapid cascade of molecular damage all around them. This can be a useful physiological response to injury, as they can act to destroy problematic cells and other issues. But this process can also be triggered inappropriately by cooking or processing of vegetable oils. Therefore, eating these activated radicals can create a damaging storm in your body that has significant negative consequences.

When oxidized PUFAs are consumed, cholesterol levels are also in the firing line. LDL and other lipoproteins can become highly damaged. So while eating PUFAs may lower your LDL, it also damages it, doing a terrible injury to your whole system.

As we talked about in Chapter 10, oxidized LDL is the true "bad cholesterol." Evidence has been available for decades to show that undamaged LDL is not really the problem.[71] Oxidized LDL, on the other hand, drives atherosclerosis, coronary heart disease, and more.

There is no good reason to consume vegetable oils and many good reasons to avoid them.

THE OMEGA-3 INDEX: THE POWER OF KNOWLEDGE

So let's say you eliminate vegetable oils, reduce your omega-6 intake, and boost your omega-3. How do you ensure that you are getting it right? A simple blood test called the omega-3 index tells you the amount of omega-3 in your cells, based on the ratios of omega-6 to omega-3 in the membranes of your red blood cells.

In Japan, the population omega-3 index is generally around 8 to 11 percent (currently accepted as optimal). Below 8 percent is increasingly being seen as problematic. Northern Europeans vary greatly around the 6 percent level. Unsurprisingly, US citizens average around 4 percent. This is acknowledged to be a really bad level.[72] Of course, the US is swimming in vegetable oils. And, again unsurprisingly, it has the worst omega-3 index numbers in the world.

The scientific data underpinning the omega-3 index is substantial and growing. One fascinating analysis used dietary and blood test data from multiple studies of coronary heart disease and compared the omega-3 indexes of the participants with their risk for major cardiac events.[73]

The team found that, when it comes to predicting sudden coronary death, the omega-3 index outgunned traditional factors by a wide margin. When the omega-3 index was greater than 8 percent, it showed nearly a 90 percent lower likelihood of death. Importantly, this applied even when the omega-3 index was statistically corrected for all of the other risk factors, so that it was a highly independent predictor.

This makes sense: while all the other glucose and cholesterol risk variables tend to be interrelated through their common links to insulin resistance, the omega-3 index reflects an independent accelerator of coronary heart disease and other chronic diseases by looking at inflammatory pathways beyond the insulin-related ones.

Food manufacturers are already scrambling to create vegetable oils high in omega-3. Japanese researchers are even trying to develop a breed of cattle whose flesh is lower in omega-6 and much higher in omega-3. Meta-analyses of big associational studies have begun to show that increased omega-6 is associated with higher mortality, while omega-3 is associated with lower mortality.[74]

There is a lot more one could say about the detrimental health effects of vegetable oil ingestion. There are also a lot of recent publications by doctors who have done the detailed research in this area and come to the same worrying conclusions.[75] The fact is that our population has overdosed on inappropriate industrial oils for generations, with huge negative consequences for chronic disease rates. We were sold on these harmful substances through the inappropriate demonization of natural, healthy fats and oils.

The war on fat sure has a lot to answer for.

ABOUT THE AUTHORS

IVOR CUMMINS, BE (Chem), CEng MIEI, is a top-class engineer with a long career in the medical device field and other industries. Although he has served in many roles as a technical leader, his specialty is leading teams in complex problem-solving efforts. Ivor trained at University College Dublin, graduating in 1990, and spent six years developing and optimizing medical devices.

In recent years, Ivor has become a Chartered Engineer (CEng) and Project Management Professional (PMP); he also completed an Innovation and Entrepreneurial Management Certificate at Stanford University. In 2015, he was shortlisted for Irish Chartered Engineer of the Year.

Most recently, Ivor has applied his technical expertise to decoding the causes of human chronic disease and obesity. He has analyzed countless scientific publications from the past century, creating a strategy to achieve health, weight loss, and longevity. Ivor speaks at conferences and conducts seminars around the world to provide actionable plans for preventing and healing chronic disease.

Ivor lives in Dublin, Ireland, with his wife and five children.

JEFFRY N. GERBER, MD, FAAFP, is a board-certified family physician and owner of South Suburban Family Medicine in Littleton, Colorado. Widely known as Denver's Diet Doctor, Dr. Gerber has been providing personalized health care to the Denver community since 1993, with an emphasis on longevity, wellness, and prevention.

For decades, Dr. Gerber has researched the science of carbohydrate and fat metabolism, insulin resistance, inflammation, and chronic metabolic disease. Frustrated with spiraling health-care costs related to the treatment of obesity, diabetes, and heart disease, Dr. Gerber decided to focus on using low-carb high-fat, ancestral, Paleo, and primal diets to treat and prevent these chronic conditions. His patients' outcomes demonstrate the benefits of these types of diets.

In 2010, Dr. Gerber received the honorary Degree of Fellow from the American Academy of Family Physicians for his commitment to family medicine and his contributions to the local community.

Jeff, his wife, and their three children love the outdoors and enjoy all that the state of Colorado has to offer.

ABOUT THE CHEF

CHEF RYAN TURNER has been a cooking devotee his whole life. As a chef and a gourmet food enthusiast, Ryan always found it difficult to remain at a healthy weight. After adopting a low-carb approach in 2013, he slimmed down and has since remained at a healthy weight without any struggle or sacrifice.

Ryan currently lives in Houston, Texas, where he runs Sola, the company he founded, which offers the signature Sola brand sweetener as well as a range of low-carb, sugar-free prepared foods. Sola is pioneering great-tasting, genuinely healthy packaged food products that are backed by clinical studies showing blood sugar and insulin responses.

NOTES

CHAPTER 1

1 K. Flegal, M. D. Carroll, B. K. Kit, and C. L. Ogden, "Prevalence of Obesity and Trends in the Distribution of Body Mass Index Among US Adults, 1999–2010," *JAMA* 307, no. 5 (2012): 491–97.

2 J. Xu, S. L. Murphy, K. D. Kochanek, and E. Arias. "Mortality in the United States, 2015," National Center for Health Statistics. Data Brief No. 267, December 2016. www.cdc.gov/nchs/data/databriefs/db267.pdf.

3 S. J. Olshansky et al., "A Potential Decline in Life Expectancy in the United States in the 21st Century," *New England Journal of Medicine* 352, no. 11 (2005): 1138–45.

4 American Heart Association, "Cardiovascular Disease: A Costly Burden for America—Projections Through 2035," 2017, www.heart.org/idc/groups/heart-public/@wcm/@adv/documents/downloadable/ucm_491543.pdf.

5 J. P. Boyle et al., "Projection of the Year 2050 Burden of Diabetes in the US Adult Population: Dynamic Modeling of Incidence, Mortality, and Prediabetes Prevalence," *Popular Health Metrics* 8 (2010): 29.

6 Impian Emas Medical Centre, "Heart Attacks, A Test Collapses," July 24, 2013, www.impianemasmedicalcentre.com/wall-street-journal-in-1982-announced-the-long-awaited-results-heart-attacks-a-test-collapses.

7 Gary Taubes, *Good Calories, Bad Calories: Fats, Carbs, and the Controversial Science of Diet and Health* (New York: Anchor, 2002).

8 A. S. Go et al., "Heart Disease and Stroke Statistics—2014 Update: A Report from the American Heart Association," *Circulation* 129, no. 3 (2014): e28–e292.

CHAPTER 2

1 This example comes from Tyler Vigen's excellent *Spurious Correlations*, www.tylervigen.com/spurious-correlations.

2 David S. Grimes, *Vitamin D and Cholesterol: The Importance of the Sun* (York, UK: Tennison Publishing, 2009).

3 J. Yerushalmy and H. E. Hilleboe, "Fat in the Diet and Mortality from Heart Disease: A Methodologic Note," *New York State Journal of Medicine* 57, no. 14 (1957): 2343–54.

4 Nina Teicholz, *The Big Fat Surprise* (New York: Simon & Schuster, 2015).

5 M. Dehghan et al., "Associations of Fats and Carbohydrate Intake with Cardiovascular Disease and Mortality in 18 Countries from Five Continents (PURE): A Prospective Cohort Study," *Lancet* 390, no. 10107 (2017): 2050–62.

6 I. D. Frantz Jr. et al., "Test of Effect of Lipid Lowering by Diet on Cardiovascular Risk: The Minnesota Coronary Survey," *Arteriosclerosis* 9, no. 1 (1989): 129–35.

7 Taubes, *Good Calories, Bad Calories.*

8 B. V. Howard et al., "Low-Fat Dietary Pattern and Risk of Cardiovascular Disease," *JAMA* 295, no. 6 (2006): 655–66.

9 US Food and Drug Administration, "Final Determination Regarding Partially Hydrogenated Oils (Removing Trans Fats)," September 29, 2017, www.fda.gov/food/ingredientspackaginglabeling/foodadditivesingredients/ucm449162.htm.

10 Danish Veterinary and Food Administration, "Trans Fatty Acid Content in Food: Danish Legislation on Industrially Produced Trans-Fatty Acids," December 21, 2015, www.foedevarestyrelsen.dk/english/Food/Trans%20fatty%20acids/Pages/default.aspx#1.

CHAPTER 3

1 Public Health Collaboration, "A Summary Table of 53 Randomised Controlled Trials of Low-Carb-High-Fat Diets of Less Than 130g Per Day of Total Carbohydrate and Greater Than 35% Total Fat, Compared to Low-Fat Diets of Less Than 35% Total Fat Compiled by the Public Health Collaboration," n.d., https://phcuk.org/wp-content/uploads/2016/04/Summary-Table-53-RCTs-Low-Carb-v-Low-Fat.pdf.

2 A. Luke and R. S. Cooper, "Physical Activity Does Not Influence Obesity Risk: Time to Clarify the Public Health Message," *International Journal of Epidemiology* 42, no. 6 (2013): 1831–36.

3 T. A. Mann et al., "Medicare's Search for Effective Obesity Treatments: Diets Are Not the Answer," *American Psychologist* 62, no. 3 (2007): 220–33.

4 A. Menke, S. Casagrande, L. Geiss, and C. C. Cowie, "Prevalence of and Trends in Diabetes Among Adults in the United States, 1988–2012," *JAMA* 314, no. 10 (2015): 1021–29.

5 J. M. Lee et al., "Prevalence and Determinants of Insulin Resistance Among U.S. Adolescents: A Population-Based Study," *Diabetes Care* 29, no. 11 (2006): 2427–32.

6 D. Eddy et al., "Relationship of Insulin Resistance and Related Metabolic Variables to Coronary Artery Disease: A Mathematical Analysis," *Diabetes Care* 32, no. 2 (2009): 361–66.

7 B. Arcidiacono et al., "Insulin Resistance and Cancer Risk: An Overview of the Pathogenetic Mechanisms," *Experimental Diabetes Research* 2012 (2012); T. Tsujimoto, H. Kajio, and T. Sugiyama, "Association Between Hyperinsulinemia and Increased Risk of Cancer Death in Nonobese and Obese People: A Population-Based Observational Study," *International Journal of Cancer* 141, no. 1 (2017): 102–11.

8 C. Li et al., "Trends in Hyperinsulinemia Among Nondiabetic Adults in the U.S.," *Diabetes Care* 29, no. 11 (2006): 2396–402; A. B. Olokoba, O. A. Obateru, and L. B. Olokoba, "Type 2 Diabetes Mellitus: A Review of Current Trends," *Oman Medical Journal* 27, no. 4 (2012): 269–73.

9 C. Y. Smith et al., "Contributions of Increasing Obesity and Diabetes to Slowing Decline in Subclinical Coronary Artery Disease," *Journal of the American Heart Association* 4, no. 4 (2015): e001524.

10 American Heart Association. "Cardiovascular Disease."

11 A. Tchernof and J. P. Déprés, "Pathophysiology of Human Visceral Obesity: An Update," *Physiology Review* 93, no. 1 (2013): 359–404.

CHAPTER 4

1 D. M. Torres and S. A. Harrison, "Diagnosis and Therapy of Nonalcoholic Steatohepatitis," *Gastroenterology* 134, no. 6 (2008): 1682–98.

2 American Heart Association. "Cardiovascular Disease."

3 Indiana University Office of Science Outreach, "Obesity, Type 2 Diabetes, and Fructose," n.d., www.indiana.edu/~oso/Fructose/Fructose.html.

4 T. Nishizawa et al., "Some Factors Related to Obesity in the Japanese Sumo Wrestler," *American Journal of Clinical Nutrition* 29, no. 10 (1976): 1167–74.

5 A. W. Oliver and E. L. Potter, "Fattening Pigs for Market," Agricultural Experiment Station, Oregon State Agricultural College, Station Bulletin 269, https://ir.library.oregonstate.edu/xmlui/bitstream/handle/1957/14694/StationBulletin269.pdf.

6 M. A. Cornier et al., "The Metabolic Syndrome," *Endocrine Reviews* 29, no. 7 (2008): 777–822.

7 P. Huang, "A Comprehensive Definition for Metabolic Syndrome," *Disease Model & Mechanisms* 2, no. 5-6 (2009): 231–37.

8 Y. M. Hong, "Atherosclerotic Cardiovascular Disease Beginning in Childhood," *Korean Circulation Journal* 40, no. 1 (2010): 1–9.

9 World Health Organization, *Guideline: Sugars Intake for Adults and Children* (2015), http://apps.who.int/iris/bitstream/10665/149782/1/9789241549028_eng.pdf.

10 US Department of Agriculture, Economic Research Service, "Dietary Assessment of Major Trends in U.S. Food Consumption, 1970–2005," Economic Information Bulletin No. 33 (March 2008), www.ers.usda.gov/publications/pub-details/?pubid=44220.

11 J. M. Lee et al., "Prevalence and Determinants of Insulin Resistance Among U.S. Adolescents." *Diabetes Care* 29, no. 11 (2006): 2427–32.

12 M. Basaranoglu, G. Basaranoglu, and E. Bugianesi, "Carbohydrate Intake and Nonalcoholic Fatty Liver Disease: Fructose as a Weapon of Mass Destruction," *Hepatobiliary Surgery and Nutrition* 4, no. 2 (2015): 109–16.

13 K. L. Stanhope and P. J. Havel, "Fructose Consumption: Potential Mechanisms for Its Effects to Increase Visceral Adiposity and Induce Dyslipidemia and Insulin Resistance," *Current Opinion in Lipidology* 19, no. 1 (Feb. 2008): 16–24.

14 T. Nakagawa et al., "A Causal Role for Uric Acid in Fructose-Induced Metabolic Syndrome," *American Journal of Physiology: Renal Physiology* 290, no. 3 (March 2006): F625–F631.

15 M. Maersk et al., "Sucrose-Sweetened Beverages Increase Fat Storage in the Liver, Muscle, and Visceral Fat Depot: A 6-Month Randomized Intervention Study," *American Journal of Clinical Nutrition* 95, no. 2 (2012): 283–89. There are far fewer of these experiments available than should be the case. This is partly because the vast majority of experimental funding was squandered in desperate attempts to blame dietary fat for health issues.

16 A. Miller and K. Adeli, "Dietary Fructose and the Metabolic Syndrome," *Current Opinion in Gastroenterology* 24, no. 2 (2008): 204–9; Stanhope and Havel, "Fructose Consumption"; K. Nomura and T. Yamanouchi, "The Role of Fructose-Enriched Diets in Mechanisms of Nonalcoholic Fatty Liver

Disease," *Journal of Nutritional Biochemistry* 23, no. 3 (2012): 203–8; M. E. Bocarsly, E. S. Powell, N. M. Avena, and B. G. Hoebel, "High-Fructose Corn Syrup Causes Characteristics of Obesity in Rats: Increased Body Weight, Body Fat and Triglyceride Levels," *Pharmacology Biochemistry and Behavior* 97, no. 1 (2010): 101–6; M. B. Vos and J. E. Lavine, "Dietary Fructose in Nonalcoholic Fatty Liver Disease," *Hepatology* 57, no. 6 (2013): 2525–31; Z. Khitan and D. H. Kim, "Fructose: A Key Factor in the Development of Metabolic Syndrome and Hypertension," *Journal of Nutrition and Metabolism* 2013 (2013).

17 F. Amin and A. H. Gilani, "Fiber-Free White Flour with Fructose Offers a Better Model of Metabolic Syndrome," *Lipids in Health and Disease* 12, no. 44 (March 2013).

18 A. A. Bremer et al., "Fructose-Fed Rhesus Monkeys: A Nonhuman Primate Model of Insulin Resistance, Metabolic Syndrome, and Type 2 Diabetes," *Clinical and Translation Science* 4, no. 4 (2011): 243–52.

19 T. L. Blasbalg et al., "Changes in Consumption of Omega-3 and Omega-6 Fatty Acids in the United States During the 20th Century," *American Journal of Clinical Nutrition* 93, no. 5 (2011): 950–62.

20 P. Deol et al., "Soybean Oil Is More Obesogenic and Diabetogenic Than Coconut Oil and Fructose in Mouse: Potential Role for the Liver," *PLoS One* 10, no. 7 (2015): e0132672.

21 A. R. Alvheim et al., "Dietary Linoleic Acid Elevates the Endocannabinoids 2-AG and Anandamide and Promotes Weight Gain in Mice Fed a Low Fat Diet," *Lipids* 49, no. 1 (2014): 59–69; A. R. Alvheim et al., "Dietary Linoleic Acid Elevates Endogenous 2-AG and Anandamide and Induces Obesity," *Obesity* 20, no. 10 (2012): 1984–94; F. Massiera et al., "A Western-Like Fat Diet Is Sufficient to Induce a Gradual Enhancement in Fat Mass over Generations," *Journal of Lipid Research* 51, no. 8 (2010): 2352–61; L. Madsen et al., "cAMP-Dependent Signaling Regulates the Adipogenic Effect of n-6 Polyunsaturated Fatty Acids," *Journal of Biological Chemistry* 283, no. 11 (2008): 7196–205; C. Madigan et al., "Dietary Unsaturated Fatty Acids in Type 2 Diabetes: Higher Levels of Postprandial Lipoprotein on a Linoleic Acid–Rich Sunflower Oil Diet Compared with an Oleic Acid–Rich Olive Oil Diet," *Diabetes Care* 23, no. 10 (2000): 1472–77; S. P. Singh, M. Niemczyk, L. Zimniak, and P. Zimniak, "Fat Accumulation in Caenorhabditis Elegans Triggered by the Electrophilic Lipid Peroxidation Product 4-hydroxynonenal (4-HNE)," *Aging* 1, no. 1 (2009): 68–80; C. M. Phillips et al., "Leptin Receptor Polymorphisms Interact with Polyunsaturated Fatty Acids to Augment Risk of Insulin Resistance and Metabolic Syndrome in Adults," *Journal of Nutrition* 140, no. 2 (2010): 238–44; A. R. Johnson et al., "Cafeteria Diet–Induced Obesity Causes Oxidative Damage in White Adipose," *Biochemical and Biophysical Research Communications* 473, no. 2 (2016): 545–50.

22 G. Spiteller and M. Afzal, "The Action of Peroxyl Radicals, Powerful Deleterious Reagents, Explains Why Neither Cholesterol nor Saturated Fatty Acids Cause Atherogenesis and Age-Related Diseases," *Chemistry: A European Journal* 20, no. 46 (2014): 14928–45.

CHAPTER 5

1 J. Wylie-Rosett et al., "Low Carbohydrate Diets Improve Atherogenic Dyslipidemia Even in the Absence of Weight Loss," *Nutrition & Metabolism* 3 (2006): 24.

2 S. J. Maw, V. R. Fowler, M. Hamilton, and A. M. Petchey, "Physical Characteristics of Pig Fat and Their Relation to Fatty Acid Composition," *Meat Science* 63, no. 2 (2003): 185-90.

CHAPTER 6

1 Alvheim et al., "Dietary Linoleic Acid Elevates Endogenous 2-AG and Anandamide and Induces Obesity"; Alvheim et al., "Dietary Linoleic Acid Elevates the Endocannabinoids 2-AG and Anandamide and Promotes Weight Gain in Mice Fed a Low Fat Diet."

2 M. Buhl et al., "Direct Effects of Locally Administered Lipopolysaccharide on Glucose, Lipid, and Protein Metabolism in the lacebo-Controlled, Bilaterally Infused Human Leg," *Journal of Clinical Endocrinology and Metabolism* 98, no. 5 (2013): 2090–99; P. D. Cani et al., "Metabolic Endotoxemia Initiates Obesity and Insulin Resistance," *Diabetes* 56, no. 7 (2007): 1761–72.

3 M. P. Lejeune, E. M. Kovacs, and M. S. Westerterp-Plantega, "Additional Protein Intake Limits Weight Regain After Weight Loss in Humans," *British Journal of Nutrition* 93, no. 2 (2005): 281–89.

4 J. S. Volek et al., "Metabolic Characteristics of Keto-Adapted Ultra-Endurance Runners," *Metabolism* 65, no. 3 (2016): 100–10.

5 H. Kahleova et al., "Eating Two Larger Meals a Day (Breakfast and Lunch) Is More Effective Than Six Smaller Meals in a Reduced-Energy Regimen for Patients with Type 2 Diabetes," *Diabetologia* 57, no. 8 (2014): 1552–60.

6 Penn Medicine, "Timing Meals Later at Night Can Cause Weight Gain and Impair Fat Metabolism" (press release), June 2, 2017, www.pennmedicine.org/news/news-releases/2017/june/timing-meals-later-at-night-can-cause-weight-gain-and-impair-fat-metabolism.

7 P. Taggart and M. Carruthers, "Endogenous Hyperlipidaemia Induced by Emotional Stress of Racing Driving," *Lancet* 1, no. 7695 (1971): 363–66.

8 K. Spiegel et al., "Sleep Loss: A Novel Risk Factor for Insulin Resistance and Type 2 Diabetes," *Journal of Applied Physiology* 99, no. 5 (2005): 2008–19.

9 D. G. Hoel, M. Berwick, F. R. de Gruijl, and M. F. Holick, "The Risks and Benefits of Sun Exposure," *Dermato-Endocrinology* 8, no. 1 (2016): e1248325.

10 S. Geldenhuys et al., "Ultraviolet Radiation Suppresses Obesity and Symptoms of Metabolic Syndrome Independently of Vitamin D in Mice Fed a High-Fat Diet," *Diabetes* 63, no. 11 (2014): 3759–69; N. Fleury, S. Geldenhuys, and S. Gorman, "Sun Exposure and Its Effects on Human Health: Mechanisms Through Which Sun Exposure Could Reduce the Risk of Developing Obesity and Cardiometabolic Dysfunction," *International Journal of Environmental Research and Public Health* 13, no. 10 (2016): 999.

11 S. Lindeberg, M. Eliasson, B. Lindahl, and B. Ahrén, "Low Serum Insulin in Traditional Pacific Islanders—The Kitava Study," *Metabolism* 48, no. 10 (1999): 1216–19.

12 S. F. Sleiman et al., "Exercise Promotes the Expression of Brain Derived Neurotrophic Factor (BDNF) through the Action of the Ketone Body ß-hydroxybutyrate," *eLife* 5 (2016): e15092.

13 G. Pyka, E. Lindenberger, S. Charette, and R. Marcus, "Muscle Strength and Fiber Adaptations to a Year-Long Resistance Training Program in Elderly Men and Women," *Journal of Gerontology* 49, no. 1 (1994): M22–M27.

14 V. Valenti et al., "A 15-Year Warranty Period for Asymptomatic Individuals Without Coronary Artery Calcium: A Prospective Follow-Up of 9,715 Individuals," *JACC: Cardiovascular Imaging* 8, no. 8 (August 2015): 900–9.

15 W. Davis, S. Rockway, and M. Kwasny, "Effect of a Combined Therapeutic Approach of Intensive Lipid Management, Omega-3 Fatty Acid Supplementation, and Increased Serum 25 (OH) Vitamin D on Coronary Calcium Scores in Asymptomatic Adults," *American Journal of Therapeutics* 16, no. 4 (July–August 2009): 326–32.

16 P. Raggi, T. Q. Callister, and L. Shaw, "Progression of Coronary Artery Calcium and Risk of First Myocardial Infarction in Patients Receiving Cholesterol-Lowering Therapy," *Arteriosclerosis, Thrombosis, and Vascular Biology* 24, no. 7 (2004): 1272–77.

17 M. Budoff, "Screening for Ischemic Heart Disease with Cardiac CT: Current Recommendations," *Scientifica* 2012 (2012), doi: 10.6064/2012/812046.

CHAPTER 7

1 James DiNicolantonio, *The Salt Fix: Why the Experts Got It All Wrong—and How Eating More Might Save Your Life* (New York: Harmony Books, 2017).

CHAPTER 8

1 Spiegel et al. "Sleep Loss."

CHAPTER 10

1 C. Franceschi et al., "Genes Involved in Immune Response/Inflammation, IGF1/Insulin Pathway and Response to Oxidative Stress Play a Major Role in the Genetics of Human Longevity: The Lesson of Centenarians," *Mechanisms of Ageing and Development* 126, no. 2 (2005): 351–61.

2 G. Reaven, "Insulin Resistance and Coronary Heart Disease in Nondiabetic Individuals," *Arteriosclerosis, Thrombosis, and Vascular Biology* 32, no. 8 (2012): 1754–59.

3 V. Gyberg et al., "Screening for Dysglycaemia in Patients with Coronary Artery Disease as Reflected by Fasting Glucose, Oral Glucose Tolerance Test, and HbA1c: A Report from EUROASPIRE IV—a Survey from the European Society of Cardiology," *European Heart Journal* 36, no. 19 (2015): 1171–77.

4 S. M. Haffner et al., "Mortality from Coronary Heart Disease in Subjects with Type 2 Diabetes and in Nondiabetic Subjects With and Without Prior Myocardial Infarction," *New England Journal of Medicine* 339, no. 4 (1998): 229–34.

5 Joseph R. Kraft, *Diabetes Epidemic and You* (Bloomington, IN: Trafford Publishing, 2008).

6 A. Menke, S. Casagrande, L. Geiss, and C. C. Cowie, "Prevalence of and Trends in Diabetes Among Adults in the United States, 1988–2012," *JAMA* 314, no. 10 (2015): 1021–29.

7 A. Ströhle and A. Hahn, "Diets of Modern Hunter-Gatherers Vary Substantially in Their Carbohydrate Content Depending on Ecoenvironments: Results from an Ethnographic Analysis," *Nutrition Research* 31, no. 6 (2011): 429–435.

8 P. D. Cani et al., "Metabolic Endotoxemia Initiates Obesity and Insulin Resistance," *Diabetes* 56, no. 7 (2007): 1761–72; Buhl et al., "Direct Effects of Locally Administered Lipopolysaccharide on Glucose, Lipid, and Protein Metabolism in the Placebo-Controlled, Bilaterally Infused Human Leg."

9 F. S. Faccini, N. Hua, F. Abbasi, and G. M. Reaven, "Insulin Resistance as a Predictor of Age-Related Diseases," *Journal of Clinical Endocrinology & Metabolism* 86, no. 8 (2001): 3574–78.

10 Kraft, *Diabetes Epidemic & You.*

11 K. Khaw et al., "Association of Hemoglobin A1c with Cardiovascular Disease and Mortality in Adults: the European Prospective Investigation into Cancer in Norfolk," *Annals of Internal Medicine* 141, no. 6 (2004): 413–20.

CHAPTER 11

1 Michael O'Riordan, "New Cholesterol Guidelines Abandon LDL Targets," *Medscape,* November 14, 2013, www.medscape.com/viewarticle/814152.

2 W. P. Castelli, "Lipids, Risk Factors and Ischaemic Heart Disease," *Atherosclerosis* 124 (1996): S1–S9.

3 Ibid.

4 Dave Feldman's website, exploring the lipoproteins as primarily an energy transport system, http://cholesterolcode.com.

5 K. Node and T. Inoue, "Postprandial Hyperglycemia as an Etiological Factor in Vascular Failure," *Cardiovascular Diabetology* 8 (2009): 23.

6 E. Ingelsson et al., "Clinical Utility of Different Lipid Measures for Prediction of Coronary Heart Disease in Men and Women," *JAMA* 298, no. 7 (2007): 776–85.

7 W. P. Castelli, "Lipids, Risk Factors and Ischaemic Heart Disease," *Atherosclerosis* 124 (1996): S1–S9.

8 A. Sachdeva et al., "Lipid Levels in Patients Hospitalized with Coronary Artery Disease: An Analysis of 136,905 Hospitalizations in 'Get with the Guidelines,'" *American Heart Journal* 157, no. 1 (2009): 111–117.e2.

9 S. A. Ahmadi et al., "The Impact of Low Serum Triglyceride on LDL-Cholesterol Estimation," *Archives of Iranian Medicine* 11, no. 3 (2008): 318–21.

10 Y. M. Park, S. Kashyap, J. Major, and R. L. Silverstein, "Insulin Promotes Macrophage Foam Cell Formation: Potential Implications in Diabetes-Related Atherosclerosis," *Laboratory Investigation* 92, no. 8 (2012): 1171–80.

11 B. G. Nordestgaard, M. Benn, P. Schnohr, and A. Tybjaerg-Hansen, "Nonfasting Triglycerides and Risk of Myocardial Infarction, Ischemic Heart Disease, and Death in Men and Women," *JAMA* 298, no. 3 (2007): 299–308.

12 J. M. Gaziano et al., "Fasting Triglycerides, High-Density Lipoprotein, and Risk of Myocardial Infarction." *Circulation* 96, no. 8 (1997): 2520–25.

13 V. Bittner et al., "The TG/HDL Cholesterol Ratio Predicts All Cause Mortality in Women with Suspected Myocardial Ischemia: A Report from the Women's Ischemia Syndrome Evaluation (WISE)," *American Heart Journal* 157, no. 3 (2009): 548–55.

14 P. L. Da Luz et al., "High Ratio of Triglycerides to HDL Cholesterol Predicts Extensive Coronary Disease," *Clinics* 63, no. 4 (2008): 427–32.

15 T. D. Wang et al., "Efficacy of Cholesterol Levels and Ratios in Predicting Future Coronary Heart Disease in a Chinese Population," *American Journal of Cardiology* 88, no. 7 (2001): 737–43.

16 P. M. Ridker et al., "Non-HDL Cholesterol, Apolipoproteins A-I and B100, Standard Lipid Measures, Lipid Ratios, and CRP as Risk Factors for Cardiovascular Disease in Women," *JAMA* 294, no. 3 (2005): 326–33.

17 J. T. Real et al., "Importance of HDL Cholesterol Levels and the Total/HDL Cholesterol Ratio as a Risk Factor for Coronary Heart Disease in Molecularly Defined Heterozygous Familial Hypercholesterolaemia," *European Heart Journal* 22, no. 6 (2001): 465–71.

18 Task Force Members et al., "2013 ESC Guidelines on the Management of Stable Coronary Artery Disease," *European Heart Journal* 34, no. 38 (2013): 2949–3003.

19 S. E. Chiuve et al., "Adherence to a Low-Risk, Healthy Lifestyle and Risk of Sudden Cardiac Death Among Women," *JAMA* 306, no. 1 (2011): 62–69.

20 L. J. Shaw, P. Raggi, T. Q Callister, and D. S. Berman, "Prognostic Value of Coronary Artery Calcium Screening in Asymptomatic Smokers and Non-Smokers," *European Heart Journal* 27 (2006): 968–69.

21 Matthew J. Budoff and Jerold S. Shinbane, eds., *Cardiac CT Imaging: Diagnosis of Cardiovascular Disease* (New York: Springer, 2010).

22 M. J. Budoff, "Screening for Ischemic Heart Disease with Cardiac CT: Current Recommendations," *Scientifica* 2012 (2012).

23 P. Raggi, T. Q. Callister, and L. J. Shaw, "Progression of Coronary Artery Calcium and Risk of First Myocardial Infarction in Patients Receiving Cholesterol-Lowering Therapy," *Arteriosclerosis, Thrombosis, and Vascular Biology* 24, no. 7 (2004): 1272–77.

24 K. Nasir et al., "Interplay of Coronary Artery Calcification and Traditional Risk Factors for the Prediction of All-Cause Mortality in Asymptomatic Individuals," *Cardiovascular Imaging* 5, no. 4 (2012): 467–73.

25 C. E. Handy et al., "The Association of Coronary Artery Calcium with Noncardiovascular Disease: The Multi-Ethnic Study of Atherosclerosis," *JACC: Cardiovascular Imaging* 9, no. 5 (2016): 568–76.

26 R. Erbel et al., "Progression of Coronary Artery Calcification Seems to Be Inevitable, but Predictable—Results of the Heinz Nixdorf Recall (HNR) Study," *European Heart Journal* 35, no. 42 (2014): 2960–71.

27 W. Davis, S. Rockway, and M. Kwasny, "Effect of a Combined Therapeutic Approach of Intensive Lipid Management, Omega-3 Fatty Acid Supplementation, and Increased Serum 25 (OH) Vitamin D on Coronary Calcium Scores in Asymptomatic Adults," *American Journal of Therapeutics* 16, no. 4 (2009): 326–32.

CHAPTER 12

1 C. Tóth, A. Dabóczi, M. Chanrai, and Z. Clemens, comment on "Systematic Review: Isocaloric Ketogenic Dietary Regimes for Cancer Patients" by Erickson et al., *Journal of Cancer Research and Treatment* 5, no. 3 (2017): 86–88.

2 R. G. Ziegler, R. N. Hoover, M. C. Pike, and M. B. Hyer, "Migration Patterns and Breast Cancer Risk in Asian-American Women," *Journal of the National Cancer Institute* 85, no. 22 (1993): 1819–27.

3 E. Igwe, A. Z. F. Azman, A. J. Nordin, and N. Mohtarrudin, "Association Between Homa-Ir and Cancer in a Medical Centre in Selangor, Malaysia," *International Journal of Public Health and Clinical Sciences* 2, no. 2 (2015): 21–34.

4 M. J. Gunter et al., "Breast Cancer Risk in Metabolically Healthy but Overweight Postmenopausal Women," *Cancer Research* 75, no. 2 (2015): 270–4.

5 Ian Sample, "Diets High in Meat, Eggs and Dairy Could Be as Harmful to Health as Smoking," *Guardian,* March 5, 2014, www.theguardian.com/science/2014/mar/04/animal-protein-diets-smoking-meat-eggs-dairy.

6 M. E. Levine et al., "Low Protein Intake Is Associated with a Major Reduction in IGF-1, Cancer, and Overall Mortality in the 65 and Younger but Not Older Population," *Cell Metabolism* 19, no. 3 (2014): 407–17.

7 A. Belfiore and R. Malaguarnera, "Insulin Receptor and Cancer," *Endocrine-Related Cancer* 18, no. 4 (2011): R125–R147; R. Huxley et al., "Type-II Diabetes and Pancreatic Cancer: A Meta-Analysis of 36 Studies," *British Journal of Cancer* 92, no. 11 (2005): 2076–83; P. Wang et al., "Diabetes Mellitus and Risk of Hepatocellular Carcinoma: A Systematic Review and Meta-Analysis," *Diabetes/Metabolism Research and Reviews* 28, no. 2 (2012): 109–22; E. Friberg, N. Orsini, C. S. Mantzoros, and A. Wolk, "Diabetes Mellitus and Risk of Endometrial Cancer: A Meta-Analysis," *Diabetologia* 50, no. 7 (2007): 1365–74; S. C. Larsson and A. Wolk, "Diabetes Mellitus and Incidence of Kidney Cancer: A Meta-Analysis of Cohort Studies," *Diabetologia* 54, no. 5 (2011): 1013–18; A. Lukanova et al., "Prediagnostic Levels of C-Peptide, IGF-I, IGFBP -1, -2 and -3 and Risk of Endometrial Cancer," *International Journal of Cancer* 108, no. 2 (2004): 262–68; G. Perseghin et al., "Insulin Resistance/Hyperinsulinemia and Cancer Mortality: The Cremona Study at the 15th Year of Follow-Up," *Acta Diabetologica* 49, no. 6 (2012): 421–28.

8 A. Djiogue et al., "Insulin Resistance and Cancer: The Role of Insulin and IGFs," *Endocrine-Related Cancer* 20, no. 1 (2013): 20, R1–R17; Belfiore and Malaguarnera, "Insulin Receptor and Cancer."

9 Djiogue et al., "Insulin Resistance and Cancer."

10 D. H. Cohen and D. LeRoith, "Obesity, Type 2 Diabetes, and Cancer: The Insulin and IGF Connection," *Endocrine-Related Cancer* 19, no. 5 (2012): F27–F45.

11 V. N. Anisimov and A. Bartke, "The Key Role of Growth Hormone-Insulin-IGF-1 Signaling in Aging and Cancer," *Critical Reviews in Oncology/Hematology* 87, no. 3 (2013): 201–23.

12 A. G. Renehan et al., "Insulin-Like Growth Factor (IGF)-I, IGF Binding Protein-3, and Cancer Risk: Systematic Review and Meta-Regression Analysis," *Lancet* 363, no. 9418 (2004): 1346–53.

13 P. F. Bruning et al., "Insulin Resistance and Breast-Cancer Risk," *International Journal of Cancer* 52, no. 4 (1992): 511–16.

14 Anisimov and Bartke, "The Key Role of Growth Hormone-Insulin-IGF-1 Signaling in Aging and Cancer."

CHAPTER 13

1 D. D. Wang et al., "Specific Dietary Fats in Relation to Total and All-Cause Mortality," *JAMA Internal Medicine* 176, no. 8 (2016): 1134–45; G. Zong et al., "Intake of Individual Saturated Fatty Acids and Risk of Coronary Heart Disease in US Men and Women: Two Prospective Longitudinal Cohort Studies," *BMJ* 355 (2016): i5796.

2 R. J. de Souza et al., "Intake of Saturated and Trans Unsaturated Fatty Acids and Risk of All Cause Mortality, Cardiovascular Disease, and Type 2 Diabetes: Systematic Review and Meta-Analysis of Observational Studies," *BMJ* 351 (2015): h3978.

3 J. Praagman et al., "The Association Between Dietary Saturated Fatty Acids and Ischemic Heart Disease Depends on the Type and Source of Fatty Acid in the European Prospective Investigation into Cancer and Nutrition–Netherlands Cohort," *American Journal of Clinical Nutrition* 103, no. 2 (2016): 356–65.

4 P. Grasgruber et al., "Food Consumption and the Actual Statistics of Cardiovascular Diseases: An Epidemiological Comparison of 42 European Countries," *Food & Nutrition Research* 60 (2016): 31694.

5 M. Dehghan et al., "Associations of Fats and Carbohydrate Intake with Cardiovascular Disease and Mortality in 18 Countries from Five Continents (PURE): A Prospective Cohort Study," *Lancet* 390, no. 10107 (2017): 2050–62.

6 A. Mente et al., "Association of Dietary Nutrients with Blood Lipids and Blood Pressure in 18 Countries: A Cross-Sectional Analysis from the PURE Study," *Lancet Diabetes & Endocrinology* 5, no. 10 (2017): 774–87.

7 C. E. Ramsden et al., "Re-evaluation of the Traditional Diet-Heart Hypothesis: Analysis of Recovered Data from Minnesota Coronary Experiment (1968–73)," *BMJ* 353 (2016): i1246; C. E. Ramsden et al., "Use of Dietary Linoleic Acid for Secondary Prevention of Coronary Heart Disease and Death: Evaluation of Recovered Data from the Sydney Diet Heart Study and Updated Meta-Analysis," *BMJ* 346 (2013): e8707; G. A. Rose, W. B. Thomson, and R. T. Williams, "Corn Oil in Treatment of Ischaemic Heart Disease," *BMJ* 1, no. 5449 (1965): 1531–33.

8 M. L. Pearce and S. Dayton, "Incidence of Cancer in Men on a Diet High in Polyunsaturated Fat," *Lancet* 1, no. 7691 (1971): 464–67.

9 J. J. DiNicolantonio, "The Cardiometabolic Consequences of Replacing Saturated Fats with Carbohydrates or Ω-6 Polyunsaturated Fats: Do the Dietary Guidelines Have It Wrong?," *Open Heart* 1, no. 1 (2014): e000032.

10 R. D. Feinman and J. S. Volek, "Low Carbohydrate Diets Improve Atherogenic Dyslipidemia Even in the Absence of Weight Loss," *Nutrition & Metabolism* 3 (2006): 24.

11 J. S. Volek et al., "Dietary Carbohydrate Restriction Induces a Unique Metabolic State Positively Affecting Atherogenic Dyslipidemia, Fatty Acid Partitioning, and Metabolic Syndrome," *Progress in Lipid Research* 47, no. 5 (2008): 307–18.

12 C. E. Forsythe et al., "Comparison of Low Fat and Low Carbohydrate Diets on Circulating Fatty Acid Composition and Markers of Inflammation," *Lipids* 43, no. 1 (2008): 65–77.

13 H. Bodkin, "Low-Carb Diet Helps Control Diabetes, New Study Suggests," *Telegraph*, May 31, 2016, www.telegraph.co.uk/news/2016/05/31/low-carb-diet-helps-control-diabetes-new-study-suggests/.

14 Public Health Collaboration, "A Summary Table of 53 Randomised Controlled Trials of Low-Carb-High-Fat Diets of Less Than 130g Per Day of Total Carbohydrate and Greater Than 35% Total Fat, Compared to Low-Fat Diets of Less Than 35% Total Fat Compiled by the Public Health Collaboration," n.d., https://phcuk.org/wp-content/uploads/2016/04/Summary-Table-53-RCTs-Low-Carb-v-Low-Fat.pdf.

15 N. Halberg et al., "Effect of Intermittent Fasting and Refeeding on Insulin Action in Healthy Men," *Journal of Applied Physiology* 99, no. 6 (2005): 2128–36.

16 A. R. Barnosky, K. K. Hoddy, T. G. Unterman, and K. A. Varady, "Intermittent Fasting vs Daily Calorie Restriction for Type 2 Diabetes Prevention: A Review of Human Findings," *Translational Research* 164, no. 4 (2014): 302–11.

17 Y. H. Youm et al., "The Ketone Metabolite β-hydroxybutyrate Blocks NLRP3 Inflammasome-Mediated Inflammatory Disease," *Nature Medicine* 21, no. 3 (2015): 263–69.

18 C. W. Cheng et al., "Fasting-Mimicking Diet Promotes Ngn3-Driven β-Cell Regeneration to Reverse Diabetes," *Cell* 168, no. 5 (2017): 775–88.e12.

19 B. Andersson et al., "Acute Effects of Short-Term Fasting on Blood Pressure, Circulating Noradrenaline and Efferent Sympathetic Nerve Activity," *Acta Medica Scandinavica* 223, no. 6 (1988): 485–90.

20 G. Li et al., "Intermittent Fasting Promotes White Adipose Browning and Decreases Obesity by Shaping the Gut Microbiota," *Cell Metabolism* 26, no. 4 (2017): 672–85.

21 K. A. Varady, "Intermittent Versus Daily Calorie Restriction: Which Diet Regimen Is More Effective for Weight Loss?," *Obesity Review* 12, no. 7 (2011): e593–601.

22 G. Fond, A. Macgregor, M. Leboyer, and A. Michalsen, "Fasting in Mood Disorders: Neurobiology and Effectiveness. A Review of the Literature," *Psychiatry Research* 209, no. 3 (2013): 253–58.

23 M. Alirezaei et al., "Short-Term Fasting Induces Profound Neuronal Autophagy," *Autophagy* 6, no. 6 (2010): 702–10.

24 F. Safdie et al., "Fasting Enhances the Response of Glioma to Chemo- and Radiotherapy," *PLoS One* 7, no. 9 (2012): e44603; A. D. Saleh et al., "Caloric Restriction Augments Radiation Efficacy in Breast Cancer," *Cell Cycle* 12, no. 12 (2013): 1955–63.

25 T. B. Dorff et al., "Safety and Feasibility of Fasting in Combination with Platinum-Based Chemotherapy," *BMC Cancer* 16 (2016): 360.

26 J. A. Mattison et al., "Caloric Restriction Improves Health and Survival of Rhesus Monkeys," *Nature Communications* 8 (2017): 14063.

27 S. F. Sleiman et al., "Exercise Promotes the Expression of Brain Derived Neurotrophic Factor (BDNF) Through the Action of the Ketone Body β-hydroxybutyrate," *eLife* 5 (2016): e15092.

28 On YouTube, there are some great interviews with D'Agostino in which he simplifies the complex topic of keto and cancer: see www.youtube.com/watch?v=Ntob6Sn06_Q.

29 Craig Thompson, "How Do People Get Cancer | Cancer Awareness | Memorial Sloan Kettering," video, 32:03, February 11, 2011, www.youtube.com/watch?v=WUlE1VHGA40.

CHAPTER 14

1 For information on the safest way to consume plant-based foods, we recommend these publications: *Carb Conscious Vegetarian* by Robin Robertson; *The Plant Paradox* by Steven R. Gundry, MD; *The Vegetarian and Vegan Guide: The Blood Sugar Solution 10-Day Detox Diet* by Mark Hyman, MD (http://10daydetox.com/resources/_downloads/10DDVegetarianVegan.pdf).

2 Joel Fuhrman, *Eat to Live: The Revolutionary Formula for Fast and Sustained Weight Loss* (New York: Little, Brown, 2005), 59.

3 US Department of Agriculture, Agricultural Research Service, USDA Food Composition Databases, https://ndb.nal.usda.gov/ndb/search/list.

4 http://www.empiri.ca/ or https://zerocarbzen.com/.

5 H. J. Leidy et al., "The Effects of Consuming Frequent, Higher Protein Meals on Appetite and Satiety During Weight Loss in Overweight/Obese Men," *Obesity* 19, no. 4 (2011): 818–24.

6 A. A. van der Klaauw et al., "High Protein Intake Stimulates Postprandial GLP1 and PYY Release," *Obesity* 21, no. 8 (2013): 1602–7.

7 T. L. Halton and F. B. Hu, "The Effects of High Protein Diets on Thermogenesis, Satiety and Weight Loss: A Critical Review," *Journal of the American College of Nutrition* 23, no. 5 (2004): 373–85.

8 Lejeune, Kovacs, and Westerterp-Plantenga, "Additional Protein Intake Limits Weight Regain After Weight Loss in Humans."

9 W. F. Martin, L. E. Armstrong, and N. R. Rodriguez, "Dietary Protein Intake and Renal Function," *Nutrition & Metabolism* 2 (2005): 25.

CHAPTER 15

1 E. Giovannucci, Y. Liu, B. W. Hollis, and E. B. Rimm, "25-Hydroxyvitamin D and Risk of Myocardial Infarction in Men: A Prospective Study," *Archives of Internal Medicine* 168, no. 11 (2008): 1174–80; M. L. Melanmed et al., "Serum 25-Hydroxyvitamin D Levels and the Prevalence of Peripheral Arterial Disease: Results from NHANES 2001 to 2004," *Arteriosclerosis, Thrombosis, and Vascular Biology* 28, no. 6 (2008): 1179–85; E. D. Gorham et al., "Optimal Vitamin D Status for Colorectal Cancer Prevention: A Quantitative Meta Analysis," *American Journal of Preventive Medicine* 32, no. 3 (2007): 201–6; C. F. Garland et al., "Vitamin D and Prevention of Breast Cancer: Pooled Analysis," *Journal of Steroid Biochemistry & Molecular Biology* 103, no. 3–5 (2007): 708–711; H. K. Joh et al., "Predicted Plasma 25-Hydroxyvitamin D and Risk of Renal Cell Cancer," *Journal of the National Cancer Institute* 105, no. 10 (2013): 726–32; E. Liu et al., "Predicted 25-Hydroxyvitamin D

Score and Incident Type 2 Diabetes in the Framingham Offspring Study," *American Journal of Clinical Nutrition* 91, no. 6 (2010): 1627–33; C. Gagnon et al., "Serum 25-Hydroxyvitamin D, Calcium Intake, and Risk of Type 2 Diabetes After 5 Years," *Diabetes Care* 34, no. 5 (2011): 1133–38.

2 J. R. Kothapally, L. Armas, M. Akhter, and J. A. Chang, "25-Hydroxyvitamin D Levels in Healthy Adults in Hawaii," *Endocrine Reviews* 32, no. 4 supplement (2011): P2–130.

3 R. Nair and A Maseeh, "Vitamin D: The 'Sunshine' Vitamin," *Journal of Pharmacology & Pharmacotherapeutics* 3, no. 2 (2012): 118–26.

4 M. F. Holick et al., "Evaluation, Treatment, and Prevention of Vitamin D Deficiency: An Endocrine Society Clinical Practice Guideline," *Journal of Clinical Endocrinology and Metabolism* 96, no. 7 (2011): 1911–30.

5 M. F. Holick et al., "Guidelines for Preventing and Treating Vitamin D Deficiency and Insufficiency Revisited," *Journal of Clinical Endocrinology and Metabolism* 97, no. 4 (2012): 1153–58.

6 L. M. Gartner and F. R. Greer, "Prevention of Rickets and Vitamin D Deficiency: New Guidelines for Vitamin D Intake," *Pediatrics* 111, no. 4 (2003): 908–10; S. Kreiter, "The Reemergence of Vitamin D Deficiency Rickets: The Need for Vitamin D Supplementation," *AMB News and Views* 7 (2001): 1, 5; L. M. Gartner et al., "Breastfeeding and the Use of Human Milk," *Pediatrics* 115, no. 2 (2005): 496–506.

7 B. W. Hollis et al., "Maternal Versus Infant Vitamin D Supplementation During Lactation: A Randomized Controlled Trial," *Pediatrics* 136, no. 4 (2015): 625–34.

8 David S. Grimes, *Vitamin D and Cholesterol: The Importance of the Sun* (York, UK: Tennison Publishing, 2009); R. P. Heaney, "Vitamin D in Health and Disease," *Clinical Journal of the American Society of Nephrology* 3, no. 5 (2008): 1535–41.

9 P. G. Lindqvist et al., "Avoidance of Sun Exposure Is a Risk Factor for All-Cause Mortality: Results from the Melanoma in Southern Sweden Cohort," *Journal of Internal Medicine* 276, no. 1 (2014): 77–86; W. B. Grant and C. F. Garland, "The Association of Solar Ultraviolet B (UVB) with Reducing Risk of Cancer: Multifactorial Ecologic Analysis of Geographic Variation in Age-Adjusted Cancer Mortality Rates," *Anticancer Research* 26, no. 4A (2006): 2687–2700; J. Moan et al., "UVA, UVB and Incidence of Cutaneous Malignant Melanoma in Norway and Sweden," *Photochemical & Photobiological Sciences* 11, no. 1 (2012): 191–98; M. Berwick, "Could Sun Exposure Improve Melanoma Survival?," *Solar Radiation and Human Health* (2008): 95–101.

10 D. G. Hoel, M. Berwick, F. R. de Gruijl, and M. F. Holick, "The Risks and Benefits of Sun Exposure 2016," *Dermato-endocrinology* 8, no. 1 (2016): e1248325.

11 N. Fleury, S. Geldenhuys, and S. Gorman, "Sun Exposure and Its Effects on Human Health: Mechanisms Through Which Sun Exposure Could Reduce the Risk of Developing Obesity and Cardiometabolic Dysfunction," *International Journal of Environmental Research and Public Health* 13, no. 10 (2016): 999.

12 R. S. Johnson, J. Titze, and R. Weller, "Cutaneous Control of Blood Pressure," *Current Opinion in Nephrology and Hypertension* 25, no. 1 (2016): 11–15; D. Liu et al., "UVA Irradiation of Human Skin Vasodilates Arterial Vasculature and Lowers Blood Pressure Independently of Nitric Oxide Synthase," *Journal of Investigative Dermatology* 134, no. 7 (2014): 1839–46.

13 S. Seneff, A. Lauritzen, R. M. Davidson, and L. Lentz-Marino, "Is Endothelial Nitric Oxide Synthase a Moonlighting Protein Whose Day Job Is Cholesterol Sulfate Synthesis? Implications for Cholesterol Transport, Diabetes and Cardiovascular Disease," *Entropy* 14, no. 12 (2012): 2492–530.

14 SPERTI Vitamin D Lamp, https://www.sperti.com/product-category/vitamin-d.

15 Lindqvist et al., "Avoidance of Sun Exposure Is a Risk Factor for All-Cause Mortality."

16 E. E. Hellerstein et al., "Influence of Dietary Magnesium on Cardiac and Renal Lesions of Young Rats Fed an Atherogenic Diet," *Journal of Experimental Medicine* 106, no. 5 (1957): 767–76.

17 N. Mahalle, M. V. Kulkarni, and S. S. Naik, "Is Hypomagnesaemia a Coronary Risk Factor Among Indians with Coronary Artery Disease?," *Journal of Cardiovascular Disease Research* 3, no. 4 (2012).

18 S. E. Chiuve et al., "Plasma and Dietary Magnesium and Risk of Sudden Cardiac Death in Women," *American Journal of Clinical Nutrition* 9, no. 2 (2011): 253–60.

19 P. M. Ridker, "Inflammation, C-Reactive Protein, and Cardiovascular Disease: Moving Past the Marker Versus Mediator Debate," *Circulation Research* 114, no. 4 (2014): 594–95.

20 D. Almoznino-Sarafian et al., "Magnesium and C-reactive Protein in Heart Failure: An Anti-inflammatory Effect of Magnesium Administration?," *European Journal of Nutrition* 46, no. 4 (2007): 230–37.

21 J. J. DiNicolantonio, M. F. McCarty, and J. H. O'Keefe, "Decreased Magnesium Status May Mediate the Increased Cardiovascular Risk Associated with Calcium Supplementation," *Open Heart* 7 (2017): e000617.

22 J. M. Geleijnse et al., "Dietary Intake of Menaquinone Is Associated with a Reduced Risk of Coronary Heart Disease: The Rotterdam Study," *Journal of Nutrition* 134, no. 11 (2004): 3100–105.

23 M. H. Knapen et al., "Menaquinone-7 Supplementation Improves Arterial Stiffness in Healthy Postmenopausal Women. A Double-Blind Randomised Clinical Trial," *Thrombosis and Haemostasis* 113, no. 5 (2015): 1135–44.

24 J. J. DiNicolantonio, J. Bhutani, and J. H. O'Keefe, "The Health Benefits of Vitamin K," *Open Heart* 2, no. 1 (2015): e000300.

25 C. Vermeer, "Vitamin K: The Effect on Health Beyond Coagulation—An Overview," *Food & Nutrition Research* 56, no. 1 (2012).

26 F. Ahad and S. A. Ganie, "Iodine, Iodine Metabolism and Iodine Deficiency Disorders Revisited," *Indian Journal of Endocrinology and Metabolism* 14, no. 1 (2010): 13–17.

27 M. B. Zimmermann, "Iodine Deficiency," *Endocrine Reviews* 30, no. 4 (2009): 376–408.

28 J. G. Hollowell et al., "Iodine Nutrition in the United States. Trends and Public Health Implications: Iodine Excretion Data from National Health and Nutrition Examination Surveys I and III (1971–1974 and 1988–1994)," *Journal of Clinical Endocrinology and Metabolism* 83, no. 10 (1998): 3401–408.

29 U. Kapil, "Health Consequences of Iodine Deficiency," *Sultan Qaboos University Medical Journal* 7, no. 3 (2007): 267–72.

30 WHO Secretariat et al., "Prevention and Control of Iodine Deficiency in Pregnant and Lactating Women and in Children Less Than 2-years-old: Conclusions and Recommendations of the Technical Consultation," *Public Health Nutrition* 10, no. 12A (2007): 1606–11.

31 J. A. Pennington and S. A. Schoen, "Total Diet Study: Estimated Dietary Intakes of Nutritional Elements, 1982–1991," *International Journal for Vitamin and Nutrition Research* 66, no. 4 (1996): 350–62; C. G. Perrine, K. Herrick, M. K. Serdula, and K. M. Sullivan, "Some Subgroups of Reproductive Age Women in the United States May Be at Risk for Iodine Deficiency," *Journal of Nutrition* 140, no. 8 (2014): 1489–94; K. L. Caldwell et al., "Iodine Status of the U.S. Population, National Health and Nutrition Examination Survey, 2005–2006 and 2007–2008," *Thyroid* 21, no. 4 (2011): 419–27.

32 M. B. Zimmermann, "Iodine Deficiency," *Endocrine Reviews* 30, no. 4 (2009): 376–408.

33 B. V. Stadel, "Dietary Iodine and Risk of Breast, Endometrial, and Ovarian Cancer," *Lancet* 1, no. 7965 (1976): 890–91; B. A. Eskin, "Iodine and Mammary Cancer," *Advances in Experimental Medicine and Biology* 91 (1977): 293–304; A. B. Slebodzinski, "Ovarian Iodide Uptake and Triiodothyronine Generation in Follicular Fluid: The Enigma of the Thyroid Ovary Interaction," *Domestic Animal Endocrinology* 29, no. 1 (2005): 97–103.

34 V. G. Bezpalov et al., "Investigation of the Drug 'Mamoclam' for the Treatment of Patients with Fibroadenomatosis of the Breast," *Voprosy Onkologii* 51, no. 2 (2005): 236–41.

35 L. C. Hartmann et al., "Benign Breast Disease and the Risk of Breast Cancer," *New England Journal of Medicine* 353, no. 3 (2005): 229–37.

36 C. Aceves, B. Anguiano, and G. Delgado, "Is Iodine a Gatekeeper of the Integrity of the Mammary Gland?," *Journal of Mammary Gland Biology and Neoplasia* 10, no. 2 (2005): 189–96; F. R. Stoddard II, A. D. Brooks, B. A. Eskin, and G. J. Johannes, "Iodine Alters Gene Expression in the MCF7 Breast Cancer Cell Line: Evidence for an Anti-estrogen Effect of Iodine," *International Journal of Medical Sciences* 5, no. 4 (2008): 189–96.

37 B. M. Gilfix, "Vitamin B_{12} and Homocysteine," *CMAJ* 173, no. 11 (2005): 1360.

38 L. A. O'Hearn, "C Is for Carnivore" (blog post), Empirica, www.empiri.ca/2017/02/c-is-for-carnivore.html.

39 The reason is explained excellently in Michael Eades's blog post "Low Carb Diets and Copper," https://proteinpower.com/drmike/2006/11/13/low-carb-diets-and-copper/.

40 A book from our cardiac-researcher friend James DiNicolantonio, *The Salt Fix*, explains in detail why the low-salt recommendations were based overwhelmingly on flawed interpretations of the science.

41 C. Y. Shan et al., "Alteration of the Intestinal Barrier and GLP2 Secretion in Berberine-Treated Type 2 Diabetic Rats," *Journal of Endocrinology* 218, no. 3 (2013): 255–62.

CHAPTER 16

1 Y. Song, M. J. Stampfer, and S. Liu, "Meta-Analysis: Apolipoprotein E Genotypes and Risk for Coronary Heart Disease," *Annals of Internal Medicine* 141, no.

2 (2004): 137–47; A. M. Bennet et al., "Association of Apolipoprotein E Genotypes with Lipid Levels and Coronary Risk," *JAMA* 298, no. 11 (2007): 1300–11.

2 For example, 23 and Me (www.23andme.com) offers a genetic test.

3 Steven Gundry, "AHS16—Steven Gundry—Dietary Management of the ApoE4," video, 38:47, August 17, 2016, www.youtube.com/watch?v=Bfr9RPq0HFg.

4 A. A. Teixeiraa et al., "Diversity of Apolipoprotein E Genetic Polymorphism Significance on Cardiovascular Risk Is Determined by the Presence of Metabolic Syndrome Among Hypertensive Patients," *Lipids in Health and Disease* 13 (2014): 174.

5 J. S. Volek et al., "Metabolic Characteristics of Keto-Adapted Ultra-endurance Runners," *Metabolism* 65, no. 3 (2016): 100–10.

APPENDIXES

1 P. Holvoet, "Relations Between Metabolic Syndrome, Oxidative Stress and Inflammation and Cardiovascular Disease," *Verhandelingen—Koninklijke Academie Voor Geneeskunde Van Belgie* 70, no. 3 (2008): 193–219.

2 A. S. Kelly et al., "Relation of Circulating Oxidized LDL to Obesity and Insulin Resistance in Children," *Pediatric Diabetes* 11, no. 8 (2010): 552–5.

3 M. Bartnik, et al., "Abnormal Glucose Tolerance—A Common Risk Factor in Patients with Acute Myocardial Infarction in Comparison with Population-Based Controls," Journal of Internal Medicine 256, no. 4 (2004): 288–97; R. W. Bergstrom et al., "Association of Plasma Triglyceride and C-Peptide with Coronary Heart Disease in Japanese-American Men with a High Prevalence of Glucose Intolerance," *Diabetologia* 33, no. 8 (August 1990): 489–96; R. Laaksonen et al., "Plasma Ceramides Predict Cardiovascular Death in Patients with Stable Coronary Artery Disease and Acute Coronary Syndromes Beyond LDL-Cholesterol," *European Heart Journal* 37, no. 25 (July 2016): 1967–76.

4 Bartnik et al., "Abnormal Glucose Tolerance."

5 M. A. Austin, C. M. Hutter, R. L. Zimmern, and S. E. Humphries, "Familial Hypercholesterolemia and Coronary Heart Disease: A HuGE Association Review," *American Journal of Epidemiology* 160, no. 5 (September 2004): 421–9.

6 E. J. Sijbrands et al., "Mortality over Two Centuries in Large Pedigree with Familial Hypercholesterolaemia: Family Tree Mortality Study," *British Medical Journal* 322, no. 7293 (2001): 1019–23; P. N. Hopkins, "Evaluation of Coronary Risk Factors in Patients with Heterozygous Familial Hypercholesterolemia," *American Journal of Cardiology* 87, no. 5 (2001): 547–53; T. A. Miettinen and H. Gylling, "Mortality and Cholesterol Metabolism in Familial Hypercholesterolemia. Long-Term Follow-Up of 96 Patients," *Arteriosclerosis* 8, no. 2 (1988): 163–7; J. S. Hill, M. R. Hayden, J. Frohlich, and P. H. Pritchard, "Genetic and Environmental Factors Affecting the Incidence of Coronary Artery Disease in Heterozygous Familial Hypercholesterolemia," *Arteriosclerosis and Thrombosis* 11, no. 2 (1991): 290–7; J. Ferrières, J. Lambert, S. Lussier-Cacan, and J. Davignon, "Coronary Artery Disease in Heterozygous Familial Hypercholesterolemia Patients with the Same LDL Receptor Gene Mutation," *Circulation* 92 (1995): 290–5.

7 Hopkins, "Evaluation of Coronary Risk Factors in Patients with Heterozygous Familial Hypercholesterolemia."

8 M. Sebestjen, B. Zegura, B. Guzic-Salobir, and I. Keber, "Fibrinolytic Parameters and Insulin Resistance in Young Survivors of Myocardial Infarction with Heterozygous Familial Hypercholesterolemia," *Wiener Klinische Wochenschrift* 113, nos. 3–4 (February 2001): 113–8.

9 J. Besseling, "Severe Heterozygous Familial Hypercholesterolemia and Risk for Cardiovascular Disease: A Study of a Cohort of 14,000 Mutation Carriers," *Atherosclerosis* 223, no. 1 (March 2014): 219–23.

10 D. Gaudet et al., "Relationships of Abdominal Obesity and Hyperinsulinemia to Angiographically Assessed Coronary Artery Disease in Men with Known Mutations in the LDL Receptor Gene," *Circulation* 97 (1998): 871–7.

11 J. T. Real et al., "Importance of HDL Cholesterol Levels and the Total/HDL Cholesterol Ratio as a Risk Factor for Coronary Heart Disease in Molecularly Defined Heterozygous Familial Hypercholesterolaemia," *European Heart Journal* 22, no. 6 (2001): 465–71.

12 M. J. Veerkamp, J. de Graaf, and A. F. H. Stalenhoef, "Role of Insulin Resistance in Familial Combined Hyperlipidemia," *Arteriosclerosis, Thrombosis, and Vascular Biology* 25 (2005): 1026–31.

13 G. Collier, A. McLean, and K. O'Dea, "Effect of Co-ingestion of Fat on the Metabolic Responses to Slowly and Rapidly Absorbed Carbohydrates," *Diabetologia* 26, no. 1 (1984): 50–4.

14 C. Desmarchelier et al., "Diet-Induced Obesity in Ad Libitum–Fed Mice: Food Texture Overrides the Effect of Macronutrient Composition," *British Journal of Nutrition* 109, no. 8 (April 2013): 1518–27.

15 K. S. Juntunen et al., "Postprandial Glucose, Insulin, and Incretin Responses to Grain Products in Healthy Subjects," *American Journal of Clinical Nutrition* 75, no. 2 (2002): 254–62.

16 M. H. Shanik et al., "Insulin Resistance and Hyperinsulinemia: Is Hyperinsulinemia the Cart or the Horse?," *Diabetes Care* 31, suppl. 2 (2008): S262–8; C. T. Kelly et al., "Hyperinsulinemic Syndrome: The Metabolic Syndrome Is Broader Than You Think," *Surgery* 156, no. 2 (August 2014): 405–11; W. Cao, J. Ning, X. Yang, and Z. Liu, "Excess Exposure to Insulin Is the Primary Cause of Insulin Resistance and Its Associated Atherosclerosis," *Current Molecular Pharmacology* 4, no. 3 (2011): 154–66; U. Smith, "Impaired ('Diabetic') Insulin Signaling and Action Occur in Fat Cells Long Before Glucose Intolerance—Is Insulin Resistance Initiated in the Adipose Tissue?," *International Journal of Obesity* 26 (2002): 897–904.

17 P. M. Moraes-Vieira, A. Saghatelian, and B. B. Kahn, "GLUT4 Expression in Adipocytes Regulates De Novo Lipogenesis and Levels of a Novel Class of Lipids with Antidiabetic and Anti-inflammatory Effects," *Diabetes* 65, no. 7 (July 2016): 1808–15; H. Cao et al., "Identification of a Lipokine, a Lipid Hormone Linking Adipose Tissue to Systemic Metabolism," *Cell* 134, no. 6 (September 2008): 933–44.

18 A. Hammarstedt, T. E. Graham, and B. B. Kahn, "Adipose Tissue Dysregulation and Reduced Insulin Sensitivity in Non-obese Individuals with Enlarged Abdominal Adipose Cells," *Diabetology & Metabolic Syndrome* 4, no. 42 (2012); R. P. Vazirani et al., "Disruption of Adipose Rab10-Dependent Insulin Signaling Causes Hepatic Insulin Resistance," *Diabetes* 65, no. 6 (2016): 1577–89.

19 M. Seip and O. Trygstad, "Generalized Lipodystrophy, Congenital and Acquired (Lipoatrophy)," *Acta Paediatrica* 413, suppl. (1996): 2–28; O. Søvik, H. Vestergaard, O. Trygstad, and O. Pedersen, "Studies of Insulin Resistance in Congenital Generalized Lipodystrophy," *Acta Paediatrica* 413, suppl. (1996): 29–37; K. I. Rother and R. J. Brown, "Novel Forms of Lipodystrophy: Why Should We Care?," *Diabetes Care* 36, no. 8 (August 2013): 2142–5.

20 O. Gavrilova, "Surgical Implantation of Adipose Tissue Reverses Diabetes in Lipoatrophic Mice," *Journal of Clinical Investigation* 105, no. 3 (February 2000): 271–8.

21 S. E. McQuaid et al., "Downregulation of Adipose Tissue Fatty Acid Trafficking in Obesity," *Diabetes* 60, no. 1 (January 2011): 47–55.

22 S. Heinonen et al., "Adipocyte Morphology and Implications for Metabolic Derangements in Acquired Obesity," *International Journal of Obesity* 38, no. 11 (November 2014): 1423–31; S. Le Lay, G. Simard, M. C. Martinez, and R. Andriantsitohaina, "Oxidative Stress and Metabolic Pathologies: From an Adipocentric Point of View," *Oxidative Medicine and Cellular Longevity* 2014 (2014); R. Lomonaco et al., "Effect of Adipose Tissue Insulin Resistance on Metabolic Parameters and Liver Histology in Obese Patients with Nonalcoholic Fatty Liver Disease," *Hepatology* 55, no. 5 (May 2012): 1389–97.

23 O. Nov et al., "Interleukin-1ß Regulates Fat-Liver Crosstalk in Obesity by Auto-paracrine Modulation of Adipose Tissue Inflammation and Expandability," PLOS ONE, 8, no. 1 (January 2013).

24 Hammarstedt, Graham, and Kahn, "Adipose Tissue Dysregulation and Reduced Insulin Sensitivity in Non-obese Individuals with Enlarged Abdominal Adipose Cells"; H. Xu et al., "Chronic Inflammation in Fat Plays a Crucial Role in the Development of Obesity-Related Insulin Resistance," *Journal of Clinical Investigation* 112, no. 12 (2003): 1821–30.

25 N. Klöting et al., "Insulin-Sensitive Obesity," *American Journal of Physiology-Endocrinology and Metabolism* 299, no. 3 (September 2010): E506–15.

26 P. Jansson et al., "A Novel Cellular Marker of Insulin Resistance and Early Atherosclerosis in Humans Is Related to Impaired Fat Cell Differentiation and Low Adiponectin," *The FASEB Journal* 17, no. 11 (August 2003): 1434–40; N. Slutsky et al., "Decreased Adiponectin Links Elevated Adipose Tissue Autophagy with Adipocyte Endocrine Dysfunction in Obesity," *International Journal of Obesity*, January 20, 2016.

27 A. Gastaldelli, "Role of Beta-Cell Dysfunction, Ectopic Fat Accumulation and Insulin Resistance in the Pathogenesis of Type 2 Diabetes Mellitus," *Diabetes Research and Clinical Practice* 93, suppl. 1 (August 2011): S60–5; G. I. Shulman, "Ectopic Fat in Insulin Resistance, Dyslipidemia, and Cardiometabolic Disease," *New England Journal of Medicine* 371 (September 2014): 1131–41; "Letter in Reply: 'Ectopic Fat in Insulin Resistance, Dyslipidemia, and Cardiometabolic Disease,'" New England Journal of Medicine 371 (December 2014): 2236–8.

28 S. M. Kitessa and M. Y. Abeywardena, "Lipid-Induced Insulin Resistance in Skeletal Muscle: The Chase for the Culprit Goes from Total Intramuscular Fat to Lipid Intermediates, and Finally to Species of Lipid Intermediates," *Nutrients* 8, no. 8 (2016): E466; A. L. Olson, "Insulin Resistance: Cross-Talk Between Adipose Tissue and Skeletal Muscle, Through Free Fatty Acids,

Liver X Receptor, and Peroxisome Proliferator-Activated Receptor-α Signaling," *Hormone Molecular Biology and Clinical Investigation* 15 no. 3 (2013): 115–21.

29 C. Saponaro, M. Gaggini, F. Carli, and A. Gastaldelli, "The Subtle Balance Between Lipolysis and Lipogenesis: A Critical Point in Metabolic Homeostasis," *Nutrients* 7, no. 11 (2015): 9453–74; J. W. Eriksson et al., "Glucose Turnover and Adipose Tissue Lipolysis Are Insulin-Resistant in Healthy Relatives of Type 2 Diabetes Patients," *Diabetes* 48, no. 8 (August 1999): 1572–8.

30 V. T. Samuel and G. I Shulman, "The Pathogenesis of Insulin Resistance: Integrating Signaling Pathways and Substrate Flux," *Journal of Clinical Investigation* 126, no. 1 (January 2016): 12–22.

31 S. Lindeberg, M. Eliasson, B. Lindahl, and B. Ahrén, "Low Serum Insulin in Traditional Pacific Islanders—The Kitava Study," *Metabolism* 48, no. 10 (October 1999): 1216–19.

32 L. H. Kurt and B. Bronte-Stewart, "The Fatty Acids of Human Depot Fat," *Journal of Lipid Research* 5 (1964): 343–51.

33 S. J. Guyenet and S. E. Carlson, "Increase in Adipose Tissue Linoleic Acid of US Adults in the Last Half Century," *Advances in Nutrition* 6 (November 2015): 660–4.

34 B. Lands, "Historical Perspectives on the Impact of n-3 and n-6 Nutrients on Health," *Progress in Lipid Research* 55 (July 2014): 17–29.

35 G. A. Rose, W. B. Thompson, and R. T. Williams, "Corn Oil in Treatment of Ischaemic Heart Disease," *British Medical Journal* 1 (1965): 1531–3.

36 E. Patterson et al., "Health Implications of High Dietary Omega-6 Polyunsaturated Fatty Acids," *Journal of Nutrition and Metabolism* 2012 (2012).

37 A. L. Johnson, K. Z. Edson, R. A. Totah, and A. E. Rettie, "Cytochrome P450 ω-Hydroxylases in Inflammation and Cancer," *Advances in Pharmacology* 74 (2015): 223–62.

38 W. E. M. Lands, "Diets Could Prevent Many Diseases," *Lipids* 38 (May 2003): 317–21.

39 A. P. Simopoulos, J. J. DiNicolantonio, "The Importance of a Balanced Ω-6 to Ω-3 Ratio in the Prevention and Management of Obesity," *Open Heart* 3 (2016): e000385.

40 A. P. Simopoulos, "The Importance of the Ratio of Omega-6/Omega-3 Essential Fatty Acids," *Biomedicine & Pharmacotherapy* 56, no. 8 (October 2002): 365–79.

41 W. S. Harris and C. Von Schacky, "The Omega-3 Index: A New Risk Factor for Death from Coronary Heart Disease?," *Preventive Medicine* 39, no. 1 (2004): 212–20.

42 Lands, "Diets Could Prevent Many Diseases."

43 Ibid.

44 C. E. Ramsden, J. R. Hibbeln, Sharon F. Majchrzak, and John M. Davis, "N-6 Fatty Acid-Specific and Mixed Polyunsaturate Dietary Interventions Have Different Effects on CHD Risk: A Meta-Analysis of Randomised Controlled Trials," *British Journal of Nutrition* 104, no. 11 (2010): 1586–1600.

45 P. Leren, "The Oslo Diet-Heart Study," *Circulation* 42 (1970): 935–42.

46 G. Christakis, S. H. Rinzler, M. Archer, and A. Kraus, "Effect of the Anti-Coronary Club Program on Coronary Heart Disease Risk-Factor Status," *JAMA* 198, no. 6 (1966): 129–36.

47 J. M. Woodhill et al., "Low Fat, Low Cholesterol Diet in Secondary Prevention of Coronary Heart Disease," *Advances in Experimental Medicine and Biology* 109 (1978): 317–30.

48 C. E. Ramsden et al., "Use of Dietary Linoleic Acid for Secondary Prevention of Coronary Heart Disease and Death: Evaluation of Recovered Data from the Sydney Diet Heart Study and Updated Meta-Analysis," *British Medical Journal* 346 (2013): e8707.

49 M. de Lorgeril et al., "Mediterranean Diet, Traditional Risk Factors, and the Rate of Cardiovascular Complications After Myocardial Infarction: Final Report of the Lyon Diet Heart Study," *Circulation* 99 (1999): 779–85.

50 K. K. Carroll and G. J. Hopkins, "Dietary Polyunsaturated Fat Versus Saturated Fat in Relation to Mammary Carcinogenesis," *Lipids* 14, no. 2 (February 1979): 155–8.

51 M. P. Fay, L. S. Freedman, C. K. Clifford, and D. N. Midthune, "Effect of Different Types and Amounts of Fat on the Development of Mammary Tumors in Rodents: A Review," *Cancer Research* 57, no. 18 (September 1997): 3979–88.

52 M. MacLennan and D. W. Ma, "Role of Dietary Fatty Acids in Mammary Gland Development and Breast Cancer," *Breast Cancer Research* 12, no. 5 (2010): 211.

53 C. A. Daley et al., "A Review of Fatty Acid Profiles and Antioxidant Content in Grass-Fed and Grain-Fed Beef," *Nutrition Journal* 9 (2010): 10.

54 D. E. Bauman and A. L. Lock, "Conjugated Linoleic Acid: Biosynthesis and Nutritional Significance," in *Advanced Dairy Chemistry*, 3rd ed., vol. 2: Lipids, ed. P. F. Fox and P. H. McSweeney (New York: Springer, 2006): 93–126.

55 Deol et al., "Soybean Oil Is More Obesogenic and Diabetogenic Than Coconut Oil and Fructose in Mouse: Potential Role for the Liver."

56 A. R. Alvheim et al., "Dietary Linoleic Acid Elevates Endogenous 2-AG and Anandamide and Induces Obesity," *Obesity* 20, no. 10 (October 2012): 1984–94.

57 G. Ghigliotti, "Adipose Tissue Immune Response: Novel Triggers and Consequences for Chronic Inflammatory Conditions," *Inflammation* 37, no. 4 (2014): 1337–53.

58 A. A. Nanji, C. L. Mendenhall, and S. W. French, "Beef Fat Prevents Alcoholic Liver Disease in the Rat," *Alcoholism Clinical and Experimental Research* 13, no. 1 (February 1989): 15–19.

59 A. A. Nanji and S. W. French, "Dietary Linoleic Acid Is Required for Development of Experimentally Induced Alcoholic Liver Injury," *Life Science* 44, no. 3 (1989): 223–7.

60 I. A. Kirpich et al., "Alcoholic Liver Disease: Update on the Role of Dietary Fat," *Biomolecules* 6, no. 1 (March 2016): 1.

61 K. Pereira, J. Salsamendi, and J. Casillas, "The Global Nonalcoholic Fatty Liver Disease Epidemic: What a Radiologist Needs to Know," *Journal of Clinical Imaging Science* 5 (2015): 32; D. M. Torres and S. A. Harrison, "Diagnosis and Therapy of Nonalcoholic Steatohepatitis," *Gastroenterology* 134, no. 6 (2008): 1682–98.

62 S. C. Cunnane and P. Guesnet, "Linoleic Acid Recommendations—A House of Cards," *Prostaglandins, Leukotrienes and Essential Fatty Acids* 85, no. 6 (2011): 399–402.

63 B. S. Peskin and M. J. Carter, "Chronic Cellular Hypoxia as the Prime Cause of Cancer: What Is the De-oxygenating Role of Adulterated and Improper Ratios of Polyunsaturated Fatty Acids When Incorporated into Cell Membranes?," *Medical Hypotheses* 70, no. 2 (2008): 298–304.

64 Simopoulos, "The Importance of the Ratio of Omega-6/Omega-3 Essential Fatty Acids."

65 N. Teicholz, "Don't Believe the American Heart Assn.—Butter, Steak and Coconut Oil Aren't Likely to Kill You," *LA Times,* July 23, 2017, www.latimes.com/opinion/op-ed/la-oe-teicholz-saturated-fat-wont-kill-you-20170723-story.html.

66 Simopoulos, "The Importance of the Ratio of Omega-6/Omega-3 Essential Fatty Acids."

67 K. D. Brownell and J. L. Pomeranz, "The Trans-Fat Ban—Food Regulation and Long-Term Health," *New England Journal of Medicine* 370 (2014): 1773–5.

68 P. Lambelet et al., "Formation of Modified Fatty Acids and Oxyphytosterols During Refining of Low Erucic Acid Rapeseed Oil," *Journal of Agricultural and Food Chemistry* 51, no. 15 (2003): 4284–90.

69 D. Spiteller and G. Spiteller, "Oxidation of Linoleic Acid in Low-Density Lipoprotein: An Important Event in Atherogenesis," *Angewandte Chemie International Edition* 39, no. 3 (2000): 585–9.

70 G. Spiteller and M. Afzal, "The Action of Peroxyl Radicals, Powerful Deleterious Reagents, Explains Why Neither Cholesterol nor Saturated Fatty Acids Cause Atherogenesis and Age-Related Diseases," *Chemistry: A European Journal* 20, no. 46 (2014): 14928–45.

71 J. L. Witztum and D. Steinberg, "Role of Oxidized Low Density Lipoprotein in Atherogenesis," *Journal of Clinical Investigation* 88, no. 6 (December 1991): 1785–92; H. Itabe, T. Obama, and R. Kato, "The Dynamics of Oxidized LDL During Atherogenesis," *Journal of Lipids* 2011 (2011); X. Que et al., "Abstract 361: Oxidized Phospholipids Are Proinflammatory and Proatherogenic," *Arteriosclerosis, Thrombosis, and Vascular Biology* 36, suppl. 1 (2016): A361; D. Steinberg, "Low Density Lipoprotein Oxidation and Its Pathobiological Significance," *Journal of Biological Chemistry* 272, no. 34 (1997): 20963–6; S. Ehara et al., "Small Coronary Calcium Deposits and Elevated Plasma Levels of Oxidized Low Density Lipoprotein Are Characteristic of Acute Myocardial Infarction," *Journal of Atherosclerosis and Thrombosis* 15, no. 2 (2008): 75–81; C. Meisinger et al., "Plasma Oxidized Low-Density Lipoprotein, a Strong Predictor for Acute Coronary Heart Disease Events in Apparently Healthy, Middle-Aged Men from the General Population," *Circulation* 112, no. 5 (2005): 651–7; R. Zaguri et al., "'Danger' Effect of Low-Density Lipoprotein (LDL) and Oxidized LDL on Human Immature Dendritic Cells," *Clinical and Experimental Immunology* 149, no. 3 (September 2007): 543–52; S. Li et al., "Targeting Oxidized LDL Improves Insulin Sensitivity and Immune Cell Function in Obese Rhesus Macaques," *Molecular Metabolism* 2, no. 3 (August 2013): 256–69.

72 R. C. Block, W. S. Harris, and J. V. Pottala, "Determinants of Blood Cell Omega-3 Fatty Acid Content," *Open Biomarkers Journal* 1 (2008): 1–6.

73 Harris and Von Schacky, "The Omega-3 Index."

74 Ramsden, Hibbeln, Majchrzak, and Davis, "N-6 Fatty Acid-Specific and Mixed Polyunsaturate Dietary Interventions Have Different Effects on CHD Risk."

75 See Catherine Shanahan, *Deep Nutrition: Why Your Genes Need Traditional Food* (New York: Flatiron Books, 2016).

INDEX

5